W9-ARQ-040

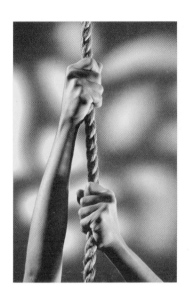

Fitness for Life

Fourth Edition

Authors

Charles B. Corbin
Professor of Physical Education
Arizona State University
Tempe, Arizona

Ruth Lindsey
Professor Emeritus of Physical Education
California State University
Long Beach, California

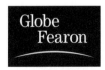

Globe
Fearon

Upper Saddle River, New Jersey
www.globefearon.com

Contributors

Reviewers and Consultants

Phil Abbadessa
Physical Education Teacher
Mountain Pointe High School
Phoenix, Arizona

Bonnie Beach
Chair, Department of Kinetic Wellness
New Trier Township High School
Winnetka, Illinois

Virginia Beech
Teacher
Gateway Senior High School
Monroeville, Pennsylvania

Lila L. Farr
Teacher
Ocean View High School
Huntington Beach, California

Dr. David R. Laurie
Professor
Kansas State University—College of Education
Manhattan, Kansas

Fred E. Leider, Ed.D.
Coordinator for Physical Education and Athletics
Austin Independent School District
Austin, Texas

Bruce MacPherson
Director of Health
Dennis/Yarmouth Schools
South Yarmouth, Massachusetts

Marilu D. Meredith, Ed.D.
Director, Management Information Services
The Cooper Institute for Aerobics Research
Dallas, Texas

Dan Ramirez
Teacher
W. E. Greiner Middle School
Dallas, Texas

Steve Swanson
Teacher/Coach
Klein Forest High School
Houston, Texas

George R. Taylor, Ed.D.
Assistant Professor, Kinesiology
The University of Texas—San Antonio
San Antonio, Texas

Adolf Yanez
Director, Physical Education Department
Dallas Independent School District
Dallas, Texas

Adapted Physical Education Consultant

Janet A. Seaman
Executive Director
American Association for Active Lifestyles and Fitness
Reston, Virginia

Acknowledgments appear on page 250.
Cover photograph by Peterson/FPG.

ISBN: 0-673-29825-6 (Hardcover)
ISBN: 0-673-29824-8 (Softcover)

Printed in the United States of America

1 2 3 4 5 6 7 8 9 10   04 03 02 01 0

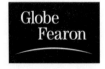

1-800-848-950
www.globefearon.co

ii

Contents

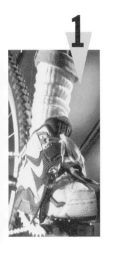
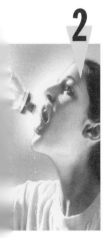
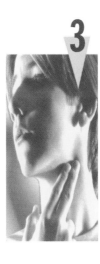
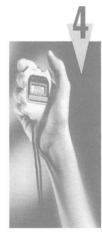

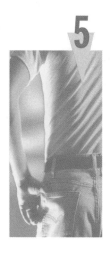

5

Benefits of Physical Activity 61

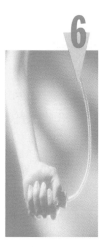

6

Cardiovascular Fitness 73

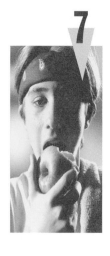

7

Physical Activity and Fat Control 87

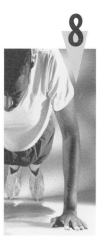

8

Muscular Endurance 103

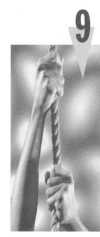

9

Strength 119

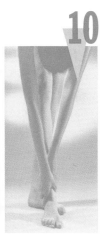
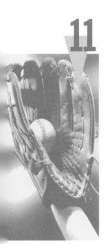
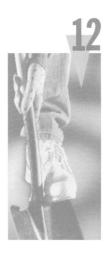
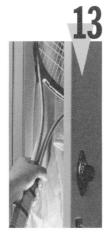
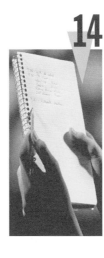

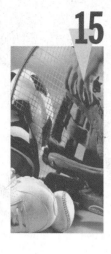

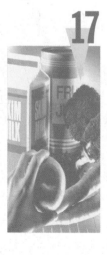

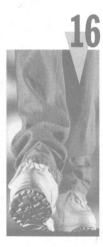

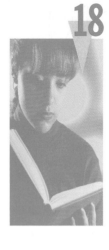

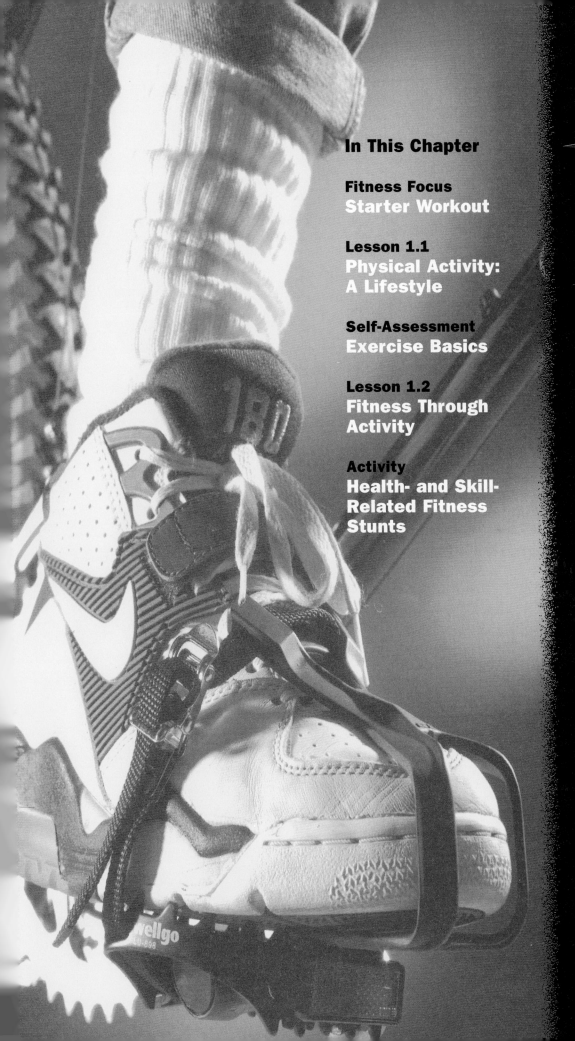

Fitness and Wellness for All

1

Starter Workout

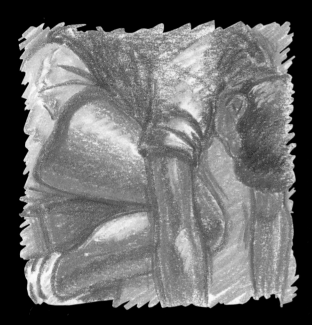

As part of this course, you will develop a personal physical activity plan that will include lifetime activities. The Fitness Focus feature at the beginning of each chapter will teach you some fitness activities that you can do on your own. You might include several of these activities in your lifetime plan.

This Starter Workout is designed to help you begin exercising. You will find the instructions for the workout on the instruction sheet your teacher will provide for you. The workout can help you prepare for the more advanced activities in the book. You probably won't find this workout difficult if you already exercise regularly. But if you don't exercise regularly, you might use it as your regular physical activity program until you can complete the larger number of repetitions shown on the chart on your instruction sheet.

Cat Back	Jog in Place
Side-Leg Raise	Forward Lunge
Pogo Hop	Bent Knee Push-Up
Knee to Nose	Rope Jump

Lesson 1.1

Physical Activity: A Lifestyle

Lesson Objectives
After reading this lesson, you should be able to:
1. Explain what physical fitness is.
2. Describe some benefits of being physically active.

Lesson Vocabulary
physical fitness, health, wellness, physical activity, exercise

Physical fitness! What is it? Do you need it? And how can you achieve it? As you read this book, you will find answers to these questions and many more. This book will help you decide what kinds of physical activities you need and help you develop a personal fitness plan for getting fit on your own. You will learn about the benefits of being fit.

Before you get started on your physical activity plan, you probably need some basic information about fitness. In this lesson you will learn the definitions of some words you will use throughout this course. You will find out what fitness, health, and wellness are. You also will learn how physical activity provides health and wellness benefits.

What Is Physical Fitness?
Look at the pictures on page 3. Some of these people are building fitness. Can you tell which ones? You might be surprised to find out that they are all involved in activities that can improve their fitness.

You might not be certain what fitness is. **Physical fitness** simply is the ability of your body systems to work together efficiently. Being efficient means being able to do daily activities with the least amount of effort. A fit person is able to carry out the typical activities of living, such as work, and still have enough energy and vigor to respond to emergency situations and to enjoy leisure time activities.

As a child you probably were very active and thought little, if any, of improving or maintaining your fitness. However, as you get older you most likely will be less active and will need to develop a plan for regular physical activity. But getting fit and staying fit can be fun. The activities you choose can be those that you like doing best and those that are best for you.

You might wonder why you should worry about getting fit at all. The Surgeon General of the United States recently published a report noting that being physically active provides many benefits to health and well-being and that being inactive presents many health risks. In fact, inactivity is a major risk factor for many diseases. Therefore, increasing physical activity should be a major health goal for people of all ages.

So what are some specific benefits of regular physical activity? Understanding the meaning of some basic words may help answer this question.

Health and Wellness **Health** is a word often associated with good fitness; it refers to "the state of optimal physical, mental, and social well-being." Early definitions of *health* focused on illness. The first medical doctors concentrated on helping sick people get well; they treated illnesses. Health was nothing more than an absence of disease. But as medical and public health experts received better training, they began to focus on the prevention of illness or disease as well as on the

treatment. This new focus led world health leaders to define *health* as more than absence from disease.

In recent years the definition of *health* has been expanded to include **wellness,** a state of being that enables you to reach your fullest potential. It includes your intellectual, social, emotional, physical, and spiritual health. Wellness has to do with feeling good about yourself and with having goals and purposes in life. Wellness is more likely to be present in individuals who assume more responsibility for their own health. So illness is the "negative" component of health that we want to treat or prevent, and wellness is the "positive" component of health that we want to promote.

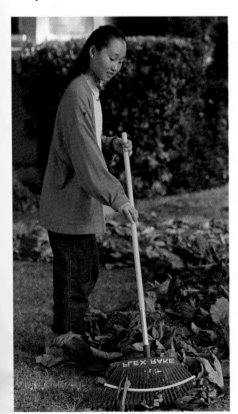
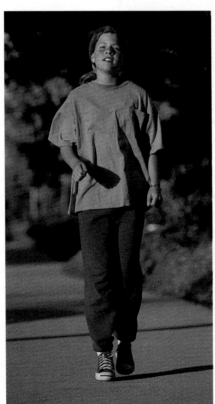
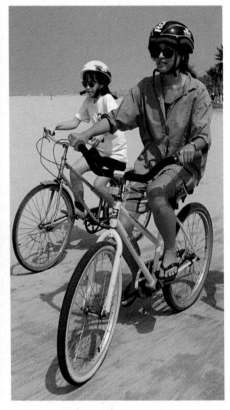

Can you tell which of these people are building fitness?

Physical Activity and Exercise The people in the photos on page 3 are all involved in **physical activity**—movement using the larger muscles of the body. *Physical activity* is a general term that includes sports, dance, and activities done at work or at home, such as walking, climbing stairs, or mowing the lawn. Physical activity may be to do a specific job, to enjoy recreation, or to improve physical fitness. Sometimes you do physical activity with a specific purpose in mind; other times you just do it with no real purpose other than enjoyment.

When people do physical activity especially for the purpose of getting fit, we say they are doing **exercise.** Even though the terms *physical activity* and *exercise* have slightly different meanings, they are sometimes used interchangeably. The thing to remember is that physical activity and exercise are important to your health and wellness.

Health and Wellness Benefits

You might not be concerned with the fact that physical activity has been shown to be effective in treating various illnesses or in preventing them. You might assume that since illness and disease are most common later in life, you don't have to worry about them now. You might even share a common attitude of many teenagers that "I am young and healthy; it can't happen to me." But evidence indicates that the disease process begins early in life. Adopting healthy lifestyles such as regular physical activity can do much to prevent disease and illness. In Chapter 5 you will learn more about the benefits of physical activity in preventing illness.

The benefits derived from physical activity do not only help you later in life. Many benefits are ones you can enjoy now. These benefits include those associated with wellness such as looking good, feeling good,

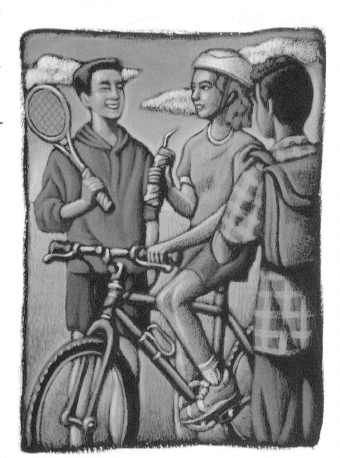

Part of having good health is enjoying life.

meeting emergencies, and being physically fit. The active people in the picture enjoy these benefits.

Looking Good Do you care about how you look? Most people do. In fact, one study showed that 94 percent of all men and 99 percent of all women would change some part of their personal appearance if they could. People are most concerned with weight (weighing too much or too little), the size of their waists and thighs, and their muscles, hair, and teeth. Experts agree that regular physical activity is one healthy lifestyle that can help you look your best. Of course, others are proper nutrition, good posture, and good body mechanics.

Feeling Good Besides looking better, people who do regular physical activity feel better. If you are active and therefore more physically fit, you can resist fatigue, are less likely to be injured, and are capable of working more efficiently. National surveys indicate that active people sleep better, generally feel better, do better on academic work, and are less depressed than people who are less active.

Enjoying Life Like most other people, enjoyment of life is probably important to your personal wellness. But what if you are too tired most days to participate in activities you really enjoy? Regular physical activity results in physical fitness which is the key to being able to do more of the things you want to do.

Meeting Emergencies Another important health and wellness benefit of activity is that it allows you to be fit enough to meet emergencies and day-to-day demanding situations. If you are fit and active, you will be able to run for help, change a flat tire, and offer assistance to others when needed.

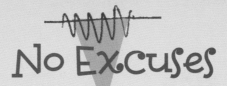

No Excuses

Building Self-Confidence

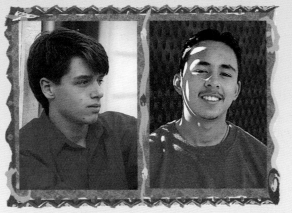

Self-confidence is having faith that you can be successful in some activity. If you think you will succeed in the activity, you have a higher level of self-confidence than if you are unsure about how well you will do. You are more likely to participate in an activity if your self-confidence level is high.

Tony is 6 feet tall and weighs 160 pounds. He looks like a natural athlete. In reality, Tony hardly ever takes part in any physical activity. Because he went through an awkward stage in his preteen years, Tony thinks that people laugh at the way he runs. "My arms and legs don't seem to work together when I run. I think that I look foolish."

Richard loves any kind of physical activity. Every day he shoots baskets or rides his bike. He is part of several teams. While Richard excels in sports, he is shy around strangers, especially when the strangers are female. "I can't think of anything witty or even half-

way intelligent to say. Even when I try to talk, I get tongue-tied. It's easier for me to just avoid talking."

Tony and Richard both lack self-confidence, but in different situations. While Tony really wants to participate in physical activity and Richard wants to socialize with some girls, they both avoid getting into any situation that might require their involvement. Both need to find a way to build their self-confidence levels and be successful in these situations.

For Discussion
People who lack self-confidence may avoid trying new activities or experiences, or they may prematurely quit an activity. What are some reasons people lack self-confidence? How can they increase their confidence levels? Fill out the questionnaire for this chapter to see how self-confident you are about taking part in physical activities.

Being Physically Fit Being physically active can build physical fitness which, in turn, provides you with many health and wellness benefits. If you experience health and wellness benefits, you are likely to enjoy physical activities. As the diagram shows, being active sets up a cycle of wellness that can be beneficial throughout your life.

Don't be tempted to wait until you are older to begin a lifetime fitness program. If you don't have a fitness plan, begin now! You will enjoy the benefits both now and later in life.

By doing the Self-Assessment for this chapter, you will learn some basics of physical activity to get you started on a lifetime of physical activity and fitness. In the next lesson, you will learn about each of the parts of physical fitness and the health and wellness benefits of each.

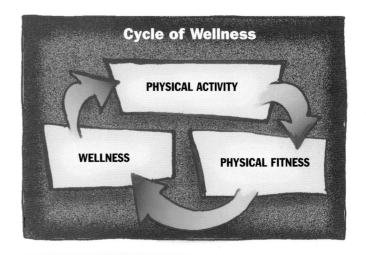

Lesson Review
1. **What is physical fitness?**
2. **What are some benefits of being physically active?**

Self-Assessment 1
Exercise Basics

Safety Tips

Stretch slowly. Try to stretch the muscles slightly, but do not stretc[h] too far. Avoid stretching until you [feel] pain. Do not bounce or jerk

In each chapter of this book, you will find a Self-Assessment to help you determine your own fitness level. The record sheet that your teacher will provide for each Self-Assessment will help you record and analyze your assessment results.

This Self-Assessment will teach you some basics you will need to know in order to do activities in the following chapters. You will learn how to count your heart rate and how to do a warm-up and a cool-down. In Chapter 4 you will learn some of the reasons why a warm-up and cool-down are recommended before and after your physical activity sessions. You also will learn how to plan your own personal warm-up and cool-down. However, you will be doing some physical activities before you've read Chapter 4. For this reason you will learn how to do a basic warm-up and cool-down that you can perform with the activities you will do before you read Chapter 4.

Part 1: The Warm-Up and Stretch

Try the warm-up activities described here. You can use them to warm up for future activities. Keep these guidelines in mind:

• Do the exercises on a soft surface, such as carpeting, a mat, a towel, or on grass. Do not do them on a very soft surface, such as a bed.

• Do each stretch 1 to 3 times.

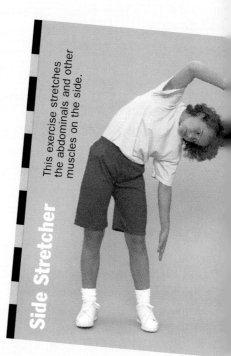

Side Stretcher

This exercise stretches the abdominals and other muscles on the side.

Heart Warm-Up

1 Walk slowly for 1 minute and then jog slowly for 1 minute.

2 If you do not have enough room to jog or walk, jog in place for 2 minutes.

3 Complete the heart warm-up both before and after your muscle stretch.

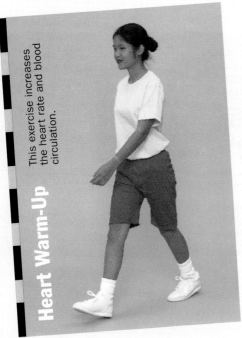

Heart Warm-Up

This exercise increases the heart rate and blood circulation.

Side Stretcher

1 Stand with your feet about shoulder-width apart.

2 Lean to your left.

3 Reach down with your left hand. Reach over your head with your right arm. Hold for a count of 15. **Caution: Do not twist or lean your body forward.**

4 Repeat on your right side.

Knee-to-Chest

1 Lie on your back. Lift one leg off the floor with your knee bent.

2 Hug the thigh of the lifted leg with your hands.

3 Slowly straighten your leg as much as you can. You can pull with your arms if you can fully straighten your leg.

4 Try to keep your other leg straight and flat on the floor. Hold for a count of 15.

5 Repeat with your other leg.

Calf Stretcher

1 Face a wall and stand 2 or 3 feet away.

2 Reach forward. Touch the wall with your hands.

3 Slowly bend your arms and let your body lean forward. Keep your knees straight and your heels on the floor. **Caution: Do not arch your back.**

4 Turn your toes in slightly. Hold for a count of 15.

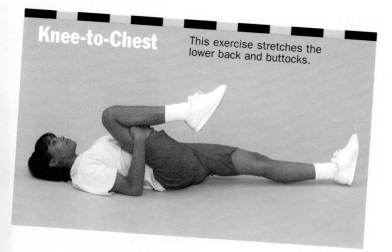

Knee-to-Chest This exercise stretches the lower back and buttocks.

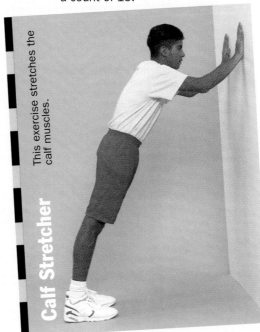

This exercise stretches the calf muscles.

Calf Stretcher

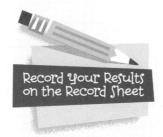

Record Your Results on the Record Sheet

Back and Hip Stretcher

1 Lie on your back. Bend your knees and bring them up to your chest.

2 Reach behind your knees and hug your thighs with your arms.

3 Lift your head and shoulders off the floor as you pull your legs to your chest. Hold for a count of 15.

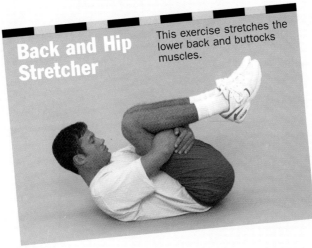

Back and Hip Stretcher This exercise stretches the lower back and buttocks muscles.

Part 2: Counting Heart Rate

To perform many of the activities that you will do in future weeks, you will need to be able to determine your one-minute heart rate. These activities will teach you how.

Counting Resting Heart Rate

Your resting heart rate is the number of times your heart beats when you are relatively inactive. Follow these instructions to learn how to determine your resting heart rate:

1 Sit and take your heart rate by using the first and second fingers of your hand to find a pulse at your wrist. Do not use your thumb. This is your radial pulse. Practice so that you can locate the pulse quickly.

2 Count the number of pulses for 1 minute. Record your one-minute heart rate on your record sheet.

3 Take your resting (seated) heart rate again, this time counting the pulse at the neck. This is your carotid pulse. Record your results.

4 Try taking your pulse using three other simple methods. First, count the heart rate for 15 seconds; then multiply the number by 4. Next, count the number of beats in 10 seconds and multiply by 6. Finally, count your pulse for 6 seconds; then add a 0 to get your minute heart rate. These methods are good for counting your one-minute heart rate after exercise. Make sure you count each pulse. If you miss one pulse on a 6-second count, your pulse count will be off by 10 beats.

5 Now take both your wrist and neck pulse while you are standing. Try it twice using two of the different methods described. Compare your results. Usually your standing pulse is faster than your sitting pulse. Record your results.

6 Take the pulse of a partner while a partner takes your pulse (standing). Compare your self-counted heart rate with your heart rate determined by your partner. You may use different methods of counting but use the same one as your partner when making comparisons. Record your results.

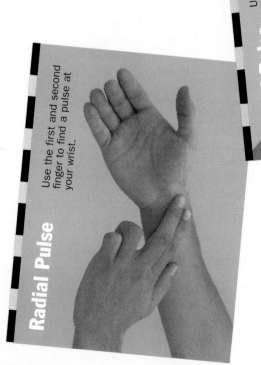

Carotid Pulse
Use the first and second finger to find a pulse at your neck.

Radial Pulse
Use the first and second finger to find a pulse at your wrist.

Counting Exercise Heart Rate

Counting your pulse during activities such as jogging can be difficult, but you can get a good estimate of your exercise heart rate by determining your heart rate immediately after exercising. To do this, follow these instructions:

1 Walk at a fast pace for 1 minute.

2 Immediately after the walk, locate your pulse (within 5 seconds) and use one of the methods described to determine your heart rate. You may want to continue to walk slowly while you count your heart rate, because slow walking can help you recover faster. If you have trouble counting your heart rate while walking, stand still when you count. Your heart rate should be faster than it was at rest. Record your results on your record sheet.

3 Jog or run at a moderate pace for 1 minute. Immediately after the jog determine your heart rate while you continue to walk slowly or stand still. Your heart rate should be even faster than it was after walking. Record your results.

4 Play an active fitness game. After the game, count your heart rate. If it was a vigorous game, your heart rate will be higher than after the run. Record your results on your record sheet.

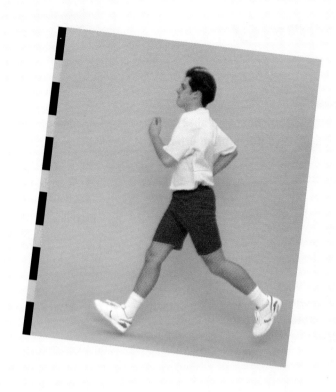

Part 3: The Cool-Down

A cool-down after activity helps you recover. Until you learn to plan your own cool-down, you can use the same exercises as you used for the warm-up to cool-down. Repeat the exercises again to get additional practice in doing them properly.

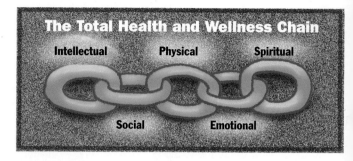

The Total Health and Wellness Chain

Intellectual Physical Spiritual

Social Emotional

1.2 Fitness Through Activity

Lesson Objectives

After reading this lesson, you should be able to:
1. Name and describe the five parts of health-related physical fitness.
2. Name and describe the six parts of skill-related physical fitness.
3. Explain how to use the Stairway to Lifetime Fitness.

Lesson Vocabulary

health-related fitness, skill-related fitness, hypokinetic condition, cardiovascular fitness, strength, muscular endurance, flexibility, body fatness, agility, balance, coordination, power, reaction time, speed

Look at the total health and wellness chain at the top of the page. Notice that each link in the chain represents a different part of health and wellness—social, emotional, spiritual, intellectual, and physical. To have a strong chain that will not break, all of the links have to be strong. Physical fitness is the physical part of the chain. People with good physical fitness have less risk of disease, and they possess wellness components. Without a strong physical fitness link, the rest of the chain will be weakened.

In this lesson you will learn about the eleven parts of physical fitness that contribute to a strong health and wellness chain. You will also learn about the steps you can take to begin building a lifetime of activity and fitness.

The Parts of Physical Fitness

When you see a person who is good at sports, such as the swimmer in the photo, do you assume that the person is physically fit? You might be surprised to know that this is not always true. It is true that a person who excels in sports needs a certain degree of physical fitness. However, being good at specific skills may not be a good indicator of total physical fitness; some sports require only certain parts of fitness.

Physical fitness is made up of eleven parts; five parts are health related and six parts are skill-related. As the terms imply, **health-related fitness** helps you

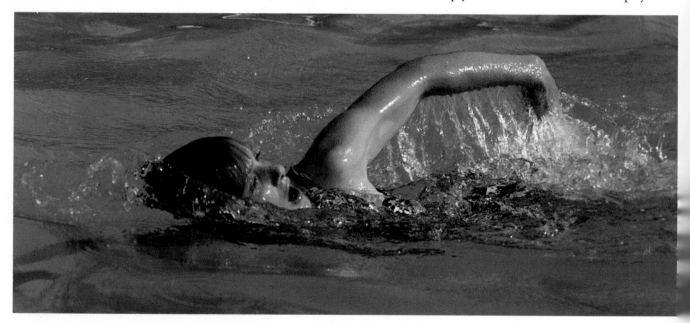

Different activities require different parts of fitness. This swimmer needs good muscular endurance.

stay healthy, while **skill-related fitness** helps you perform well in sports and activities that require certain skills. The Activity at the end of this chapter will help you better understand the differences among the eleven parts. Each part of physical fitness also will be discussed in later chapters.

Health-Related Physical Fitness Think about the swimmer again. She probably can swim long distances without tiring. She has good fitness in at least one area of health-related fitness. But does she have good fitness in all five parts? Swimming does not guarantee that she will be fit in all areas of health-related fitness. Like the swimmer you may be more fit in some parts of health-related fitness than in others. As you read about the parts below, ask yourself how fit you think you are in each.

• **Cardiovascular fitness** is the ability to exercise your entire body for long periods of time. Cardiovascular fitness requires a strong heart, healthy lungs, and clear blood vessels to supply the cells in your body with the oxygen they need.

• **Strength** is the amount of force your muscles can produce. Strength is often measured by how much weight you can lift. People with good strength can perform daily tasks efficiently—that is, with the least amount of effort.

• **Muscular endurance** is the ability to use your muscles many times without tiring. People with good muscular endurance are likely to have better posture and fewer back problems. They are also better able to resist fatigue. The soccer players in the picture need good muscular endurance.

• **Flexibility** is the ability to use your joints fully through a wide range of motion. You are flexible when your muscles are long enough and your joints are free enough to allow movement. People with good flexibility have fewer sore or injured muscles.

• **Body fatness** is the percentage of body weight that is made up of fat when compared to other body tissue, such as bone and muscle. For example, a person who weighs 100 pounds, of which 20 pounds is fat, is said to have a body fat composition of 20 percent. People who are in a healthy range of body fatness are more likely to avoid illness and even have lower death rates than those outside the healthy range. The extreme ranges are the most dangerous; too little body fat, like too much, can cause health problems.

How much of each of the five health-related parts of fitness do you think you have? To be healthy, you should have some of each. If you do, you are less likely to develop a **hypokinetic condition**—a health problem caused partly by lack of exercise. Examples include heart disease, high blood pressure, backache, colon cancer, and being overfat. You will learn more about hypokinetic conditions in Chapter 5.

People who are fit feel better, look better, and have more energy. You do not have to be a great athlete to have good health and feel fit. Regular physical activity can improve anyone's health-related fitness.

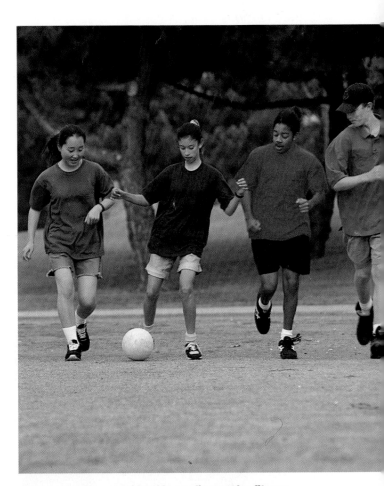

Soccer requires considerable cardiovascular fitness and muscular endurance.

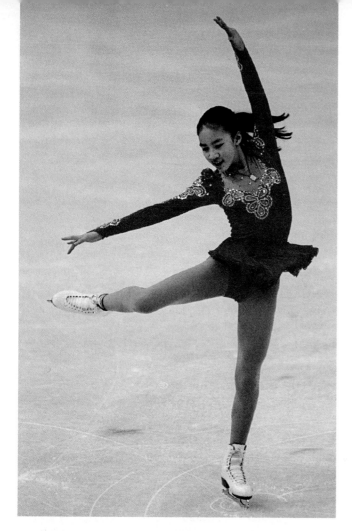

Ice skating requires balance, agility, and coordination.

Skill-Related Physical Fitness Just as the swimmer may not possess a high rating in all parts of health-related fitness, she also may not possess the same amount of fitness in all parts of skill-related fitness. Different sports require different parts of skill-related fitness. Most sports require several parts.

• **Agility** is the ability to change the position of your body quickly and to control your body's movements. People with good agility are likely to be good at activities such as wrestling, diving, soccer, and ice skating.

• **Balance** is the ability to keep an upright posture while standing still or moving. People with good balance are likely to be good in activities such as gymnastics and ice skating.

• **Coordination** is the ability to use your senses together with your body parts, or to use two or more body parts together. People with good eye-hand or eye-foot coordination are

good at hitting and kicking games such as baseball, soccer, and golf.

• **Power** is the ability to use strength quickly. It involves both strength and speed. People with good power might have the ability to put the shot, throw the discus, high jump, play football, and speed swim.

• **Reaction** time is the amount of time it takes to move once you realize the need to act. People with good reaction time are able to make fast starts in track or swimming, or to dodge a fast attack in fencing or karate. Good reaction time is necessary for your own safety while driving or walking.

• **Speed** is the ability to perform a movement or cover a distance in a short period of time. People with leg speed can run fast, while people with good arm speed can throw fast or hit a ball that is thrown fast.

Remember most sports require different parts of skill-related fitness. For example, a skater might have good agility, but may not possess good power. Some people have more natural ability in skill areas than others. No matter how you score on the skill-related parts of fitness, you can enjoy some type of physical activity. Keep in mind that good health does not come from being good in skill-related fitness. Good health comes from doing activities designed to improve your health-related fitness and can be had by people who consider themselves poor athletes as well as by those who see themselves as great athletes.

The Stairway to Lifetime Fitness

You are probably quite active now; most teens are. But will you be as active as you grow older? Will you do the same kinds of activities you do now? If you answered "no" to either of these questions, you need to

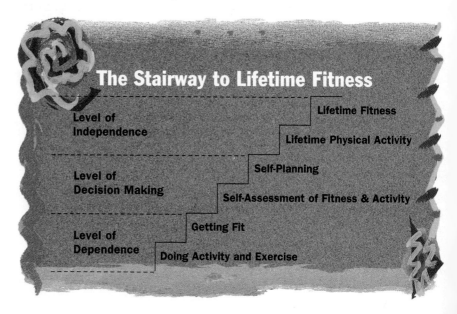

The Stairway to Lifetime Fitness

Level of Independence

Lifetime Fitness

Lifetime Physical Activity

Self-Planning

Level of Decision Making

Self-Assessment of Fitness & Activity

Getting Fit

Level of Dependence

Doing Activity and Exercise

Have you Heard?

One important national health goal is to increase the number of teens who do vigorous physical activity for 20 minutes at least three times a week.

begin learning now for lifetime fitness and activity. One way to accomplish this is to climb the Stairway to Lifetime Fitness. As you can see in the diagram, when you climb the stairway, you move from a level of dependence to a level of independence, allowing you to make good decisions about lifetime physical activity.

Step 1: Doing Physical Activity Think about the various physical activities you are involved in. If you are like many people your age, much of your activity results from community or school activities. You also have other opportunities to do physical activity, such as in physical education classes. As you become an adult, school programs will no longer serve as your incentive to exercise, and other opportunities for physical activity will probably decrease. Doing activity planned by others is a good first step, but it is important to keep climbing the stairway.

Step 2: Getting Fit Because getting fit depends on physical activity and exercise patterns, fitness is something that people often planned for you when you were young. For example, coaches prescribe exercises to get kids fit for sports, and physical education teachers plan activities to get students fit. But when do young people learn to get or keep fit without depending on others? Moving up the stairway means learning to become responsible for your own fitness. When you move to the third step in the stairway, you begin to make your own decisions.

Step 3: Self-Assessment Before you can make good decisions about your own personal fitness and activities, you need to know your own personal fitness level. You may have had your fitness tested before, but probably it was something someone else did for you, rather than something you did for yourself. When you learn to self-assess your own fitness, you will have

reached the third step on the Stairway to Lifetime Fitness. You can use the skills of self-assessment all your life to help in self-planning for lifetime activity and fitness. You will find a Self-Assessment in each chapter of this book.

Step 4: Self-Planning When you have learned to self-assess your own fitness, you are ready to progress to self-planning. You use your own fitness results (a personal fitness profile) to help plan your own fitness and activity program. No two people will have identical fitness needs and no two people will have exactly the same program. The information you learn from this book and in this class will help you do self-planning.

Step 5: Lifetime Activity When you climb to Step 5, you will have moved from the level of decision making and problem solving to the level of lifetime activity. This means you have learned WHY activity is important, WHAT your fitness needs are, and HOW to plan for a lifetime. You will be a lifetime activity participant. This step is much like Step 1 in the stairway, but now you are making your own decisions.

Step 6: Lifetime Fitness When you reach the top level of the stairway, you will have taken responsibility for your own lifetime fitness. You'll have moved from dependence on others to keep you fit. Throughout your life, you will use the skills you learn to reevaluate your fitness needs and to adjust your physical activity program as needed to maintain your fitness.

A major purpose of this book and this class is to help you to achieve lifetime fitness as a result of a healthy lifestyle, including regular lifetime physical activity. In the chapters that follow, you will learn how to climb the stairway and reach this highest step.

Lesson Review
1. Name and describe the five parts of health-related physical fitness.
2. Name and describe the six parts of skill-related physical fitness.
3. Use the Stairway to Lifetime Fitness to explain how you can develop a lifetime habit of fitness.

Activity 1
Health- and Skill-Related Fitness Stunts

At the end of each chapter of this book, you will find an Activity which will help you apply what you learn. Your teacher will provide you with a record sheet for each Activity where you can record your results. Many of these activities can be used as part of your lifetime fitness plan.

You might find it difficult to understand the difference between the parts of health-related and skill-related physical fitness. Use this activity to get a better understanding of the eleven parts. The activities are not intended to test your fitness; future Self-Assessments in the book will help you do that. Remember to warm up before and cool down after doing the activity.

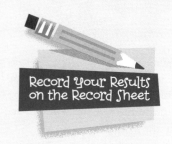

Record Your Results on the Record Sheet

Part 1: Health-Related Fitness

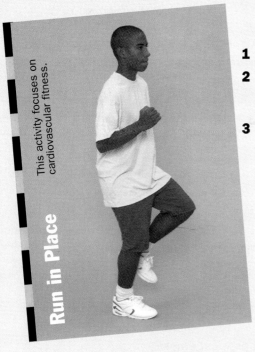

This activity focuses on cardiovascular fitness.

Run in Place

Run in Place
(Cardiovascular Fitness)

1 Find your pulse.

2 Run 120 steps in the same place for 1 minute. A step is every time a foot hits the floor.

3 Rest for 1 minute. Count your heart rate for 30 seconds. A low heart rate after exercise is an indicator of good cardiovascular fitness.

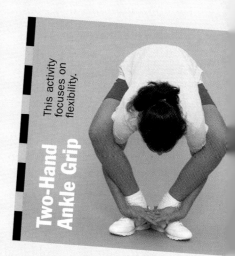

This activity focuses on flexibility.

Two-Hand Ankle Grip

Two-Hand Ankle Grip
(Flexibility)

1 With your heels together, bend forward and reach with your hands between your legs and behind your ankles.

2 Clasp your hands in front of your ankles.

3 Interlock your hands for the full length of your fingers. You must keep your feet still.

4 Hold for 5 seconds.

Single Leg Raise
(Muscular Endurance)

1 Position your upper body on a table so your feet touch the floor. Extend one leg straight out.

2 Complete several leg raises. Performing more than 8 is an indicator of muscular endurance. For this stunt, stop when you reach 25. You can use an ankle weight to make this activity more difficult.

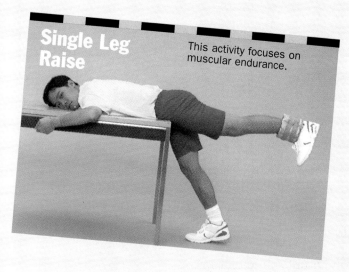

Single Leg Raise

This activity focuses on muscular endurance.

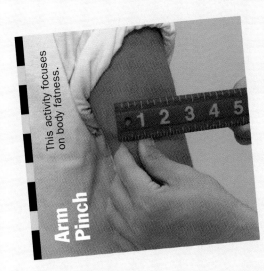

This activity focuses on body fatness.

Arm Pinch

Arm Pinch
(Body Fatness)

1 Let your right arm hang relaxed at your side. Have a partner pinch the skin and fat under the skin on the back of your arm. Pinch halfway between your elbow and shoulder.

2 Have your partner use a ruler to measure the skin thickness. Thicker skinfolds generally mean a greater amount of total body fatness.

Half Push-Up
(Strength)

1 Lie facedown, hands on the floor outside of your shoulders.

2 Keep your body straight. Push up until your upper arms are parallel to the floor.

3 Lower your body until your nose touches the floor. Only your toes and hands may touch the floor.

4 Stronger people can do more repetitions. Once you are able to do 10 push-ups, this stunt becomes an indicator of muscular endurance.

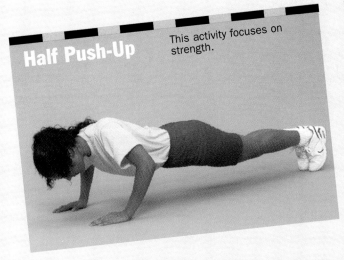

Half Push-Up

This activity focuses on strength.

Part 2: Skill-Related Fitness

Line Jump
(Agility)

1 Balance on your right foot on a line on the floor.

2 Leap onto the left foot so that it lands to the right of the line.

3 Leap across the line onto the right foot; land to the left of the line.

4 Leap onto the left foot, landing on the line.

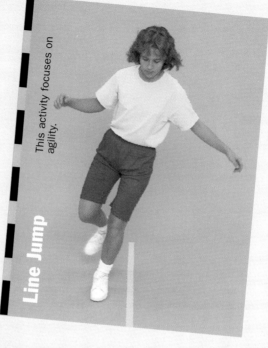

This activity focuses on agility.

Line Jump

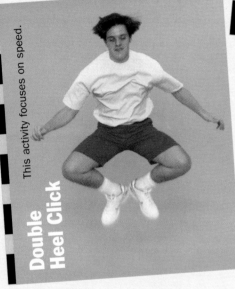

This activity focuses on speed.

Double Heel Click

Double Heel Click
(Speed)

1 Jump into the air and click your heels together twice before you land.

2 Your feet should be at least 3 inches apart when you land.

Backward Hop
(Balance)

1 With your eyes closed, hop backward on one foot for 5 hops.

2 After the last hop, hold your balance for 3 seconds.

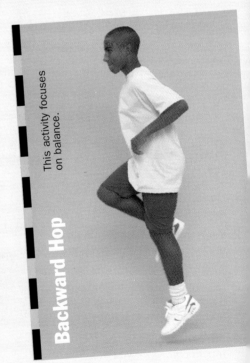

This activity focuses on balance.

Backward Hop

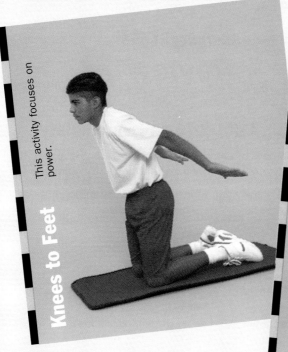

This activity focuses on power.

Knees to Feet

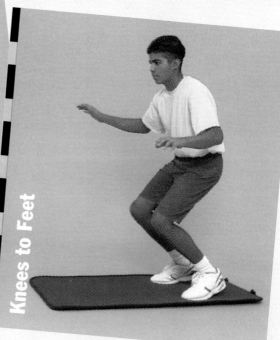

Knees to Feet

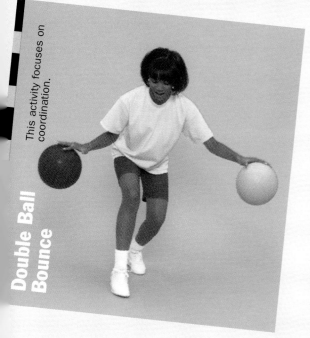

This activity focuses on coordination.

Double Ball Bounce

Knees to Feet
(Power)

1 Kneel so that your shins and knees are on a mat. Hold your arms back. Point your toes straight backward.

2 Without curling your toes under you or rocking your body backward, swing your arms upward and spring to your feet.

3 Hold your position for 3 seconds after you land.

Double-Ball Bounce
(Coordination)

1 Hold a volleyball in each hand. Beginning at the same time with each hand, bounce both balls at the same time, at least knee high.

2 Bounce both balls 3 times in a row without losing control of them.

Coin Catch
(Reaction Time)

1 Point your right elbow in front of you. Your right hand, palm up, should be by your right ear. If you are left-handed, do this activity with your left hand.

2 Place a coin as close to the end of your elbow as possible.

3 Quickly lower your elbow and grab the coin in the air with your right hand before it touches the ground. Drop the coin from your elbow; do not throw it.

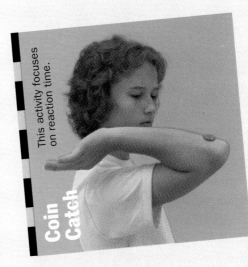

This activity focuses on reaction time.

Coin Catch

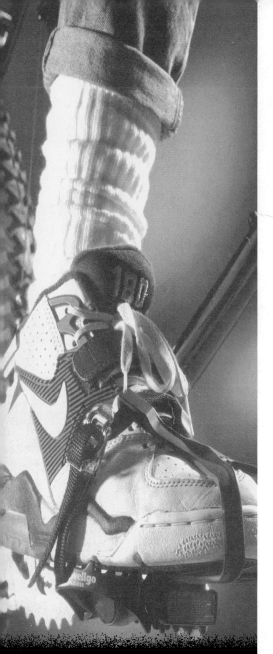

1 ▸ Chapter Review

Reviewing Concepts and Vocabulary

Copy the number of each statement on a sheet of paper. Next to each number, write the word or words that correctly complete the sentence.

1. Physical activity done for the purpose of getting fit is called _____.

2. The _____ is a series of steps to help you achieve lifetime fitness.

3. Cardiovascular fitness is one part of _____ fitness.

4. A hypokinetic condition is a health problem caused by _____ .

5. Body fatness is _____ .

Number your paper. Next to each number, choose the letter of the best answer.

Column I	Column II
6. muscular endurance	a. movement of body using larger muscles
7. flexibility	b. ability to use body parts together
8. agility	c. ability to cover a distance quickly
9. balance	d. positive component of health
10. coordination	e. ability to use joints through a wide range of motion
11. reaction time	f. ability to change body position quickly
12. speed	g. ability to keep an upright position
13. physical activity	h. ability to use muscles continuously without tiring
14. wellness	i. amount of time to start moving

On your paper, write a short answer for each statement or question.

15. What is physical fitness?

16. Why is fitness important for everyone?

17. How do health-related fitness and skill-related fitness differ?

18. Explain why a sports star may not possess the same levels of fitness in all areas of physical fitness.

19. What is the difference between power and strength?

20. Explain how the definition of health has changed over time.

Thinking Critically

Write a paragraph to answer the following question.

A friend of yours tells you she sees no reason to develop a plan for lifetime physical activity because she gets plenty of activity in school. She is on the basketball team and the track team. She also has physical education classes five times a week. What would you tell her? Explain your answer.

Project

Interview several healthy older adults about their health-related fitness. Ask questions such as: What kinds of activity do you do for cardiovascular fitness? How has your fitness and physical activity changed over the years? Are you more fit or more active now? Use the data to discuss how teenagers can use exercises they learn now throughout their lives.

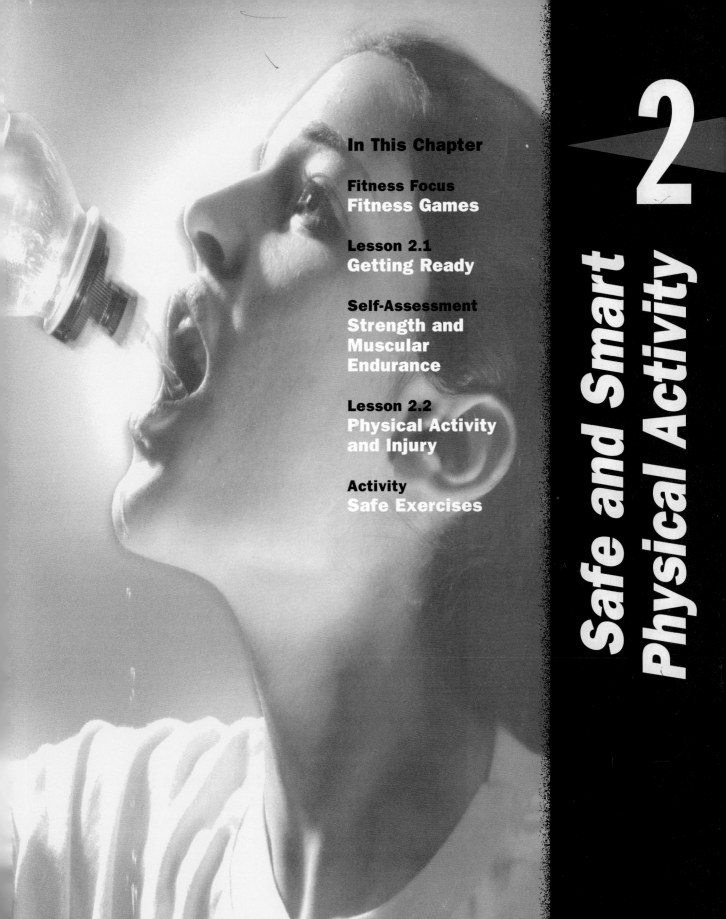

2

Safe and Smart Physical Activity

Fitness Games

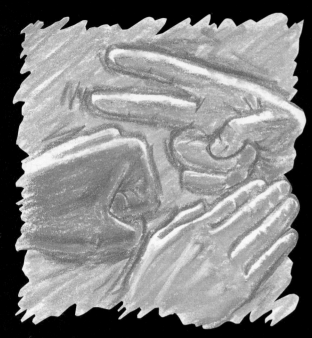

One of the most important forms of activity is games. Generally young people play more games than adults, but games can be a way of being physically active to build fitness.

Many of the fitness games you see on your instruction sheet may not be ones you will use later in life. But try some of them just for fun. They can help you achieve fitness right now.

Parachute Warm-Up
Parachute Ball
Parachute Tug-o-War
Group Tag
Train Tag
Active Rock, Paper, Scissors
Mind the Store

Lesson 2.1 Getting Ready

Lesson Objectives
After reading this lesson, you should be able to:
1. Explain how to prepare yourself for physical activity.
2. Explain how the environment affects physical activity.
3. Explain how learning self-assessment helps you prepare for a lifetime of physical activity.

Lesson Vocabulary
heat exhaustion, heat stroke, frostbite, hypothermia

Whether you're a beginner in physical activity or you've been exercising for some time, it's important for you to be prepared to exercise and to know how to exercise safely in all conditions. If you're a beginner, a first step is to be medically ready. As a young person you probably won't have a problem with physical readiness, but you should answer some simple questions about yourself just to be sure. Also, you should be ready for a variety of environmental conditions such as heat, cold, pollution, and altitude that may require a change in your exercise habits. Avoiding injuries and being ready to cope with injuries that may occur are also important.

In this lesson you will learn how to prepare yourself for physical activity. You also will learn about self-assessments and how they can help you prepare for a lifetime of physical activity.

Medical Readiness
If you are going to participate in an interscholastic sport or a program of similar intensity, such as preparing to participate in community sports or rigorous personal challenges, a medical examination is recommended. Medical exams help make sure that you are free from disease and can help prevent future health problems.

If you are interested in starting a regular physical activity program for health and wellness, it would be wise to assess your medical and physical readiness.

Your teacher can provide you with a questionnaire to help you do your assessment. Also, discuss your plans for activity with your parents or guardians so they can help you make a determination about readiness.

Readiness for Extreme Environmental Conditions

Weather plays an important role in determining when and how strenuously you exercise. Whether you are just beginning a physical activity program or you have been exercising for a while, understanding how environmental conditions can affect your body during

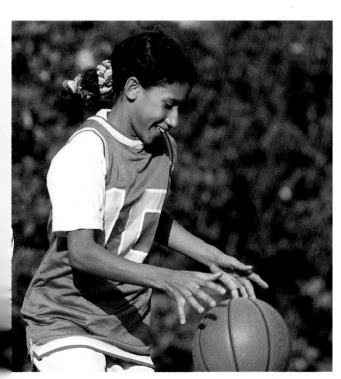

When exercising in hot weather, wear light porous clothing.

exercise is important. If you follow simple guidelines, you can reduce the risk of developing heat-related conditions.

Hot, Humid Weather

Hot, humid weather causes your body temperature to rise more quickly than it might in cooler weather. Be careful when exercising in hot weather. Heat-related medical conditions can occur if your body temperature rises too high. **Heat exhaustion** is a condition caused by excessive exposure to heat and is characterized by cold, clammy skin and symptoms of shock. **Heat stroke** is a more serious condition that is caused by exposure to excessive heat. The symptoms of heat stroke include high body temperature and dry skin. A more detailed list of symptoms for each condition is shown in the chart above. Follow these guidelines to prevent heat-related conditions:

- **Begin gradually.** As your body becomes accustomed to physical activity in hot weather, it becomes more resistant to heat-related injuries. Start with short periods of activity and gradually increase the time.

- **Drink water.** During hot weather your body perspires more than normally to cool itself. You need to drink plenty of water to replace the water your body loses through perspiration.

- **Wear proper clothing.** Wear porous clothing that allows air to pass through it to cool your body. Wear light-colored clothing; lighter colors reflect the sun's heat, while darker colors absorb heat.

- **Rest frequently.** Physical activity creates body heat. Periodically stop and rest in a shady area to help your body lower its temperature.

- **Avoid extreme heat and humidity.** You can use the chart on the next page to determine if weather is too hot. You should do physical activity in the caution

Heat-Related Conditions

Heat Exhaustion:
- Approximately normal body temperature
- Pale, clammy skin
- Profuse perspiration
- Tiredness, weakness
- Headache, perhaps cramps
- Nausea, dizziness, possible vomiting
- Possible fainting

Heat Stroke:
- High body temperature (might be 106°F or higher)
- Skin is hot, red, and dry
- Pulse is rapid and strong
- Victim may be unconscious

Heat Index

As humidity increases, air can feel hotter than it actually is.
This chart shows how hot it feels as humidity rises.

Relative Humidity (%)											
100	72	80	91	108	132						
90	71	79	88	102	122						
80	71	78	86	97	113	136					
70	70	77	85	93	106	124	144				
60	70	76	82	90	100	114	132	149			
50	69	75	81	88	96	107	120	135	150		
40	68	74	79	86	93	101	110	123	137	151	
30	67	73	78	84	90	96	104	113	123	135	148
20	66	72	77	82	87	93	99	105	112	120	130
10	65	70	75	80	85	90	95	100	105	111	116
0	64	69	73	78	83	87	91	95	99	103	107
	70	75	80	85	90	95	100	105	110	115	120

Air Temperature (Degrees F)

Caution Zone
Danger Zone

zones only if you have adapted to hot environments and follow the basic guidelines. The amount of time it takes to adapt to conditions varies with each person.

Cold, Windy, Wet Weather

Exercising during cold, windy weather can be dangerous also. Extreme cold can result in two serious conditions. A condition called **frostbite** results when body tissues become frozen. Often a person with frostbite feels no pain, making this condition more dangerous. Another condition related to cold weather is **hypothermia.**
With hypothermia, the body temperature becomes abnormally low. The chart above gives more information about frostbite and hypothermia. Be sure to keep the following guidelines in mind when exercising in cold weather:

Cold-Related Conditions

Frostbite:
- Skin becomes white or grayish-yellow; looks glossy
- Pain sometimes felt early, but subsides later (often no pain at all)
- Blisters may appear later
- Affected area feels intensely cold and numb

Hypothermia:
- Shivering
- Numbness
- Low body temperature
- Drowsiness
- Marked muscular weakness
- Victim acts confused or disoriented, seems apathetic

• **Avoid extreme cold and wind.** Before dressing for physical activity, use the chart on the next page to determine the wind-chill factor. Exercising when the temperature is cold and the wind is blowing is especially dangerous because the air feels colder. If the wind-chill factor is in the great danger zone, activity should be postponed. If you are active when the wind-chill factor is in the increasing danger zone, be sure to dress properly and be aware of the symptoms of frostbite and hypothermia.

• **Dress properly.** Wear several layers of lightweight clothing rather than a heavy jacket or coat. The clothing closest to your body should be made of absorbent material. The outer layers should be nylon or other material that will stop the wind. Avoid nonporous jackets—they do not let your body release heat. Wear a knit cap, ski mask, and mittens, as needed. Mittens keep your hands warmer than gloves.

• **Avoid exercising in icy or wet and cold weather.** Special problems can occur during icy or wet and cold weather. Your shoes, socks, and pant legs can get wet, increasing the risk of foot injuries and falls.

Other Environmental Conditions Conditions other than weather, including air pollution and altitude, can influence the effectiveness and safety of exercise.

High levels of air pollution affect your breathing ability. Radio and television stations usually issue warnings when air-pollution levels are high. Avoid exercising during these times.

People who live in high-altitude locations are able to exercise with little trouble; however, people who live at lower altitudes might have trouble adjusting to higher altitudes. Even if you are physically fit, allow your body to adjust to higher altitudes by first exercising for short periods of time. For example, snow skiers should avoid hard skiing for a day or two in order to become accustomed to the higher altitude.

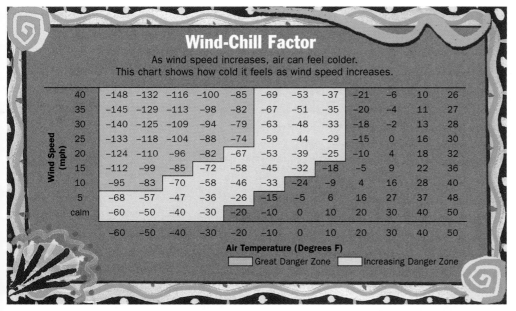

Wind-Chill Factor

As wind speed increases, air can feel colder.
This chart shows how cold it feels as wind speed increases.

Wind Speed (mph)	-60	-50	-40	-30	-20	-10	0	10	20	30	40	50
40	-148	-132	-116	-100	-85	-69	-53	-37	-21	-6	10	26
35	-145	-129	-113	-98	-82	-67	-51	-35	-20	-4	11	27
30	-140	-125	-109	-94	-79	-63	-48	-33	-18	-2	13	28
25	-133	-118	-104	-88	-74	-59	-44	-29	-15	0	16	30
20	-124	-110	-96	-82	-67	-53	-39	-25	-10	4	18	32
15	-112	-99	-85	-72	-58	-45	-32	-18	-5	9	22	36
10	-95	-83	-70	-58	-46	-33	-24	-9	4	16	28	40
5	-68	-57	-47	-36	-26	-15	-5	6	16	27	37	48
calm	-60	-50	-40	-30	-20	-10	0	10	20	30	40	50

Air Temperature (Degrees F)

☐ Great Danger Zone   ☐ Increasing Danger Zone

Readiness for Self-Assessments

In the weeks that follow, you will be learning to do several different physical fitness assessments. For example, to assess cardiovascular fitness you will do the PACER, the walking test, and the step test or the mile run. If you are not prepared, these tests will seem difficult and may result in soreness. To avoid these consequences, you should begin now to do regular physical activity. Walking, jogging, cycling, and swimming will help you prepare. Later you will be doing strength and flexibility self-assessments. You will do some activities in class to prepare for these assessments. Doing some additional activities outside of class would be good.

Why Do Self-Assessments? You learned in Chapter 1 that self-assessment is an important tool to use when planning for a lifetime of physical activity. The reasons below will help you understand why self-assessment is so important.

• **Determining your current level of fitness.** How much health-related fitness do you have? Self-assessment can help you answer this important question. When you have completed all of the self-assessments in this book, you will be able to create a fitness profile that will tell you how fit you are. You can use that profile as a basis for planning your physical activity program planning.

• **Learning to make your own assessments.** Most likely any fitness tests that you have taken already were given by your teachers. As you get older, you will need to learn to make assessments on your own because teachers will not always be there to help you. It is important to learn how to assess your own fitness throughout life. Knowing your current fitness level is essential to planning a good fitness program.

• **Learning to rate each fitness part.** Fitness test scores have little meaning unless you know how to interpret them. In Chapter 3 you will learn to use charts to help you rate your fitness scores. A worthy long-term goal is to achieve fitness in the good fitness zone for all parts of health-related fitness. For now you should not worry about setting fitness goals. Instead focus on doing some regular activity and doing self-assessments on all health-related fitness parts.

Why Do More Than One Self-Assessment for Each Fitness Part? As you move through this book, you might notice that for each of the health-related physical fitness parts you will perform more than one self-assessment. There are several reasons for this:

• **Some assessments are better suited to some individuals than others.** For example, the PACER and the walking test are probably best for beginners. But the mile run is probably best for people interested in assessing high-performance fitness.

• **Some assessments are easy to do but may have more error.** Using height and weight to assess your body composition is easy because most people have access to a yardstick and a scale. But height-weight measures are not good for measuring body fatness. On the other hand, skinfold tests help you better understand body fatness but require special equipment. If you learn to do more than one test, you have more than one choice of assessments.

• **Having a choice of assessments may help you avoid some types of problems.** Motivation is a problem in tests such as the mile run or push-ups. Motivation is less of a problem with a test such as the Step

No Excuses

Making Activity Convenient

Have you ever decided not to exercise because you couldn't get a ride to the gym? Or your old basketball has lost its bounce? Or it's too dangerous to jog in your neighborhood? If you choose activities that are convenient and practical, you won't be tempted to use these excuses.

"How was swim club today, Hope?" Judy asked over the phone.

"The water was kind of cold, but we had a good workout. Why don't you try out for the club, Judy? You're a good swimmer, and you could use some exercise."

"I'd like to, but I have no car and the pool is too far away," Judy replied.

"You could take the bus from the school to the pool, like the rest of us," Hope suggested.

"But how would I get home?" she asked. "You and the rest of the team can walk home, because you live near the pool or the school. But I live way over here in Broadhurst, on the other side of town. My dad works

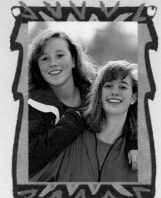

until 6:00, so he can't pick me up at 5:00 when practice ends. I'd have to wait for him forever."

"I think Karla lives out your way, and she has a car," Hope suggested. "Why don't you ask her for a ride home?"

"I don't think she lives that close to me. What if she says no?"

"Let's wait to see what Karla says first. You never know till you ask!"

For Discussion

Why is joining the swim club not convenient for Judy? What else might Judy do to make exercise more convenient? What are some other things that might make exercise and physical activity inconvenient for everyone? What are some ways to deal with these inconveniences in order to still be physically active? Fill out the questionnaire to analyze how convenient it is for you to exercise or otherwise be physically active.

Test or measuring the circumference of your waist and hips. By learning several assessments you can overcome motivational problems if they occur.

• **Several assessments are usually better than one.** If you do only one assessment and make an error, you may make incorrect assumptions about your fitness. If you do several assessments, you can consider all of them to get a better indicator of your fitness. Of course, when you do several assessments, there is a chance that results on one assessment may differ from the results of another assessment. One of the skills of a good physical activity planner is interpreting assessments accurately. With practice in self-assessment you can learn this skill.

Lesson Review

1. Explain how to prepare yourself for physical activity.
2. How does the environment affect physical activity?
3. How can self-assessment help you prepare for a lifetime of physical activity?

Self-Assessment 2
Strength and Muscular Endurance

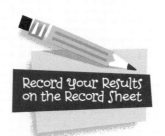

Record your Results on the Record Sheet

The Prudential FITNESSGRAM® is a group of physical fitness assessments developed specifically for youth. In this activity you will perform two of the FITNESSGRAM assessments, the curl-up and the push-up. These two assessments are designed to measure strength and muscular endurance. You will perform the remaining FITNESSGRAM assessments in Chapters 3 and 4.

For the FITNESSGRAM tests in this chapter and in Chapter 3, you will record your scores and ratings on your record sheets. Later in Chapter 3 you will learn to interpret your ratings. Then in Chapter 4, you will chart your results for all your FITNESSGRAM assessments to provide a fitness profile. You can use this profile for personal fitness planning.

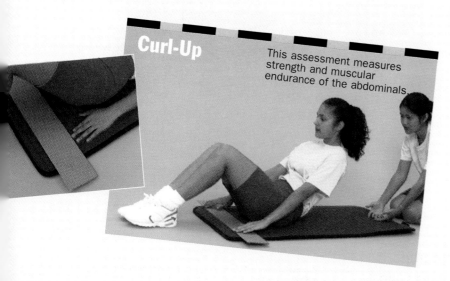

Curl-Up

This assessment measures strength and muscular endurance of the abdominals.

Curl-Up

1 Lie on your back on a mat. Bend your knees half way between straight and 90 degrees. Your feet should be slightly apart and your arms straight down to your sides.

2 Place your head in a partner's hands or on a small pillow. Place a cardboard strip under your knees so that the fingers of both hands just touch the near edge of the strip. A partner can stand on the strip to keep it stationary or you can tape it down.

3 Keeping your heels on the floor, curl your shoulders up slowly and slide your arms forward so that the fingers move across the cardboard strip. Curl up until the fingertips reach the far side of the strip.

4 Slowly lower your back until your head rests in your partner's hands or on the pillow.

5 Repeat the procedure so that you do one curl-up every 3 seconds. A partner could help you by saying "up-down" every 3 seconds. You are finished when you can not do another curl-up, when you fail to keep up with the 3-second count, or when you have completed 25 curl-ups.
Note: To avoid soreness you may want to stop at 25 curl-ups. If you want to see if you are in the high performance zone, you can retake the test when you have been active on a regular basis.

6 Record the number of curl-ups you have completed on your record sheet. Then find your rating in the chart.

Rating Chart: Curl-Up

	13 years old		14 years old		15 years old or above	
	males	females	males	females	males	females
High Performance	41+	33+	46+	33+	48+	36+
Good Fitness	21–40	18–32	24–45	18–32	24–47	18–35
Marginal Fitness	18–20	15–17	20–23	15–17	20–23	15–17
Low Fitness	17–	14–	19–	14–	19–	14–

Adapted from FITNESSGRAM

Push-Up

1 Lie face down on a mat or carpet with your hands under your shoulders, your fingers spread, and your legs straight. Your legs should be slightly apart and your toes should be tucked under.

2 Push up until your arms are straight. Keep your legs and back straight. Your body should form a straight line.

3 Lower your body by bending your elbows until they are at a 90-degrees angle. Do one push-up every 3 seconds. You may want to have a partner say "up-down" to help you. You are finished when you fail to do a push-up with proper form for the second time or when you reach a score of 15 for females or 25 for males.
Note: To avoid soreness you may wish to stop at 15 if you are female or 25 for males. If you want to see if you are in the high performance zone, you can retake the test when you have been active on a regular basis.

4 Record the number of push-ups you performed on your record sheet. Then find your score in the rating chart.

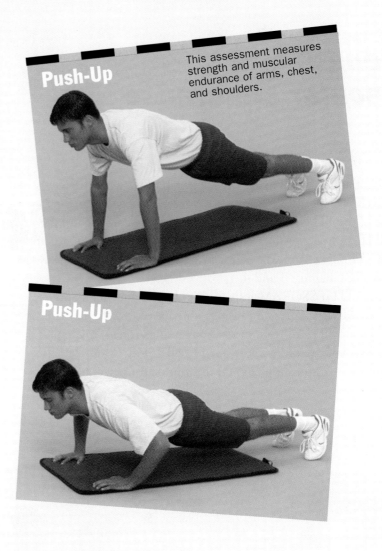

Push-Up

This assessment measures strength and muscular endurance of arms, chest, and shoulders.

Push-Up

Rating Chart: Push-Up

	13 years old		14 years old		15 years old		16 years old or above	
	males	females	males	females	males	females	males	females
High Performance	26+	16+	31+	16+	36+	16+	36+	16+
Good Fitness	12–25	7–15	14–30	7–15	16–35	7–15	18–35	7–15
Marginal Fitness	10–11	6	12–13	6	14–15	6	16–17	6
Low Fitness	9–	5–	11–	5–	13–	5–	15–	5–

Adapted from FITNESSGRAM

Physical Activity and Injury

Lesson Objectives
After reading this lesson, you should be able to:
1. List and describe some exercise-related physical injuries.
2. List some guidelines for preventing injuries during physical activity.
3. Explain how to apply the RICE formula to the treatment of physical injuries.
4. Identify different types of risky exercises.

Lesson Vocabulary
overuse injury, side stitch, microtrauma, joint, ligament, tendon, biomechanical principles

Have you Heard?
A sprain is an injury to ligaments and muscles. If a ligament is stretched, swelling and pain around the joint can result. A strain, or muscle pull, is an injury to a tendon or muscle. A strain also can result in muscle pain and swelling.

You know that physical activity has many advantages to your health and general well-being. But if physical activity is not done properly, injury can sometimes result. Most injuries are minor but can be prevented if care is taken.

Before you start a physical activity program, be sure you are prepared to exercise and know how to exercise safely. In this lesson you will learn about some of the common minor injuries, as well as some basic precautions that you should take to avoid them. Some exercises are considered to be risky because they can lead to injury. You will learn about some of these risky exercises and about safer alternatives that you can use.

Common Injuries
If you have ever suffered an injury related to sports or exercise, you know that it can be quite painful even if it's not serious. Some of the more common minor injuries related to sports and exercise are sprains, strains, blisters, bruises, cuts, and scrapes. More serious but less common injuries include joint dislocations and bone fractures. The most common parts of the body injured in physical activity are the skin, feet, ankles, knees, and leg muscles. Injuries to the head, arms, body, and internal organs such as the liver and kidneys are less likely.

Some injuries are called **overuse injuries.** These injuries occur when you repeat a movement so much that wear and tear occur to your body. You are most likely familiar with one very common overuse injury—a blister. Another example is a shin splint, which is a soreness in the front of the lower leg. It is probably caused by small muscle tears or muscle spasms from overuse of the muscles. Runner's heel is another overuse injury that results in a soreness in the heel. The soreness is usually caused by running or jumping activities that require the heel to repeatedly hit the ground. These injuries are especially common among long-distance runners and people whose activities cause repeated impact on the feet.

A **side stitch** is a pain in the side of the lower abdomen that people often experience in sports, especially running activities. Side stitches are most common among people who are not accustomed to vigorous activity. A side stitch is not really an injury because the pain goes away if you stop the activity or continue at a more moderate pace. Unless the pain is extreme or persistent, a stitch is nothing to worry about. To help relieve a side stitch, press firmly at the point of the pain with your hand while bending forward or backward.

Another type of injury is called **microtrauma**. *Micro* means "small"—so small it may not show up on an X ray or exam—and *trauma* is another word for *injury*. So a *microtrauma* is "an invisible injury." Often these injuries do not cause immediate pain or soreness, but with repeated use damage eventually appears. Many adults today are now experiencing back problems, neck aches, and stiff, painful joints caused by microtrauma done when they were younger. Some risky exercises that can be the cause of microtrauma are discussed later in the chapter.

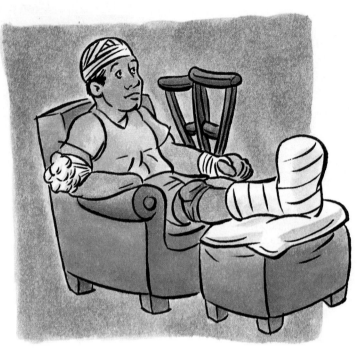

Following proper exercise guidelines can help you avoid injuries.

Preventing Injuries

You might wonder why you should exercise at all if so many injuries are related to being active. However, you don't have to end up looking like the guy in the cartoon above. By understanding how your body works and by following some simple guidelines, you can reduce the risk of common injuries.

You probably know that your body is made up of about 206 bones that connect at **joints.** You can see in the diagram below that **ligaments** hold the bones together at the joint. Ligaments are made of tough tissues. The other tissues you see in the picture are **tendons,** tissues that connect muscles to bones.

When your muscles contract, they pull your tendons and make your bones move. The bones act as levers and work with your muscles to allow body movement. But when your muscles move the bones in your body, they exert a force on those bones. These forces can cause medical problems if you don't use correct techniques when doing physical activity.

The same principles used in physics and engineering to study

forces can be applied to help living organisms function efficiently. These principles, called **biomechanical principles,** can help you use the levers of your body (your bones) to move efficiently and avoid injury to the joints and other body parts.

One important principle you should remember is that you should not force your joints to move in a way that they were not designed to move. For example, you should avoid any movement that rotates your elbow or knee; the structure of these joints does not safely allow that kind of movement.

Another principle to keep in mind as you exercise is that your movements should not overstress bones, tendons, ligaments, or muscles. Bending over and trying to touch your toes while both legs are straight has the possibility of injuring your back.

A third principle to remember as you do physical activity is that you should balance the muscle development around a joint so that all the muscles are developed properly. For example, look below at the diagram of an upper arm. If you overdevelop your biceps muscle with no attention to your triceps, eventually you might be unable to fully extend your arm; your triceps will not be strong enough. Also you increase the risk of straining your triceps muscle because this weak muscle will be overstressed by the pull of the strong biceps.

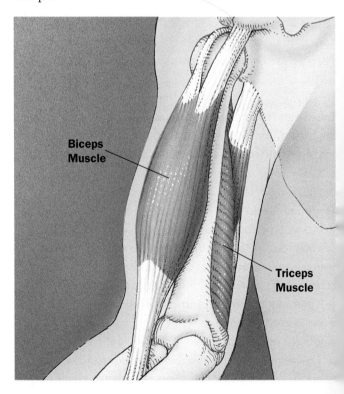

To avoid problems, balance the muscle development around a joint.

As you perform your regular physical activity keep those important biomechanical principles in mind, as well as the additional guidelines that follow.

- **Start slowly.** The greatest number of injuries occur in beginners. If you haven't been exercising regularly, be sure to start slowly and gradually build up to more vigorous activity.

- **Listen to your body.** Injuries can occur when you ignore the signs and symptoms your body is giving you. If you experience pain, pay attention to it. Until you know what is causing the pain, slow your exercise or stop altogether. Most blisters and shin splints could be avoided if people would listen to their bodies.

- **Warm up before activity and cool down after activity.** Most experts believe that a warm-up before physical activity and a cool-down after you exercise will help reduce the risk of injury. You will learn more about how to do a proper warm-up and cool-down in Chapter 4.

- **Be fit!** One of the best ways to avoid injury is to be physically fit. A person with a fit heart and lungs and long, strong muscles is less likely to be injured than one who is unfit. Proper physical activity builds total physical fitness which aids in injury prevention.

- **Use moderation.** Overuse is the cause of many minor injuries in physical activity. About 40 percent of regular runners and 50 percent of aerobic dancers experience injuries at some time. Injuries are usually caused by using a body part too much (too intensely) or for too long a period of time.

- **Dress properly.** Sometimes injuries are caused by improper dress. Poor shoes and socks can cause blisters or runner's heel. Make sure you dress properly, wear proper shoes, and replace them when they begin to wear down.

Simple Treatment of Minor Injuries

When injuries occur, it is often necessary to seek medical help. However, you can take immediate steps to reduce the pain or prevent complications of the injury. It's good to know first aid so that you know what steps to take when injuries occur. For muscle strains, sprains, and bruises, which are common in sports and other activities, you can follow the RICE formula, which you can see to the right. Each letter in the formula represents a step taken to treat a minor injury.

The RICE Formula for Treating Injury

R is for rest.
After first aid has been given for the injury, the body part should be immobilized for two to three days to prevent further injury. In some cases longer rest periods are required.

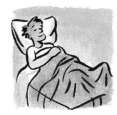

I is for ice.
A sprain or strain should be immersed in cold water or covered with ice in a towel or plastic bag. Do this for 20 minutes immediately after the injury to help reduce swelling and pain. Ice or cold should be applied several times a day for one to three days. Rubbing ice on the front of your leg can help relieve the pain of shin splints.

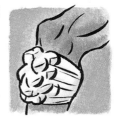

C is for compression.
Use an elastic bandage to wrap the injury. This helps to limit the swelling. For a sprained ankle keep the shoe laced and the sock on the foot until compression can be applied with a wrap. The shoe and sock compress the injury. The compression should not be too tight and should be taken off periodically so as not to restrict blood flow.

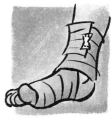

E is for elevation.
Raising the body part above the level of the heart helps reduce the swelling.

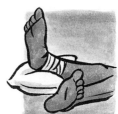

Risky Exercises

Some exercises are considered risky because they cause the body to move in ways that violate basic biomechanical principles. Doing these exercises may not cause immediate injury and pain. However, if they are done repeatedly over a period of time, these exercises put you at risk for microtrauma. They can result in pain; joint problems; "wear and tear" injuries such as inflammation of tendons, bursa, or joints; and a wearing away of the joint cartilage. Microtrauma caused by doing risky exercises over time can result in crippling arthritis or back and neck pain, a leading medical complaint in our country.

In general, the exercises listed below should be avoided. In the Activity with this chapter you will learn some safe alternative exercises. Some athletes might find it impossible to avoid potentially harmful exercises. For example, gymnasts must perform stunts that require back arching. Softball and baseball catchers must do full squats. It is especially important that these people do extra flexibility and strength exercises to prepare their bodies for these activities. They should carefully warm up and cool down. If pain occurs when exercising, medical attention should be obtained immediately.

Hyperflexion Exercises to Avoid Hyperflexion exercises bend your joints too far and overstretch the ligaments. *Hyper* means "too much"; *flexion* means "to bend." The deep knee bend is an example of hyperflexion or overflexion of the knee. Basically hyperflexion exercises cause you to use the joint in a way that it was not intended to be used. Other hyperflexing

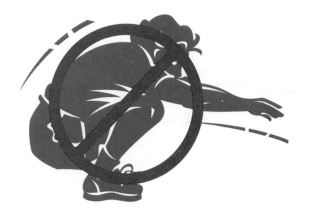

Avoid deep knee bends.

exercises to avoid include duckwalks, bicycles (also called shoulder stand), yoga ploughs, hands-behind-the-neck sit-ups, and knee pull-downs.

Back Hyperextension Exercises to Avoid

Hyperextension is the opposite of hyperflexion. Arching the lower back more than normal is called hyperextension. Some back arching exercises tend to stretch your abdominal muscles and can injure your spinal disks and joints. In addition, these exercises may shorten your back muscles which are already too

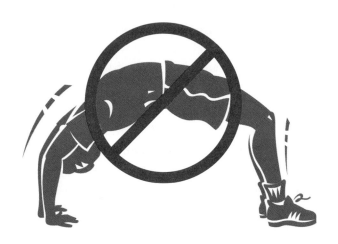

Avoid exercise that makes the lower back arch.

short in most people. People with swayback, weak abdominal muscles, protruding abdomen, and back problems should be particularly cautious. Risky exercises in this category include straight-leg sit-ups, back bends, rocking horses, cobras, prone swan positions, excessive upper-back lifts, and incorrect weight lifting with the back arched.

Other Hyperextension Exercises to Avoid Some other exercises which hyperextend the spine include rear double-leg lifts, donkey kicks, landing from a jump with the back arched, wrestler's bridges, neck hyperextensions, neck circling to the rear, and backward trunk circling.

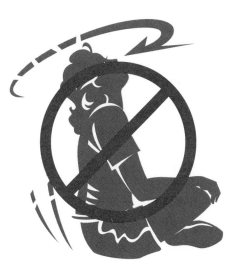

Avoid neck circling to the rear.

Joint Twisting, Compression, and Friction Exercises to Avoid Exercises that cause the joints to bend too far or to bend in a way that they were not intended to move are also risky. They can result in injury to the joint and tissues around the joint. Some exercises also cause certain structures to rub against others, creating friction that causes wear and tear. Some exercises included in this category include hurdle sits, heroes, double-leg lifts, sit-ups, standing straight leg toe touches, standing windmill toe touches, and arm circling with palms down.

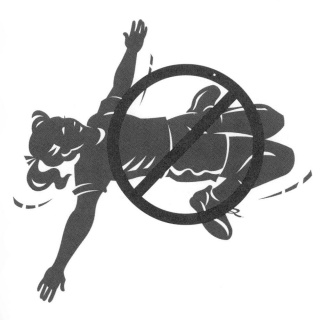

Avoid heroes and other exercises that bend joints abnormally.

Improper Strengthening or Stretching Exercises

Some exercises can result in muscle imbalance because they build muscles that are not especially in need of development rather than the muscles needed for good health and wellness. They are not risky but poor choices. Forward arm circling is an example because it develops already strong pectorals. Backward arm circles with palms up would be better because they work on the weaker back muscles. Other improper exercises

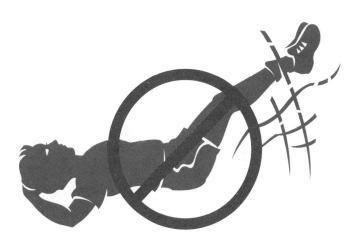

Some exercises strengthen muscles that are already too strong.

strengthen the already too strong muscles that go across the front of the hip joint. These exercises also can cause injury to the disks, abdominal tears, tendon tears, and loose ligaments. Examples of this type of risky exercise include double leg lifts and straight-leg sit-ups.

Lesson Review
1. List and describe some exercise-related physical injuries.
2. What are some guidelines for preventing injuries during physical activity?
3. How can the RICE formula be used to treat physical injuries?
4. What are some different types of risky exercises?

Activity 2
Safe Exercises

You now know some risky exercises. If you have been doing any of them, you should substitute exercises such as the ones shown and described in this Activity. If done properly, these exercises are safe to perform and give you the benefits of risky exercises without the risk.

The exercises pictured below are only a few of many safe exercises that you can substitute for risky ones. Additional safe exercises are described on your record sheet and throughout this book. Try each exercise, carefully following the directions.

Curl-Up

The curl-up, sometimes referred to as the crunch, is a good substitute for the straight-leg sit-up, bent-knee sit-up, and hands-behind-the-head sit-up.

1 Lie on your back with your knees bent and your feet close to your buttocks.

2 Hold your hands and arms straight in front of you and curl your head and shoulders up only until your shoulder blades leave the floor.

3 Slowly roll back to the starting position.
Caution: Your feet should not be held while doing a trunk curl.

Note: As you improve, you might hold your arms across your chest. When you become very good, you might place your hands on your cheeks.

Reverse Curl

The reverse curl is a good substitute for the double leg-lift.

1 Lie on your back. Bend your knees, placing your feet flat on the floor. Place your arms at your side.

2 Lift your knees to your chest, raising your hips off the floor.

3 Return to the starting position. **Caution: Do not lower your legs to the floor or hold your breath.**

This exercise can be made more difficult for the advanced exerciser by doing it on an inclined board with your head elevated.

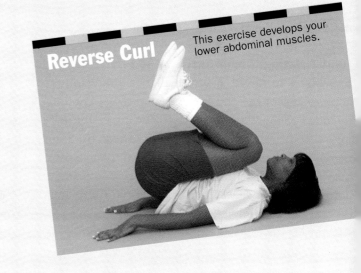
Reverse Curl
This exercise develops your lower abdominal muscles.

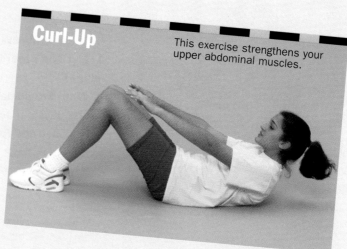
Curl-Up
This exercise strengthens your upper abdominal muscles.

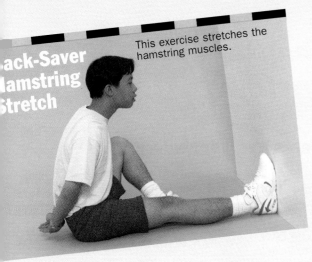
This exercise stretches the hamstring muscles.

Back-Saver Hamstring Stretch

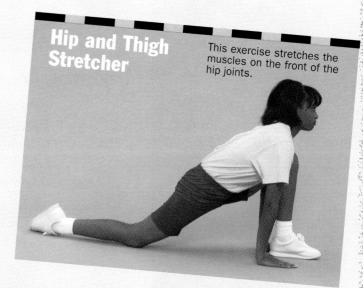
This exercise stretches the muscles on the front of the hip joints.

Hip and Thigh Stretcher

Back-Saver Hamstring Stretch

This is a safe exercise that can be substituted for the standing toe touch or the double-leg sit-and-reach.

1 Sit with your right leg against a wall and your left knee bent with your foot flat on the floor.

2 Clasp your hands behind your back and bend forward, keeping your lower back as straight as possible. Allow your bent knee to move sideway so that your trunk can move forward.

3 Stretch and hold.

Record Your Results on the Record Sheet

Hip and Thigh Stretcher

This exercise is a good substitute for the quadriceps stretcher or back arching holding on to toes.

1 Kneel with your left knee directly above your left ankle.

2 Stretch your right leg backward so that your knee touches the floor. If necessary, place your hands on the floor for balance.

3 Press your pelvis forward and downward and hold for several seconds.

4 Repeat on the left side. **Caution: Do not bend your front knee more than 90 degrees.**

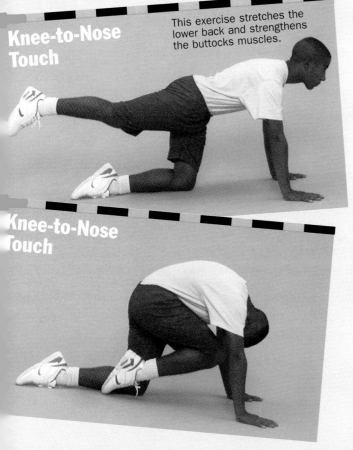
Knee-to-Nose Touch
This exercise stretches the lower back and strengthens the buttocks muscles.

Knee-to-Nose Touch

Knee-to-Nose Touch

This exercise is a good substitute for the donkey kick.

1 Kneel on "all fours."

2 Pull your right knee toward your nose.

3 Extend your right leg and head to a horizontal position. **Caution: Do not lift your leg higher than your hips. Do not hyperextend your neck and lower back.**

4 Return to the starting position. Repeat with your left leg.

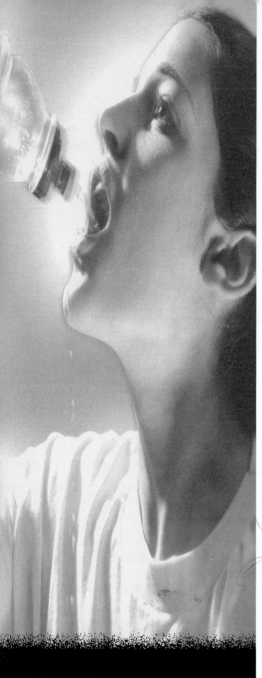

2 Chapter Review

Reviewing Concepts and Vocabulary

Copy the number of each statement on a sheet of paper. Next to each number, write the word or words that correctly complete the sentence.

1. The rules of biology and physics that can be used to prevent injury to your body joints are called _____.

2. Symptoms of frostbite include _____.

3. Invisible damage to the body resulting from repeating a movement often is a _____.

4. Some injuries related to sports and exercise include _____.

5. Numbness, shivering, low body temperature, and confusion are symptoms of _____.

Number your paper. Next to each number, choose the letter of the best answer.

Column I	Column II
6. joint	a. connects muscle to bone
7. ligament	b. place where bones connect
8. tendon	c. pain in the lower abdomen
9. side stitch	d. holds bones together at a joint
10. hypothermia	e. body temperature becomes extremely low

On your paper, write a short answer for each statement or question.

11. What are precautions you should take when getting ready to exercise in hot, humid weather?

12. What are the guidelines for exercising in wet, cold, or icy weather?

13. Why are self-assessments important tools when you plan for lifetime activity?

14. Explain how to follow the RICE formula when treating a minor injury.

15. What are some symptoms of heat exhaustion and heat stroke?

Thinking Critically

Write a paragraph to answer the following question.

You are about to begin an exercise program with a group of friends. The leader of your group has selected some exercises for you to do. How can you determine if the exercises are safe?

Project

Look through current magazines for articles that feature exercises. Evaluate each exercise to determine if you think it is safe. Report your findings to your class, telling what criteria you used to make each evaluation.

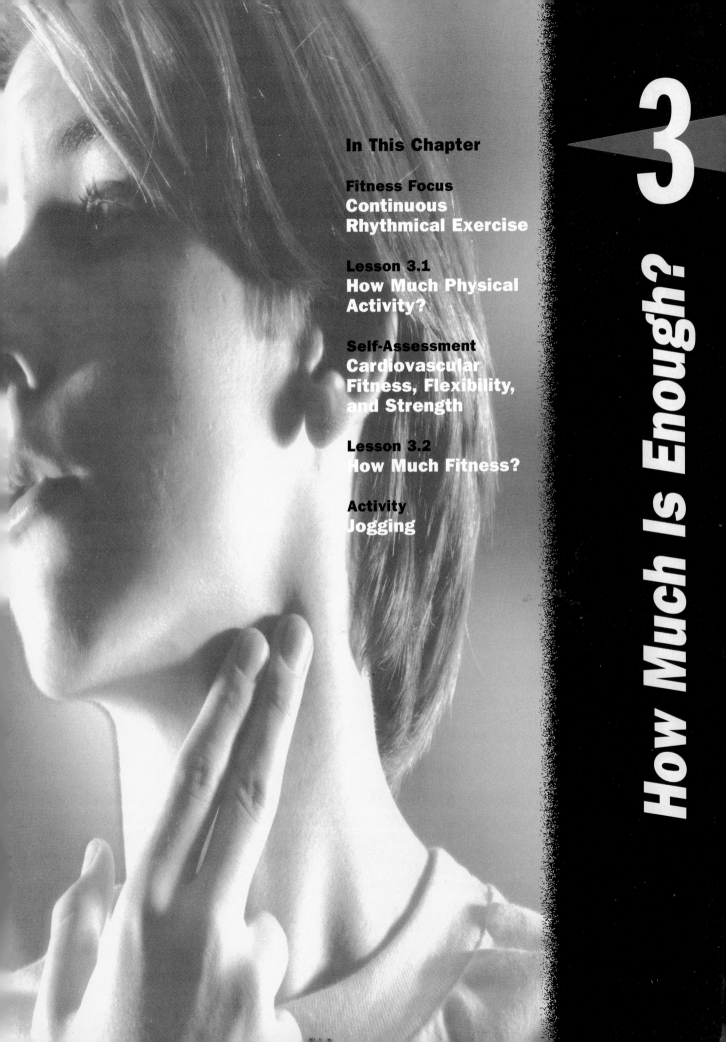

How Much Is Enough?

3

Continuous Rhythmical Exercise

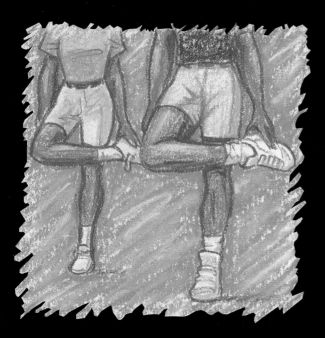

Whether you want to increase cardiovascular fitness, develop your muscular endurance, or control body fat, the exercises in this program can help. Your goal when doing the exercises is to keep your heart rate elevated during the entire program by continually moving. To do this, jog or slowly run in place between exercises. A sample program of exercises is shown on your instruction sheet. This sample program lasts about 10 minutes, but you can lengthen it by repeating the cycle of exercises or by substituting exercises from Chapters 6 through 10. When substituting other exercises, be sure to include exercises for all parts of fitness. You will learn about the parts of fitness in this chapter.

Side Stretcher	Knee Dip
Stride Step	Partner Pull-Up
Curl-Up	Side Leg Raise
Standing Heel Touch	Lateral Shuffle

Lesson 3.1
How Much Physical Activity?

Lesson Objectives
After reading this lesson, you should be able to:
1. Name and discuss the three basic principles of exercise.
2. Explain how the FITT formula helps you build fitness.
3. Explain how to use the Physical Activity Pyramid to plan a physical activity program.

Lesson Vocabulary
principle of overload, principle of progression, threshold of training, target ceiling, target fitness zone, principle of specificity, FITT formula, frequency, intensity

How much physical activity is enough? This question might seem very simple, but the answer can be complicated, especially if you are just beginning a physical activity program. In this lesson you will develop an understanding of several basic exercise principles as a good first step in answering the "how much is enough" question.

The Basic Principles of Exercise

Mia has been exercising for several months. Every day she does the same physical activities for about 15 minutes. Her activity program has not changed since she started. Initially Mia saw some positive results from her program. She no longer was tired at the end of her exercise, and a self-assessment showed that her cardiovascular fitness had improved. However, lately Mia is disappointed because her cardiovascular fitness does not seem to be improving like it did at first. She also has noticed that some areas of her flexibility and strength have not improved at all. Mia would like to know if she is doing something wrong. A look at the three basic principles of exercise might give some clues about what Mia might do differently.

The Principle of Overload The **principle of overload,** the most basic law of exercise, states that the only way to produce fitness and health benefits through physical activity is to require your body to do more than it normally does. An increased demand on your body (overload) forces it to adapt. Your body was designed to be active; so if you do nothing (underload), your fitness decreases and your health suffers.

If Mia is not overloading when she exercises, she will not gain fitness and health benefits. Mia will need to increase the amount of her physical activity if she expects to continue improving her cardiovascular fitness.

The Principle of Progression The **principle of progression** states that the amount and intensity of your exercise should be increased gradually. After a while your body adapts to an increase in physical activity (load) and your activity becomes too easy. When this happens, increase your activity slightly.

Notice in the diagram below that the minimum amount of overload you need to build physical fitness is your **threshold of training**. Activity above your threshold builds fitness and promotes health and wellness benefits. Having exercised for several months at the same level, Mia might now be exercising below her threshold of training for some of the parts of fitness.

It is possible to exercise too much and to go above your upper limit of activity, also called your **target ceiling**. Ideally you should do exercise that is above your threshold of training and below your target ceiling. This correct range of physical activity is called your **target fitness zone.**

When you do physical activity in your target fitness zone, you build fitness and other benefits.

However, when you go above your target ceiling, you increase the chances of injury and you can develop muscle soreness. The principle of progression provides the basis for rejecting the "no pain, no gain" theory. If you have pain when you exercise, you are probably overloading too fast for your body to adjust.

The Principle of Specificity The **principle of specificity** states that the specific type of exercise you do determines the specific benefit you receive. Different kinds and amounts of activity produce very specific and different benefits. For example, Mia is probably doing primarily activities for cardiovascular fitness and not doing stretching exercises that improve flexibility or resistance exercises that improve strength. An activity that promotes health benefits in one part of health-related fitness may not be equally good in promoting high levels of fitness in another part of fitness. Finally, exercises for specific body parts, such as the calf muscles, may provide benefits only for those body parts. For example, if Mia started doing an exercise that stretched the muscles of the back of her leg, she would not build flexibility of the muscles on the front of her leg—unless she did exercises designed to improve the flexibility of that specific area of her body.

The FITT Formula

You know that you must do more physical activity than normal to build fitness. You also know that you should gradually increase your physical activity in order to stay within your target fitness zone. But how much physical activity do you need?

You can use the **FITT formula** to help you apply the basic principles of exercise. Each letter in the word FITT represents one of four important factors that are important in determining how much physical activity is enough.

• **Frequency** refers to how often you do physical activity. For physical activity to be beneficial, you must do it several days a week. As you will see later, frequency depends on the type of activity you are doing and the part of fitness you want to develop. For example, to develop strength you might need exercise two days a week, but to lose fat daily activity is recommended.

• **Intensity** refers to how hard you perform physical activity. If the activity you do is too easy, you will not build fitness and gain other benefits. But remember— extremely vigorous activity can be harmful if you do not work up to it gradually. Intensity is determined

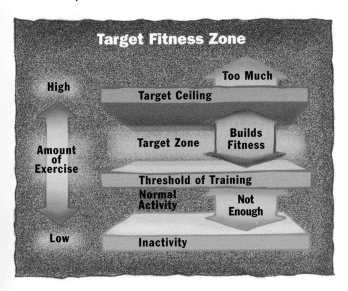

Target Fitness Zone

High
Amount of Exercise
Low

Target Ceiling
Too Much

Target Zone
Builds Fitness

Threshold of Training

Normal Activity
Not Enough

Inactivity

differently depending on the types of activity you do and the fitness you want to build. For example, counting Calories and counting heart rate can be used to determine the intensity of activity for building cardiovascular fitness, while the amount of weight you lift is used to determine intensity for building strength.

• **Time** refers to how long you do physical activity. The length of time you should do physical activity depends on the type of activity you are doing and the part of fitness you want to develop. For example, to build flexibility you should exercise for 10 to 15 seconds for each muscle group, while to build cardiovascular fitness you need to be active continuously for a minimum of 15 to 30 minutes.

• **Type** refers to the kind of activity you do to build a specific part of fitness or to gain a specific benefit.

Throughout this book, you will learn how to apply the FITT formula to specific activities to build specific parts of fitness. In the following chapters, to help you understand the correct frequency, intensity, and time for each type of exercise, we will use the phrase *FIT formula*. For simplicity the final *T* will not be used.

The Physical Activity Pyramid

The Physical Activity Pyramid on this page can help you understand the concept of specificity and will help you see which types of activity are best for the health and wellness benefits you are looking for. Different types of activity in the pyramid build different parts of fitness and produce different health and wellness benefits. For optimal benefits you should perform activities from all parts of the pyramid each week. As you can see from the frequency chart on the next page, those activities at or near the bottom of the pyramid need to be done more frequently than those near the top of the pyramid.

Lifestyle Physical Activity Lifestyle physical activity, the bottom area of the pyramid, should be performed daily or nearly every day. Examples of this kind of activity include doing yard work or climbing stairs. This kind of activity is associated with many of the benefits of activity described in Chapter 5. It is helpful in controlling body fatness and building cardiovascular fitness.

Aerobic Activity Aerobic activity, which you will learn about in Chapter 6, is also associated with many of the benefits described in Chapter 5. It is especially beneficial to building high levels of cardiovascular fitness and help in controlling body fatness. You should perform aerobic activity three to six times a week.

Active Sport Active sport is associated with many health and wellness benefits if done moderately to vigorously. It is helpful in maintaining many parts of fitness and in building skills. You can substitute active sport for some of the aerobic activity you do three to six times a week.

Exercise for Flexibility To build and maintain flexibility, you should perform flexibility exercises at least three days a week. Exercising in this way builds flexibility and produces such benefits as better performance, improved posture, and reduced risk of injury.

Exercise for Strength and Muscle Endurance To develop strength, exercise for muscle fitness at least two days a week. You will need to exercise at least three days a week to improve muscular endurance. The exercises you do for strength and muscular endurance also produce such benefits as better performance, improved body appearance, a healthier back, good posture, and stronger bones.

The Physical Activity Pyramid

Rest or Inactivity
watching TV
reading

Exercise for Flexibility
stretching

Exercise for Strength & Muscular Endurance
weight training
calisthenics

Aerobic Activity
aerobics
jogging
biking

Active Sport
tennis
basketball
raquetball

Lifestyle Physical Activity
walk rather than ride
climb the stairs
do yard work

No Excuses

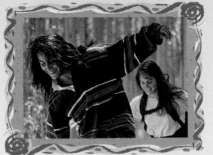

Adjusting to Noncontrollable Factors

When some people face a problem beyond their control, they use it as an excuse for not being physically active. Someone might say, "I'm too short to be a basketball player, so I'm not going to try out for any sports." To be physically active, focus on what you can do—not what you can't change.

Juana stood at the window, shaking her head. "It's pouring out there! How can we go hiking today?"

Monica sighed. "I guess we're stuck spending the afternoon here, playing cards or something."

Yesterday it was too hot to go hiking; now it was too rainy. It seemed as if they were never going to have good weather so they could exercise. Yet, good weather wasn't always the answer either. The last time they tried hiking at the state park, it was sunny, but the paths were too crowded.

"I bet Miguel is at the athletic club right now," Monica said. "He can exercise no matter what the weather is. I wish we could afford memberships there!"

Juana glanced down at her sweats. "I'd need to buy more than a membership before I could go there. They wear really expensive exercise clothes at that club. I'd get laughed out of the place in these clothes."

Monica smiled. "You don't look so bad—and the rain's starting to let up now. What if we put on even older clothes, take along some rain gear, and hike around the park for a while?"

"You're right! So what if we get a little damp?"

For Discussion

What reasons do Juana and Monica give for not being active? Which of these problems can they control? They've decided not to let the weather stop them today. What other ways could they cope with the problems they've identified? Fill out the questionnaire to see how well you can distinguish between controllable and noncontrollable factors.

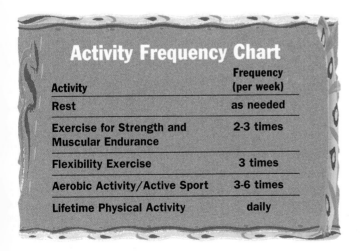

Activity Frequency Chart

Activity	Frequency (per week)
Rest	as needed
Exercise for Strength and Muscular Endurance	2-3 times
Flexibility Exercise	3 times
Aerobic Activity/Active Sport	3-6 times
Lifetime Physical Activity	daily

Rest or Inactivity Proper rest is important. We need to take time to recover from daily stresses and prepare for new challenges. But general inactivity or sedentary living is discouraged. Choices from other areas of the pyramid should exceed those from this area. The chart summarizes the amount of time you should perform activity from each area of the pyramid.

In the chapters that follow you will learn more about the Physical Activity Pyramid and how much physical activity from each area of the pyramid you need to build specific fitness and benefits to health and wellness. You will see that the frequency, intensity, and time of activity will vary for each type of activity.

Lesson Review
1. What are the three basic principles of exercise?
2. How does the FITT formula help you build physical fitness?
3. Explain how to use the Physical Activity Pyramid to begin planning a physical activity program.

Self-Assessment 3
Cardiovascular Fitness, Flexibility, and Strength

In Chapter 2 you performed two Prudential FITNESSGRAM® assessments to measure strength and muscular endurance. In this assessment you will perform two more FITNESSGRAM tests to measure cardiovascular fitness and the strength and flexibility of your back and trunk muscles.

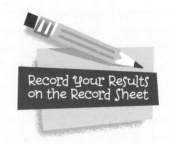

Record Your Results on the Record Sheet

The PACER

PACER stands for **P**rogressive **A**erobic **C**ardiovascular **E**ndurance **R**un and is a test of cardiovascular fitness. You will need a tape recorder and a special audiotape to perform the test. Because the test requires this special equipment, it may not be as easy to do as other cardiovascular assessments you will do later. However, by taking this test you can see if you meet the national health-related cardiovascular fitness standard. The objective of the test is to run back and forth across a 20-meter distance as many times as you can.

1 When the audiotape beeps, run across the 20-meter area and touch the line before the tape beeps again. Turn around.

2 At the sound of the beep, run back to the other side. (You must wait for the beep before running in the opposite direction.) The beeps will come faster and faster causing you to run faster and faster. The test is finished when you twice fail to reach the opposite side before the beep.

3 Your score is the number of times you can run the 20-meter distance before your test is finished. Record this number on your record sheet. Then find your fitness rating on the chart on the next page.

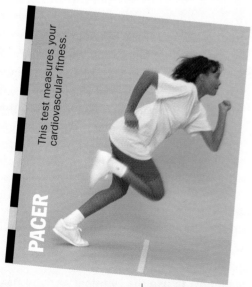

This test measures your cardiovascular fitness.

PACER

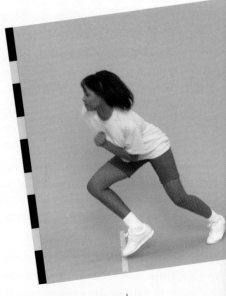

|← 20 meters →|

Rating Chart: Trunk Lift

High Performance	11–12
Good Fitness	9–10
Marginal Fitness	7–8
Low Fitness	6 or less

Adapted from FITNESSGRAM

Trunk Lift
(Upper Back)

1 Lie facedown with your arms to your side and your hands under your thighs.

2 Lift the upper part of your body very slowly so that your chin, chest, and shoulders come off the floor. Lift your trunk as high as possible to a maximum of 12 inches. Hold this position for 3 seconds while a partner measures the distance your chin lifts off the floor. Hold the ruler at least one inch in front of your chin. Look straight ahead so that your chin is not tipped upward abnormally. **Caution: Do not place the ruler directly under your chin in case you have to lower your trunk unexpectedly.**

3 Do the trunk lift 2 times and record the number of inches you could lift and hold your chin. Do not record scores above 12 inches. Use the chart above to determine your fitness rating. Record your results.

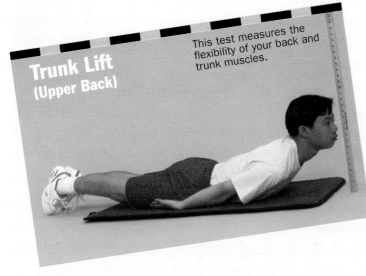

Trunk Lift (Upper Back)

This test measures the flexibility of your back and trunk muscles.

Rating Chart: PACER

	13-years old or below		14-years old		15-years old		16-years old		17-years old or above	
	males	females	males	females	males	females	males	females	males	females
High Performance	55+	51+	60+	53+	65+	55+	69+	57+	78+	61+
Good Fitness	35–54	15–30	41–60	18–32	46–64	23–37	52–69	28–42	57–73	34–49
Marginal Fitness	30–34	13–14	36–40	16–17	41–45	21–22	47–51	25–27	52–56	30–33
Low Fitness	29–	12–	35–	15–	40–	20–	46–	24–	51–	29–

Adapted from FITNESSGRAM

3.2

How Much Fitness?

Lesson Objectives
After reading this lesson, you should be able to:
1. Discuss fitness ratings and how they apply to your physical activity program.
2. Identify factors that contribute to fitness.
3. Explain why everyone should be physically active.

Lesson Vocabulary
maturation

You now know that you probably don't need the same kinds and amount of physical activity as your friends. But do you all need the same amount of fitness? In this lesson you will learn some ways to decide how much fitness is enough for you.

Fitness Rating Categories
Sometimes people judge their fitness by comparing themselves to others. If they score higher on a fitness test than most other people, they consider themselves fit. This type of comparison creates several problems. First, it suggests that only a few can be fit. Second, it suggests that only high test scores are adequate.

Most experts agree that you should judge your fitness using standards of health and wellness, also called criterion-referenced standards, rather than using standards that require you to compare yourself to others. Health and wellness standards require you to have enough fitness to:
• reduce risk of health problems,
• achieve wellness benefits,
• work effectively and meet emergencies,
• be able to enjoy your free time.

During this course you will learn to do self-assessments that you can use to determine whether your fitness is as good as it should be and whether you are fit enough to meet the goals listed above. You will use one of the four following categories to rate each of the five parts of health-related fitness. If you achieve the good fitness category, you will have achieved basic health and wellness standards of physical fitness.

Low Fitness Experts believe that people who have low ratings for health-related fitness have an above-average risk of certain health problems. If you are in the low fitness category, you might not look your best, feel your best, or work and play most efficiently.

Marginal Fitness Moving from the low to the marginal rating shows important progress in fitness. However, if you have marginal ratings you should continue to work to progress to the good fitness category in order to meet the fitness goals.

Good Fitness A good fitness rating indicates that you probably have the necessary amounts of fitness needed to live a full, healthy life. In fact, achieving good fitness is the goal of most people. However, to maintain this level of fitness you will have to continue to be physically active.

High Performance Most experts agree that a high performance rating is not necessary for good health, meeting normal daily emergencies, and daily activities. However, some people who want to achieve an exceptional physical task work to achieve a high performance fitness rating. For example, if you wanted to be a skilled gymnast, achieving such a rating could increase your chances of success.

Factors to Consider
Physical activity is the most important thing you can do to improve and maintain health-related physical fitness. Physical activity is something that you can control. You can choose the kinds of activities you want to do and schedule a regular time to do them. But as the diagram on the next page shows, physical activity is not the only factor that contributes to physical fitness. Other important factors contributing to physical fitness are maturation, age, heredity, and other lifestyles, including nutrition and stress management. You will learn more about nutrition in Chapter 17 and stress management in Chapter 18.

Maturation Physical maturation refers to becoming physically mature or fully grown and developed. In the early teens, maturation begins because of hormones that promote growth and development of such tissues as muscle and bone. Some people mature earlier than others. Early developers often do better on physical fitness tests than those who mature later.

Age Age is important because the older you are, the more mature you are likely to be. If you are older than most students in your grade and if you also began to mature earlier than others your age, you probably will have an advantage on physical fitness tests.

Heredity Heredity plays a role in determining the physical characteristics we inherit from our parents that influence how we do on different tests of physical fitness. For example, some people have more of the muscle fibers that help them run fast. Others have more of the muscle fibers that help people run a long time without fatigue. Still others have more fat cells because of heredity. Fortunately, fitness is composed of many different parts. Most of us inherit characteristics that make it relatively easy to have certain types of fitness, although we also inherit characteristics that may make it harder to get fit on other parts.

Anyone Can Succeed

Since many factors contribute to physical fitness, it is possible for some people who do relatively little physical activity to achieve relatively good fitness scores while they are in their teens. These people probably matured early and have inherited physical characteristics that help them to do well on physical fitness tests. They may conclude that they do not need to do physical activity. This idea may be true when these people are young, but it will not be true for a lifetime. As people get older, physical maturation and age no longer result in a fitness advantage. Sooner or later physical inactivity starts to catch up with even those who have a hereditary advantage. Regular physical activity and healthy lifestyles are absolutely necessary if fitness, health, and wellness are to occur for a lifetime.

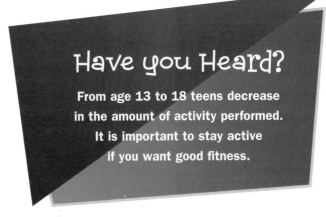

Just as some people have fitness advantages because of age, maturation, and heredity, others have disadvantages. Even if these people do physical activity, they may find it hard to get high fitness scores and, therefore, they become discouraged. If you are one of these people, avoid comparing yourself to others. Try to achieve the good fitness zone—something that all people can accomplish. Studies show that people who were good in sports in school but are not active later in life die earlier and are less healthy than those who do regular activity all of their lives, even if they were not especially good performers when they were young.

Anyone can do physical activity. No matter who you are, physical activity is important to good health and wellness as well as fitness development. With regular physical activity all people can achieve the good fitness zone in all parts of fitness.

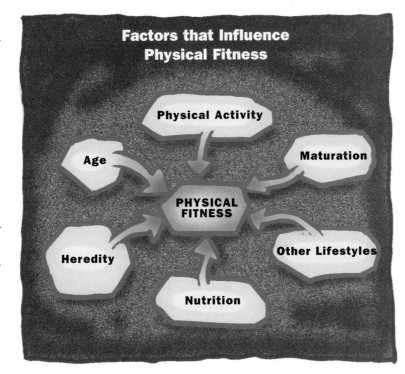

Factors that Influence Physical Fitness

Physical Activity

Age

Maturation

PHYSICAL FITNESS

Heredity

Other Lifestyles

Nutrition

Lesson Review

1. What are the four fitness ratings? How do they apply to your physical activity program?
2. Identify factors that contribute to fitness.
3. Explain why everyone should be physically active.

Activity 3
Jogging

Record Your Results on the Record Sheet

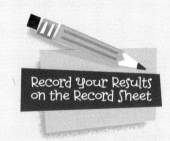

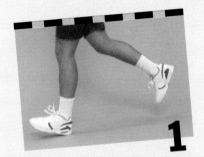

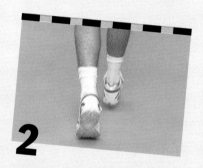

Principles and Guidelines

If you are looking for an excellent cardiovascular activity that requires little skill and no equipment except a good pair of running shoes, jogging might be for you. More than 6 million people in the United States are joggers. Many more could learn to enjoy this activity if they knew how to jog properly. If you plan to start jogging, be sure to consider the following biomechanical principles and guidelines.

1. The foot action for jogging is not the same as for fast running. In fast running, your weight is mainly on the front of your foot. In jogging, you land on your heel or on the entire foot. Then you rock forward and push off with the ball of the foot, followed by the toes. Jogging improperly can cause injuries, such as sore shins, sore calves, or even a sore back. (see photo 1)

2. Swing your legs and feet straight forward. Do not let your feet turn out to the sides. Feet and legs out of alignment cause unnecessary strain on your joints and muscles. When jogging, step farther than your normal walking step. (see photo 2)

3. Swing your arms straight forward and backward; do not swing them across your body. Keep your arms bent at the elbows, and hands relaxed. Try to keep your shoulders relaxed. If you jog with a "floppy jaw," your upper body will relax more. (see photo 3)

4. Keep your trunk fairly erect when jogging. Do not lean forward as you would when starting to run fast. (see photo 3)

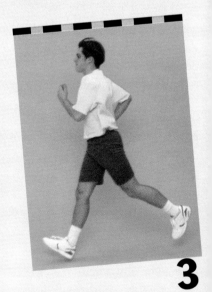

5. Learn your own best pace. Learn how fast or slow you should jog to raise your heart rate to the appropriate level. A correct jogging pace differs for each person. Find your own pace; do not try to jog at someone else's pace, especially if it is faster than your own pace.

6. Avoid running on hard surfaces. If possible, jog on a running track, grassy places, or dirt paths. These surfaces have more "give" than concrete sidewalks and put less stress on your feet and legs. If you jog indoors, try to jog on a wooden floor rather than on concrete.

7. Breathe easily. If you are jogging with a friend, you should be able to carry on a conversation as you jog. If you are jogging alone, you should be able to breathe comfortably. If you are panting or gasping for breath, you are jogging too fast.

Part 1: Jogging Practice

Work with a partner to practice the jogging techniques discussed on page 44. Jog about 100 yards while your partner stands behind you and checks your techniques. Have your partner answer these questions to check your feet and legs:

1. Does your heel or whole foot hit the ground first?

2. Do you push off with the ball of your foot?

3. Do your legs and feet swing and land straight ahead?

4. Is your stride longer than your walking stride?

Now do a second 100-yard jog and have your partner look at you from a side view and answer these questions to check your arms and body:

1. Are your elbows bent properly (90°) with your hands relaxed?

2. Do your arms swing straight forward and backward?

3. Are your head and chest up?

4. Is your body leaning only slightly?

Discuss your assessment with your partner. Then have your partner jog twice while you evaluate his or her technique. Try to correct your technique and have your partner check you again. Do the same for your partner. Both you and your partner may jog more than twice if necessary.

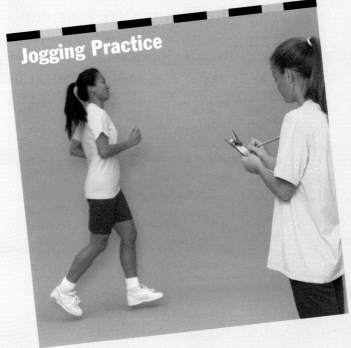
Jogging Practice

Part 2: Jogging Workout

After you have practiced your jogging technique, try this workout.

Beginner's Workout

1 Begin your workout by taking your resting heart rate using the procedure you learned in the Self-Assessment in Chapter 1.

2 Use your resting heart rate and the chart to determine your correct target heart rate for your workout.

3 Run for 5 minutes trying to get your heart to the target level. Use your watch to keep track of how long you run. How long you run is more important than how far. By using time instead of distance, you can jog anywhere. Set your own course. Try to jog half the time away from your starting point and the other half returning to your starting point. If you are not somewhere near your starting point at the end of 5 minutes, walk back to it.

4 At the end of 5 minutes, count your heart rate to get your one-minute exercise heart rate. Record this score on your record sheet. Determine if your exercise heart rate was in your target heart rate zone.

5 Repeat the 5-minute run again. This time jog faster if your exercise heart rate was lower than your target heart rate on your first jog. Jog slower if your exercise heart rate was higher than your target rate. Jog at the same speed if your exercise heart rate was in the target zone during the first jog. Count your exercise heart rate again after the second run. Record your score on the record sheet. This activity helps you learn about how fast to jog to get a fitness benefit. You will learn more about target heart rate in Chapter 6.

Target Heart Rates
(beats per minute)

Resting Heart Rate	Beginner	Regular
Below 50	127–143	143–182
51–70	132–147	147–183
71 and over	140–153	153–185

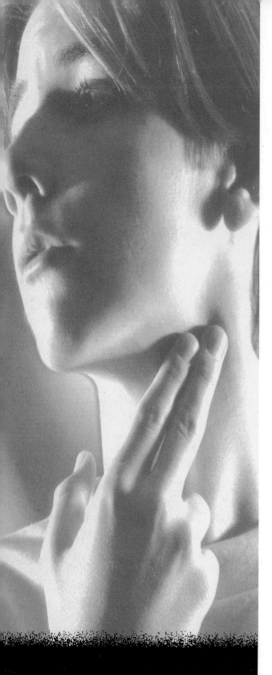

3 Chapter Review

Reviewing Concepts and Vocabulary

Copy the number of each statement on a sheet of paper. Next to each number, write the word or words that correctly complete the sentence.

1. For optimal benefits you should perform activities from _____ parts of the Physical Activity Pyramid each week.

2. The minimum amount of overload needed to achieve physical fitness is called _____.

3. If you are exercising in your target fitness zone, you are between your threshold of training and your _____.

4. If you achieve a _____ fitness rating, you probably have the necessary amounts of fitness needed to live a full, healthy life.

Number your paper. Next to each number, choose the letter of the best answer.

Column I

5. target ceiling c
6. frequency d
7. intensity a
8. progression b
9. specificity f
10. overload e

Column II

a. how hard you perform physical activity
b. increasing exercise gradually
c. the upper limit of your physical activity
d. how often you exercise
e. doing more exercise than you normally do
f. exercise for one fitness part

On your paper, write a short answer for each statement or question.

11. How do age and maturation affect physical fitness?

12. Why should you develop a lifetime physical activity plan even if you are in the good fitness zone now?

13. Explain why your physical activity program should include activities from all parts of the Physical Activity Pyramid.

14. Why should you not exercise above your target ceiling?

15. Explain why you should not compare yourself to others when assessing your fitness levels and needs.

Thinking Critically

Write a paragraph to answer the following question.

A friend tells you that he thinks it is important for everyone to attain a high performance fitness rating. He says that if a good rating is the goal for all people, then a high performance must be even better for everyone. How would you respond? Explain your answer.

Project

Keep a record of your daily activities for one week. At the end of the week review your calendar. When during the day do you seem to have the most time and energy? During what times would it be easiest for you to participate in regular physical activity? Make a new schedule for the coming week incorporating a physical activity schedule into your plan.

4

Getting Started in Physical Activity

Cooper's Aerobics

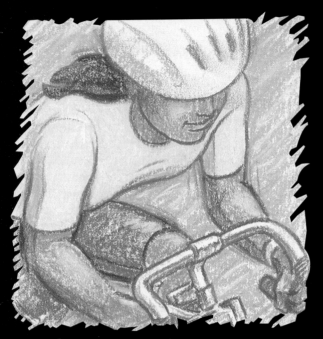

Aerobics is a physical activity program that was originally developed by Dr. Kenneth Cooper for use by the U.S. Air Force. Now the program is widely used by people of all ages and includes many kinds of activities. In Cooper's Aerobics, points are earned for various activities, such as the ones listed below. See the instruction sheet for information on how to plan Cooper's Aerobics workouts. Remember to warm up before your workout and cool down afterwards.

Walking	Basketball
Running	Racquetball
Cycling	Stationary Running
Swimming	Rope Jumping
Handball	

Lesson 4.1
Exercise Stages

Lesson Objectives
After reading this lesson, you should be able to:
1. Name the three stages of a safe exercise session and describe each.
2. Explain why your heart and muscles need a warm-up and a cool-down.
3. Use the Physical Activity Pyramid diagram to plan three different physical activity programs.
4. List general guidelines for physical activity.

Lesson Vocabulary
warm-up, heart warm-up, muscle warm-up, muscle stretch, workout, cool-down, heart cool-down

The time you spend doing physical activity on any given day is your daily physical activity session, or exercise session. A good, safe activity session includes three stages: a warm-up, a workout, and a cool-down. In this lesson, you will learn about each stage. By preparing properly, you will get more benefits from your physical activity.

Stage 1: The Warm-Up
A **warm-up** is a series of activities that prepares your body for more vigorous physical activity and helps prevent injury. A warm-up usually consists of a heart warm-up, a muscle warm-up, and a muscle stretch.

The heart is a muscle—one of the most important in your body. It needs to be warmed up. A **heart warm-up** consists of several minutes of walking, slow jogging, or a similar activity that prepares your heart for more vigorous activity.

A **muscle warm-up** consists of exercises that gently contract your muscles to warm them. Warm muscles contract and relax more efficiently than cool muscles. The **muscle stretch** consists of exercises that slowly stretch the muscles to loosen and relax them. Warm, relaxed muscles are less likely to be strained or "pulled" than short, tight muscles.

The sample warm-up and stretch on pages 6–7 is useful for people doing moderate activity. People who participate in vigorous activities, especially

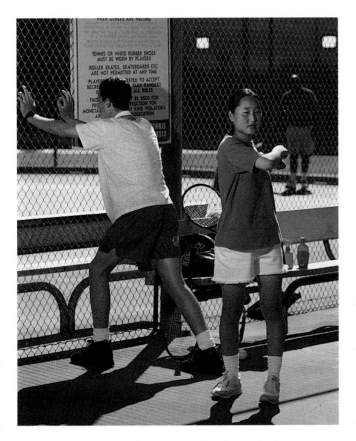

Perform a warm-up before your workout.

sports, should design a personal warm-up to prepare them for the activity. Many lifestyle activities, such as walking, do not need a warm-up. However, you should do a warm-up for any lifestyle activity that is vigorous or requires a lot of muscle stretching. These guidelines will help you develop your own warm-up.

• Your heart warm-up should last between one and three minutes. It might include walking, slow jogging, slow swimming, slow bicycling, or a similar activity. Your goal is to gradually increase your heart rate.

• Some experts think that a heart warm-up should be done both before and after a muscle warm-up. A muscle warm-up before a workout increases the blood supply to the muscles, thus raising muscle temperature. Stretching exercises then are more effective because warm muscles relax more easily than cool muscles. After the muscle warm-up, a heart warm-up prepares the heart for vigorous activity.

• Your stretch should include some gentle stretching exercises for each muscle group you will use in your workout. Stretch slowly and easily. Do not bounce or jerk or try to stretch too far. This is not the time for a flexibility workout.

• Your muscle warm-up should include a few slow, easy movements that are similar to the activity you will do. For example, if you are going to pitch for a baseball game, you should warm up your throwing arm. Start by making a few easy, short throws. Gradually work up to longer, harder throws as your arm muscles become warmer and more limber.

Stage 2: The Workout

The **workout** is the part of your physical activity program during which you do activities to improve your fitness. For optimal fitness, include activities from each part of the Physical Activity Pyramid each week. You can include activities from each part of fitness at each workout. Or you can do activities for different parts of fitness on different days. Or you can do lifestyle activities daily, adding activities for each area of fitness. The following plans show sample workouts. As you learn more about fitness, you can develop a plan that works for you.

Plan A: All parts at each workout Plan A, illustrated below, includes flexibility exercises, exercises for muscular strength and muscular endurance, and aerobics or sports at each workout. For example, Lea warms up, does weight training, jogs or rides a bicycle, and does flexibility exercises and then cools down.

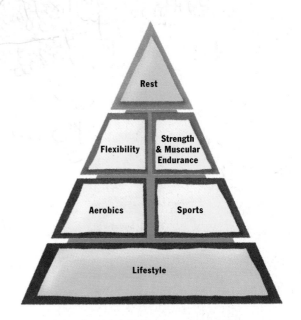

Plan B: Different parts at different workouts In this plan, a person does an aerobic activity or sport at least three days a week, exercises for muscular strength and muscular endurance at least two days a week, and

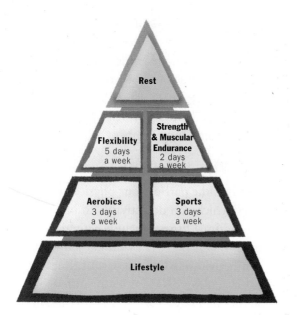

does flexibility exercises after each workout. For example, Derrick warms up before each workout; he plays tennis on Mondays and Wednesdays, jogs on Fridays, trains with weights on Tuesdays and Thursdays, and does flexibility exercises and cools down after each workout. Plan B is illustrated above.

Plan C: Lifestyle-plus workout In this plan, illustrated in the diagram below, the main source of the aerobic workout is from activities done during the day. This plan is called "Lifestyle-plus" because supplemental activities are done to develop all parts of fitness. For total fitness, exercises for flexibility, muscular strength, and muscular endurance are added to regular lifestyle activities. For example, Marla does stretches and calisthenics every morning; she walks to and from school

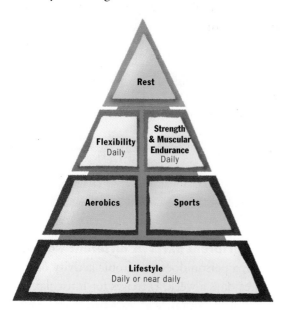

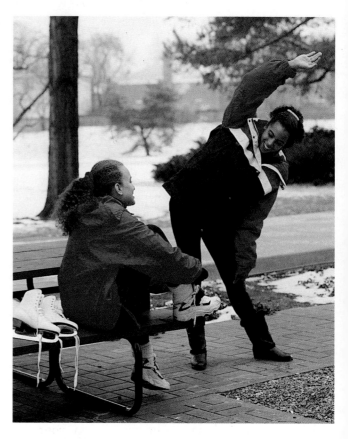

A cool-down should follow your workout.

each day, walks dogs every day after school, and bicycles to visit friends on weekends.

Stage 3: The Cool-Down

After a workout, your body needs to recover from the demands of physical activity. A **cool-down** usually consists of a heart cool-down and a muscle cool-down and stretch.

A **heart cool-down** consists of movements done at a slower pace than the workout. The heart cool-down helps prevent dizziness and fainting. Hard exercise causes an increased flow of blood to your muscles. For example, running causes more blood to be pumped to your arms and legs than to your head. If you stop running suddenly, the blood "pools" in the legs, so that the heart has less blood to pump to the brain. As a result, you may feel dizzy or faint. If you continue walking after a hard run, your muscles squeeze the veins of the legs. This helps the blood return to the heart. Then the heart has more blood to pump to the brain, and you're less likely to feel dizzy or faint.

Many experts think that a *muscle cool-down* and stretch are beneficial after a workout. The muscle cool-down and stretch consists of gradually cooling down the muscles by continuing to move around so the blood does not pool in the legs, followed by slowly stretching the muscles used during the workout. Since the muscles are already warm, this is also a good time to do stretches to increase flexibility. Keep the following guidelines in mind when you cool down.

• Do a heart and muscle cool-down before stretching your muscles. Start your heart and muscle cool-down immediately after stopping vigorous exercise. Your cool-down should last from one to three minutes. Do not stop or sit down immediately after a vigorous workout.

• Your muscle stretch can be the same stretching exercises you did as a warm-up, except that you may increase the intensity of the stretch because the muscles are now warm. Stretch slowly without bouncing. Stretch the muscle groups that you used vigorously in your workout.

Guidelines for Physical Activity

As you can see, you can choose from a variety of safe activity programs. No matter how you design your program, following these guidelines is wise:

• **Wear comfortable clothing.** Tight clothing can restrict your blood flow or limit your motion during vigorous exercise. Your body cools itself better if your clothing fits loosely.

• **Wash exercise clothing regularly.** Clean clothing is more comfortable. It also reduces chances of fungal growth or infections.

• **Dress in layers when exercising outdoors.** You can remove layers of clothing as you become warmer while exercising and put them back on when you cool down.

• **Wear proper socks and shoes.** Thick sports socks provide a cushion, help prevent blisters, and absorb perspiration from your feet.

Most people can use a good pair of "multipurpose" exercise or sport shoes. However, if you plan to do special activities, you might prefer shoes designed for these activities.

If you have had ankle injuries, wear high-top shoes, especially for activities with quick changes in direction, such as basketball and racquetball. Ankle braces can also help prevent ankle injuries.

Try on shoes before buying them. Wear socks you normally wear and walk to see how the shoes feel. The shoes should not feel too heavy because extra weight makes exercise more tiring.

Choose leather or cloth shoes. Vinyl or plastic shoes do not let air pass through to help cool your feet. As a result, your feet perspire in those shoes.

Shoes do not have to be expensive. However, be sure to look for shoes with the features shown below.

Plan for Success

Planning a physical activity program at which you will likely be successful is important. The following guidelines can help you:

• **Exercise with friends.** Friends can encourage each other to exercise. Remember that each person should exercise at his or her own level. Do not make exercise into a contest.

Wedge sole at least one-half inch higher at the heel than toe

Firm heel cup to hold your foot securely

Sole at least as wide as upper part of shoe

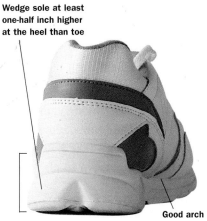
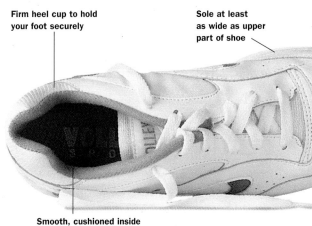

Good arch support

Smooth, cushioned inside

Characteristics of proper shoes.

No Excuses

Building Positive Attitudes

Many people have both positive and negative feelings about exercise and physical activity. Some use negative feelings as an excuse to avoid being active. To become and stay physically active, they need to increase their positive feelings and decrease any negative feelings.

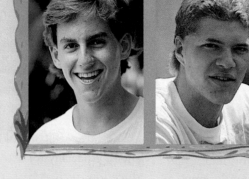

"Allen, I don't want to play tennis now." Matt put the tennis rackets down. Then he led Allen into the family room. "Anyway," he said, "a good T.V. show is on."

"I think you just don't want to lose to me in tennis again," Allen said.

"You're right," Matt admitted. "I hate losing."

"You win sometimes, Matt. The competition is what makes tennis fun."

"Not when I lose," Matt replied.

Allen thought for a minute. "How about taking a jog around the block?" he asked. "There will be no winner or loser."

"I don't want to get all sweaty," Matt replied. "I'd rather relax watching TV."

"Oh, come on, Matt. Jogging will help you relax. We need to stay in shape."

Matt smiled at Allen. "I guess I could stand to get sweaty once in a while. It does make me feel more alive." He jumped up and headed for the front door. "C'mon! Let's go for a run!"

For Discussion

What does Allen like about being physically active? What does Matt like and not like about physical activity? How could Matt change his negative attitudes and become more active? What are some positive attitudes that keep people active? What are some other negative attitudes that keep people from being active, and how can those attitudes be changed? Fill out the questionnaire to find out more about your own attitudes toward physical activity.

• **Choose activities you enjoy.** You can design your physical activity plan to include mostly activities you enjoy, although you may need to do some exercises you do not enjoy as well. Have fun with your activity program. Then you will be more likely to continue it.

• **Plan variety.** Try a new or different activity occasionally to avoid boredom and keep yourself interested in your physical activity program.

• **Select a time that is good for you.** You might prefer exercising in the morning when you feel fresh. Or you might find that exercising before a light lunch can help you feel more energetic. Some people prefer to exercise before an evening meal to help renew their energy and reduce stress. Others like to exercise in the evening. The best time of day for exercise and physical activity is the time that works best for you.

• **Set a regular time for physical activity.** If you set an appointment with yourself for exercise, and keep this appointment regularly, exercise will become a habit that is easy to keep.

Lesson Review

1. What are the three stages of a safe exercise session, and what do you need to do during each?
2. Why do your heart and muscles need a warm-up and a cool-down?
3. Explain how to use the Physical Activity Pyramid diagram to plan three different physical activity programs.
4. List general guidelines for physical activity.

Self-Assessment 4
Body Composition and Flexibility

In this Self-Assessment you will perform two additional assessments from The Prudential FITNESSGRAM:® the body mass index and the backsaver sit and reach. The body mass index is an indicator of your body composition. It is one of two methods for assessing body composition in The Prudential FITNESSGRAM.® You will do this assessment now so that you can complete your report, but you will also measure skinfolds when you study body fatness later. The backsaver sit and reach measures flexibility of the lower back and the muscles on the back of the thigh (hamstrings). After you record your results on the record sheet, complete your record sheet.

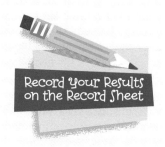

Record your Results on the Record Sheet

Body Mass Index

1 Measure your height in inches without shoes.

2 Measure your weight without shoes. If you are wearing street clothes (as opposed to light-weight gym clothing), you can subtract 2 pounds from your weight.

3 Use the Body Mass Index Chart to determine your body mass index (BMI). Place a ruler so that it cuts across the left vertical line at the mark for your height and across the right vertical line at the mark for your weight. Your BMI is the number where the ruler intersects the middle line.

4 Consult the Rating Scale for Body Mass Index. Record the results on your record sheet.

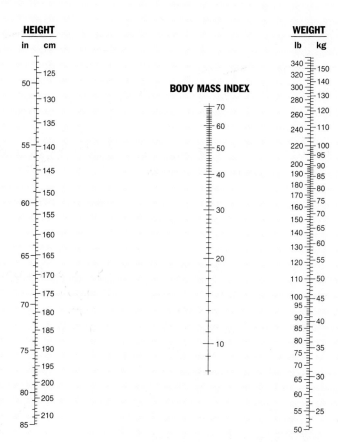

Rating Chart: Body Mass Index

	13 years old		14 years old		15 years old		16 years old		17 years old		18 years old	
	males	females	males	females	males	females	males	females	males	females	males	females
High Performance	16.6–19.9	17.5–21.0	17.5–20.9	17.5–21.5	18.1–21.5	17.5–21.5	18.5–22.0	17.5–21.5	18.8–21.9	17.5–21.5	19.0–22.4	18.0–21.9
Good Fitness	20.0–23.0	21.1–24.5	21.0–24.5	21.6–25.0	21.6–25.0	21.6–25.0	22.1–26.5	21.6–25.0	22.0–27.0	21.6–26.0	22.5–27.5	22.0–27.3
Marginal Fitness	23.1–26.0	24.6–27.0	24.6–26.5	25.1–27.5	25.1–27.0	25.1–27.5	26.6–27.5	25.1–27.5	27.1–28.0	26.1–27.5	27.6–28.5	27.4–28.0
Low Fitness	26.1+	27+	26.6+	27.6+	27.1+	27.6+	27.6+	27.6+	28.1+	27.6+	28.6+	28.1+

Backsaver Sit and Reach

1. Place a yardstick on top of a 12-inch high box. Have the yardstick extend 9 inches over the box with the lower numbers toward you.

2. To measure flexibility of the right leg, fully extend it and place the right foot flat against the box. The left leg is bent with the knee turned out and the foot 2 to 3 inches to the side of the straight right leg.

3. Extend the arms forward over the measuring stick. Place the hands, one on top of the other, with the palms facing down. The middle fingers should be together with the tips of one finger exactly on top of the other.

4. Lean forward and reach with the arms and fingers four times. On the fourth reach, hold for 3 seconds and observe the inch mark below your fingertips. Then record your score to the nearest inch.

5. Repeat the test with the left leg straight. Write the results on your record sheet.

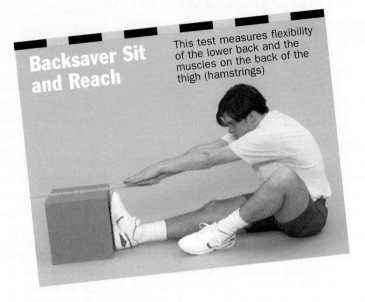

Backsaver Sit and Reach

This test measures flexibility of the lower back and the muscles on the back of the thigh (hamstrings)

Rating Chart: Backsaver Sit and Reach

	13-14 years old		15 years old and above	
	males	**females**	**males**	**females**
High Performance	10+	12+	10+	14+
Good Fitness	8–9	10–11	8–9	12–13
Marginal Fitness	6–7	8–9	6–7	10–11
Low Fitness	5 or less	7 or less	5 or less	9 or less

Based on FITNESSGRAM

4.2 Attitudes

Lesson Objectives
After reading this lesson, you should be able to:
1. List some negative attitudes about physical activity and describe how to change them into positive attitudes.
2. List some reasons why people like to exercise.
3. Explain how you can help others have a positive attitude toward physical activity.

Lesson Vocabulary
attitude

Attitude is another word for your feelings. Your attitude about physical activity can affect your well-being throughout life. In this lesson, you will learn about attitudes people have about physical activity and how to change negative attitudes to positive ones. Having a positive attitude is the key to success in fitness.

Change Negative Attitudes
The following list shows you some ways to change negative attitudes into positive attitudes.

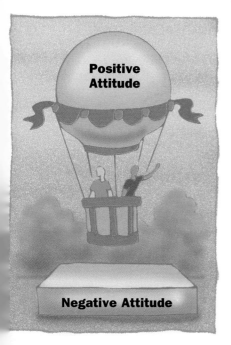

"I don't have the time" becomes "I will plan a time for physical activity." If you planned time for physical activity, you would feel better, function more efficiently, and actually may have more time to do other things you want to do.

Active people have more positive than negative attitudes.

"I don't want to get all sweaty" becomes "I'll allow time to wash up afterwards." Sweating is a natural by-product of a good workout. Allow yourself time to change before exercising, and shower and change afterwards. Focus on how good you will feel.

"People might laugh at me" becomes "I don't care what people think. When they see how fit I get, they'll wish they were exercising, too." Don't let other people's opinions affect you. Find friends who are interested in getting fit. Those who do laugh may be jealous of your efforts and results.

"None of my friends work out, so neither do I" becomes " I'll ask my friends to join me and we'll all work out together." Talk with your friends. Some of them may be interested in working out or doing lifestyle activities together.

"I get nervous and feel tense when I am in sports and games" becomes "Everyone gets nervous. I'll stay calm and do the best I can." Many athletes need to learn techniques to reduce their stress levels. You will learn some of these techniques in Chapter 18.

"I'm already in good condition" becomes "Physical activity will help keep me in good condition." Use the self-assessments in this book, and then take an honest look at yourself. Are you as fit as you thought? Physical activity can help you get in shape and stay in shape.

"I'm too tired" becomes "I'll just do a little to get started, and as I get more fit, I'll do more." You'll probably find that physical exertion actually gives you more energy. Begin slowly and gradually increase the amount of activity you do.

Increase Positive Attitudes
Following is a list of reasons why people like to be physically active. Think about these attitudes and how you might make some of them your own.

"Physical activities are a great way to meet people." Many activities provide opportunities to meet people and strengthen friendships. Aerobic dance and team sports are examples of good social activities.

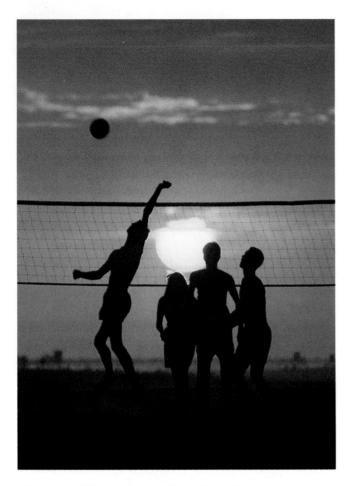

Physical activity can be an enjoyable social event.

"I think physical activity is really fun." Many teenagers do activities because they are fun. Participating in activities you enjoy also helps reduce stress.

"I enjoy the challenge." Sir Edmund Hillary was asked why he climbed Mt. Everest. "Because it was there," he replied. Many people welcome challenges.

"I like the rigor of training." Some people enjoy doing intense training. Winning and competition can be secondary for people who enjoy training.

"I like competition." If you enjoy competition, sports and other physical activities provide ways to test yourself against others. You can even compete against yourself by trying to improve your score or your time in an activity.

"Physical activities are my way of relaxing." After doing school work, physical activity can help you relax mentally or emotionally after a difficult day.

"I think physical activity improves my appearance." Physical activity can help build muscle and control body fat. However, remember that regular activity cannot completely change your appearance.

"Physical activity is a good way to improve my health and wellness." As you will learn in Chapter 5, regular physical activity helps you resist illness and improves your general sense of well-being.

"Physical activity just makes me feel good." Many people just feel better when they exercise and have a sense of loss or discomfort when they do not.

Sensitivity to Others

The way others react can affect a person's feelings about physical activity. Your positive reactions can help others change negative feelings about physical activity.

Instead of laughing, provide encouragement. Do you remember how difficult it is to start something new or different? You can encourage others by saying such words as "Good to see you exercising. Way to go!"

Try to make new friends through participation in physical activities. Introduce yourself to others and offer to help other people when it seems appropriate. Don't hesitate to ask for help from others.

Start or join a sport or exercise club. You and your friends can combine socializing with physical activity by starting or joining an activity club. Check with your school's activity coordinator concerning the rules for setting up an activity club.

Lesson Review
1. Give examples of some negative attitudes toward physical activity, and explain how you would change them into positive attitudes.
2. Give several reasons why people enjoy physical activity.
3. Explain how you can help others have a positive attitude toward physical activity.

Activity 4
Circuit Training Workout

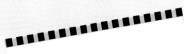

Safety Tips

While doing the Side Stretch, do not twist your body, bend forward, or push your hips sideways.

Circuit training consists of several different exercises done consecutively. You move from one exercise station to the next. At each station, you complete an exercise. When you have completed the exercises at all stations, you have completed the exercise "circuit." There are many kinds of exercise circuits. This one is designed to help you build all parts of health-related fitness.

You can use circuit training to increase your exercise overload. As you improve in a certain exercise, you can increase the number of times you complete it. In other words, you can increase the repetitions. If you try to complete the circuit more quickly, take extra care to do each exercise properly.

For a total fitness circuit such as this one, exercises for all parts of fitness and all body parts should be included. A variety of equipment can be used at the exercise stations. If no special equipment is available, you can perform calisthenics at each exercise station. Circuit training is usually planned by an exercise specialist, but you can learn to plan your own circuit course. Try the sample total fitness circuit-training workout described here. Record your results on your record sheet.

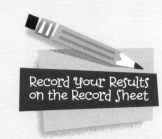

Record your Results on the Record Sheet

Side Stretch

1 Stand with feet shoulder width apart.

2 Clasp your hands behind your neck.

3 Bend your trunk sideways to the left as far as possible.

4 Repeat to the right.

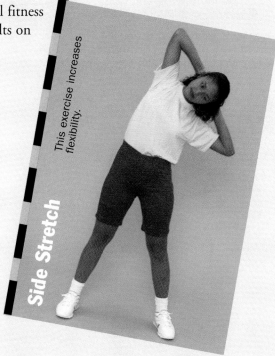

This exercise increases flexibility.

Side Stretch

Circuit Training Workout

Exercise	Repetitions
Side Stretch	15 within 2 minutes
Jump Rope	60 jumps per minute for 2 minutes
Bench Step	50 within 2 minutes
Curl-Up	5 to 10 within 2 minutes
Sprint the Line	6 within 2 minutes
Inch Worm	5 to 15 within 2 minutes
Knee Lift	5 per leg within 2 minutes
Jog in Place	120 steps per minute for 2 minutes

Jump Rope

Use either the jog step or the two-foot hop.

1 For the two-foot hop, hop on both feet simultaneously with each rope swing. Beginners should hop twice with each rope swing. This second hop is a small bounce.

2 For the jog step, jog or step from one foot to the other foot.

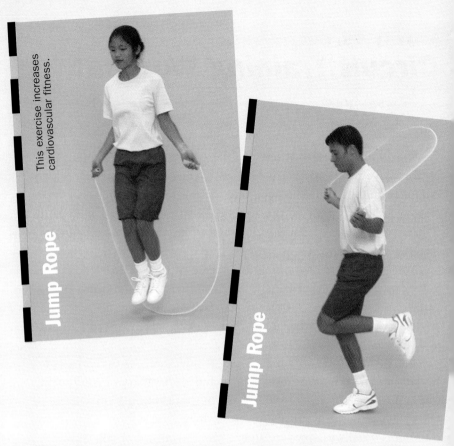

This exercise increases cardiovascular fitness.

Jump Rope

Jump Rope

Bench Step

1 Step up with your right foot, then up with your left foot.

2 Step down with your right foot and down with your left foot.

3 Repeat this 4-count (up, up, down, down) stepping at an even rhythm about 25 times per minute.

Curl-Up

1 Lie on your back with your hands folded across your chest.

2 Bend your knees at a 90° angle.

3 Flatten your back then roll your head and shoulders forward and upward. Roll far enough to feel tension in the abdominal muscles. Your shoulder blades should come up off the floor, but do not lift your back off the floor.

4 Return to the starting position.

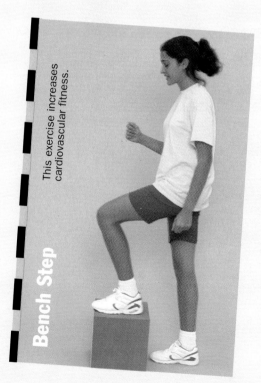

This exercise increases cardiovascular fitness.

Bench Step

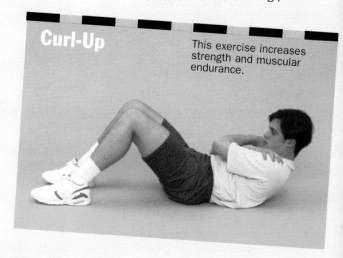

Curl-Up

This exercise increases strength and muscular endurance.

Sprint the Line

1 Run from one line to another 10 yards away.

2 Walk back and repeat.

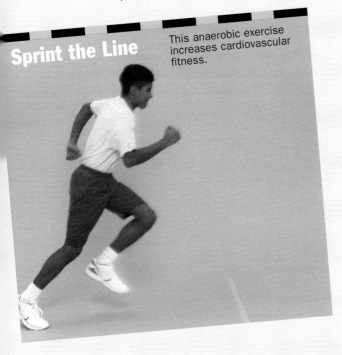

Sprint the Line

This anaerobic exercise increases cardiovascular fitness.

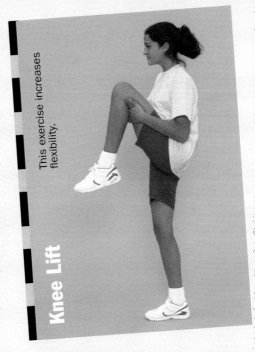

This exercise increases flexibility.

Knee Lift

Knee Lift

1 Stand with your feet together and arms at your sides.

2 Raise your left knee as high as possible, grasping your thigh with your hands.

3 Pull your knee against your body while keeping your back straight.

4 Return to starting position and repeat with your right knee.

Inch Worm

1 Support your body with your arms and feet in a push-up position.

2 Slowly walk your feet forward as far as possible while the hands remain stationary on the floor.

3 Then slowly walk your hands forward, away from your feet, until you are again in the push-up position.

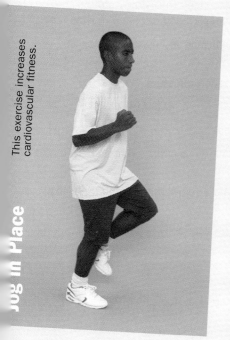

This exercise increases cardiovascular fitness.

Jog in Place

Jog in Place

Jog in place at a rate of 120 steps per minute.

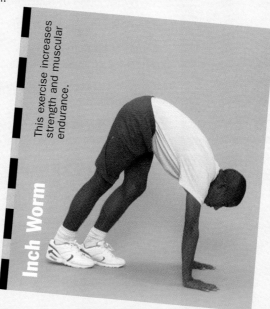

This exercise increases strength and muscular endurance.

Inch Worm

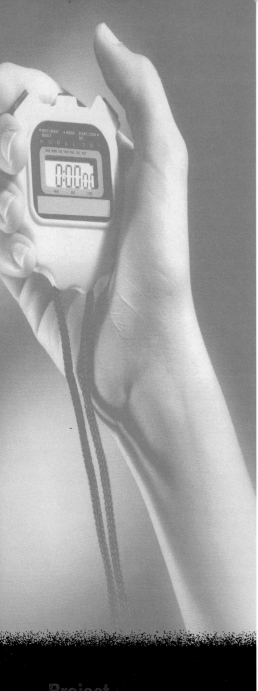

Reviewing Concepts and Vocabulary

Copy the number of each statement on a sheet of paper. Next to each number, write the word or words that correctly completes the sentence.

1. To get your heart ready for more vigorous activity, you do a _____.

2. A _____ helps prevent injury.

3. If you don't do a _____ after vigorous activity, you might get dizzy.

4. Muscles that are _____ and _____ contract, relax, and stretch more easily than muscles that are short, tight, and cool.

5. You can change your _____ about physical activity from negative to positive.

6. The _____ diagram can be used to help you make good activity choices for your physical activity program.

Number your paper. Next to each number, choose the letter of the best answer.

Column I	Column II
7. muscle stretch	a. exercises that gently contract your muscles to warm them.
8. cool-down	b. activities to help your body recover after a workout
9. workout	c. exercises that slowly stretch the muscles and increase muscle length
10. muscle warm-up	d. activities to improve fitness

On your paper, write a short answer for each question.

11. What kinds of activities can you do to warm up before a workout?

12. How long should a heart warm-up last?

13. Why do some experts think you should do a heart warm-up before and after a muscle warm-up and stretch?

14. What sorts of things can you do to help yourself stick with a physical activity program?

15. How can positive attitudes toward physical activity help you become fit?

Thinking Critically

Write a paragraph to answer the following question.

You're walking past the track and see your friend, Sam, running laps. He stops running and sits on the grass. You join him and he tells you that he just finished running two miles and he's feeling dizzy and has a leg cramp. What could you suggest to help him avoid dizziness and cramps after working out?

Project

What do the people you know think about physical activity? Develop a list of questions and ask at least six people to answer them. Try to ask people from several different age groups. Analyze your results. Then develop a plan to improve any negative attitudes you found.

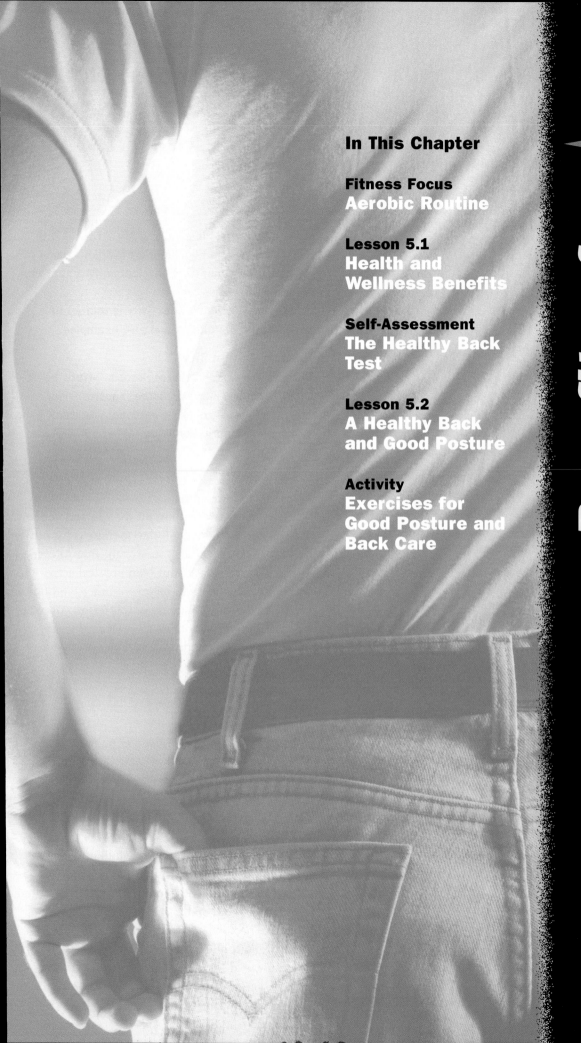

Benefits of
Physical Activity

5

Aerobic Routine

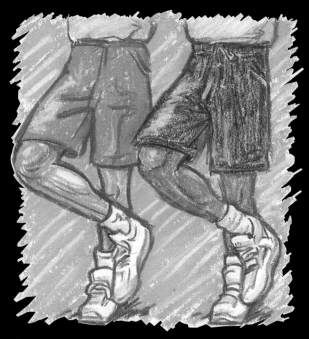

Aerobic dance is a type of exercise routine that is also a form of aerobic exercise. Aerobic dance routines are developed by combining a variety of steps and arm movement performed to music. The key to getting a good aerobic workout during the routine is to keep moving at a regular pace. Many young people enjoy aerobic dance because they can get a good workout while listening to music they enjoy.

Use the aerobic routine on your instruction sheet to acquaint yourself with this type of exercise. Later you may want to develop your own routine.

Step Hop
Forward Jog
Jumping Jack
Backward Jog
Jesse Polka
Grapevine
High Kick

Lesson 5.1 Health and Wellness Benefits

Lesson Objectives

After reading this lesson, you should be able to:
1. Describe some hypokinetic conditions.
2. List some benefits of physical activity that contribute to wellness.
3. Explain how physical activity is related to hyperkinetic conditions and give examples.

Lesson Vocabulary

primary risk factor, atherosclerosis, artery, heart attack, stroke, blood pressure, hypertension, cancer, diabetes, obesity, osteoporosis, peak bone mass, hyperkinetic condition, activity neurosis

Perhaps you are not convinced that a lifetime plan for physical activity is important for you and your well-being. You might think that exercise is for others, not for you. Whether you are reluctant to exercise or you already have your own physical activity program, this chapter will help you understand how important physical activity is. In this lesson you will learn more about how physical activity reduces your risk of hypokinetic conditions and increases your personal wellness.

Hypokinetic Diseases and Conditions

You know from Chapter 2 that a hypokinetic condition is one associated with, or caused by, a lack of physical activity or regular exercise. A number of serious health problems are classified as hypokinetic conditions or diseases.

Cardiovascular Diseases Did you know that since 1900 cardiovascular disease has been the leading cause of death in the United States every year but one? In recent years more than 42 percent of all deaths have been related to cardiovascular disease. Currently about one in every four Americans has one or more forms of cardiovascular disease.

Many cardiovascular diseases are hypokinetic conditions because sedentary living, or inactivity, is a **primary risk factor** for those diseases. A primary risk factor is a risk factor that is considered a major contributor to a disease.

Atherosclerosis is a disease in which certain substances including fats build up on the inside walls of the arteries. **Arteries** are the "pipelines" that carry blood from the heart to all parts of your body. You can see in the picture that this build-up narrows the openings through the arteries. As a result, the heart must work harder to pump blood. Notice how the coronary artery on the right has become so narrow that blood cannot flow properly to the heart muscle. Atherosclerosis begins early in life. Scientific evidence shows that regular physical activity reduces the fats and other substances in the blood that cause atherosclerosis.

ple who are recovering from a heart attack.

A **stroke** occurs when oxygen in the blood supply to the brain is severely reduced or cut off. A blood clot or atherosclerosis can block any artery that supplies blood to the brain, causing a stroke. A stroke also can occur when an artery to the brain bursts. Since a stroke damages the brain, it can affect a person's ability to move, think, and speak. Some strokes are severe enough to cause death. Regular physical activity can reduce some of the risk factors thought to cause a stroke. Also physical activity in the form of physical therapy can help a stroke patient regain some functions lost as a result of the stroke.

Each time your heart beats, it forces blood through your arteries, causing the blood to push against the artery walls. This force of blood against your artery walls is called **blood pressure.** When the doctor checks your blood pressure, he or she looks for two readings: your systolic blood pressure—the highest pressure exerted by the blood within your arteries—and your diastolic blood pressure—the lowest pressure exerted by your arteries.

Hypertension, or high blood pressure, is a disease in which blood pressure is consistently higher than normal. High blood pressure is a hypokinetic condition because regular physical activity is one way to help lower blood pressure.

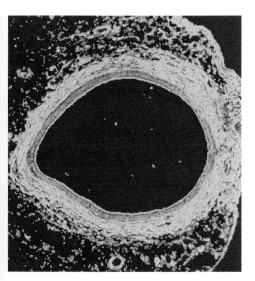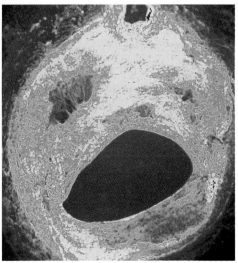

Compare the clear artery on the left with the partially-blocked artery on the right.

A **heart attack** occurs when the blood supply within the heart is severely reduced or cut off. As a result, an area of the heart muscle can die. Arteries inside the heart can be blocked by atherosclerosis, a blood clot, a spasm in the muscle of the artery, or a combination of these causes. During a heart attack, the heart may beat abnormally or even stop beating. Medicines are often used to stabilize the heartbeat of someone in distress. Also, cardiopulmonary resuscitation (CPR) often is done to restore circulation of oxygen when the heart stops beating. Studies have shown that people who participate in regular physical activity have fewer heart attacks than those who are sedentary. Medical doctors often prescribe physical activity programs to help peo-

Hypertension also is a primary risk factor because it is a major contributor to stroke, heart attack, and kidney damage. You can see the range of "normal" blood pressure in the chart below.

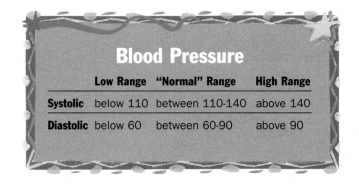

Blood Pressure

	Low Range	"Normal" Range	High Range
Systolic	below 110	between 110-140	above 140
Diastolic	below 60	between 60-90	above 90

Cancer More than 100 different diseases characterized by the uncontrollable growth of abnormal cells are catagorized as **cancer**. Cancer's uncontrolled cells invade normal cells, steal their nutrition, and interfere with the normal cell functions.

Cancer is the second leading cause of death in the United States. When diagnosed early, many forms of cancer can be treated and even cured through surgery, chemical or radiation therapy, or medication. It is not clear why physical activity helps reduce the risk of cancer. But certain forms of cancer are considered hypokinetic conditions because people who are physically active are less likely to get those cancers than people who are inactive. Colon cancer and breast cancer are examples. Many of the risk factors for heart disease are also risk factors for cancer. Regular physical exams are a good way to help prevent cancer.

Diabetes When a person's body cannot regulate the sugar level in the body, the person has a disease called **diabetes**. A person with diabetes will have excessively high blood sugar unless he or she gets medical assistance. Over time, diabetes can damage the blood vessels, heart, kidneys, and eyes. A very high level of sugar in the blood can cause coma and death. Several effective medical treatments exist to help diabetics regulate their blood sugar and lead normal lives.

One kind of diabetes—Type I—is not a hypokinetic condition. This condition is often hereditary and accounts for about 10 percent of all diabetics. Type I diabetics take insulin, a hormone made in the pancreas, to help control blood sugar levels.

The most common kind of diabetes—Type II—is a hypokinetic condition because people who are physically active are less likely to have the condition. Activity helps control this type of diabetes by controlling body fatness. Diabetes has many of the same risk factors as heart disease.

Obesity A condition in which a person has a high percentage of body fat—called **obesity**—often is the result of inactivity, although many other factors may contribute. Having too much body fatness contributes to other diseases such as heart disease and diabetes. You will learn more about obesity in Chapter 7.

Osteoporosis When the structure of the bones deteriorates and the bones become weak, a condition called **osteoporosis** exists. Osteoporosis is most common

among older people, but it has its beginnings in youth. You develop your greatest bone mass—also called your **peak bone mass**—when you are young. Those who exercise develop stronger bones than those who are sedentary. Therefore, if you are physically active when you are young, you will build a higher peak bone mass. As a result, if you lose bone mass as you get older, you will have stronger bones than if you hadn't exercised while young.

Lack of calcium in the diet, especially when a person is young, contributes to osteoporosis. Women are more likely to have osteoporosis than men because, as a result of hormonal changes that take place in women later in life, calcium absorption becomes less efficient. For bone health throughout life, good nutrition, regular activity, and hormone regulation is necessary.

Physical Activity and Wellness

As you can see, physical activity plays an important role in the prevention of hypokinetic diseases. Therefore, physical activity is important to good health. But remember—health is more than freedom from disease; it means being positively healthy. Two components of positive health identified as important national goals by the *Healthy People 2010* report are helping all people have a sense of well-being and a high quality of life. Some of the benefits of physical activity that contribute to these two factors include:

- Improved appearance
- Greater work capacity
- Greater capacity to enjoy leisure
- Improved sense of emotional well-being
- Increased opportunity for successful experiences and social interactions
- Increased opportunity for fun
- Added functional years
- Increased ability to meet emergencies

Hyperkinetic Conditions

You've probably heard the saying that "too much of a good thing can be bad." This saying can be true of physical activity too. Just because some physical activity is good does not always mean that more activity is better. In some cases people experience **hyperkinetic conditions**—health problems caused by doing too much physical activity.

Overuse Injuries You learned in Chapter 2 that overuse injuries occur when you do so much physical

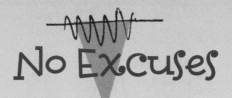

No Excuses

Reducing Risk Factors

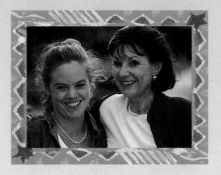

A risk factor is any action or condition that increases your chances of developing a disease. Some risk factors, such as your age, cannot be controlled or changed by you. Other non-controllable risk factors, such as whether you are a male or female, are genetically controlled. Sometimes, you are able to control individual risk factors. For example, you can control your diet and physical activity. Your actions affect the probability of your getting a disease.

Brenda's family took a trip to Colorado last summer. Plans were made to hike in the mountains, raft the rivers, and ride bikes and horses. Unfortunately, Brenda's mother did not get to enjoy all of the activities.

"I never thought my mother had any health problems because she was always busy with work and taking care of the house. She never went to the doctor. "

But Brenda's mother was a smoker. While she may have been "busy," she didn't really do much physical activity because she easily became short of breath.

Brenda's mother found that she couldn't keep up with the rest of the family. While hiking, she became so short of breath that she almost fainted. She fell far behind while trying to bike ride. In the evenings, while the rest of the family did other things, Brenda's mother went to bed.

When they returned home, Brenda's mother went to her doctor. He recommended changes in her lifestyle. She was to stop smoking and get more exercise. He warned that she was at risk for heart disease and other health problems if she continued her present activities.

For Discussion

What controllable risk factors for heart disease did Brenda's mother have? What can she do to reduce her risk? What can you do to decrease your risk for heart disease? Fill out the questionnaire to learn more about Brenda's mother's risk factors as well as your own.

---

activity that your bones, muscles, or other tissues are damaged. It is easy to see that overuse injuries are a type of hyperkinetic condition. Examples are stress fractures, shin splints, and blisters.

Activity Neurosis Neurosis is a condition that occurs when a person is overly concerned or fearful about something. Excessive fear of high places is one type of neurosis. People with an **activity neurosis** are overly concerned about getting enough exercise and are upset if they miss a regular workout. In addition, they often continue physical activity when they are sick or injured. Runners and body builders are more likely to experience activity neurosis than other exercisers.

Eating Disorders Several kinds of eating disorders result from an extreme desire to be abnormally thin. People with these conditions have dangerous eating habits and often resort to excessive activity to expend Calories for fat loss. Eating disorders that abuse exercise are considered hyperkinetic conditions. You will learn more about eating disorders in Chapter 7.

Lesson Review
1. Describe at least three hypokinetic conditions.
2. What are some wellness benefits of physical activity?
3. How is physical activity related to hyperkinetic conditions? Give examples.

Self-Assessment 5
The Healthy Back Test

Backache is a condition that is often caused by weak muscles. Use this self-assessment to test the muscles that help support your back. Each part focuses on a certain muscle group. If you do well on this assessment, you are more likely to have a healthy back.

   If possible, work with a partner. As you complete each test, note the points you earn on your record sheet. When you complete all six tests, add your points to get your total score. Then use the rating chart to determine your risk of back problems.

Single Leg Lift
(Supine)

1 Lie on your back on the floor. Lift your right leg off the floor as high as possible without bending either knee.

2 Repeat using your left leg. Score 1 point if you can lift your right leg to a 90-degree angle to the floor. Score 1 additional point if you can lift your left leg to a 90-degree angle.

Knee-to-Chest

1 Lie on your back on the floor. Make sure your lower back is flat on the floor.

2 Keep your left leg straight and touching the floor. Bring your right knee up until you can hold it tight against your chest. Grasp the back of the thigh.

3 Repeat using your left leg.

4 Score 1 point if you can keep your left leg touching the floor while you hold your right leg against your chest. Score 1 additional point if you can keep your right leg touching the floor while holding the left leg against your chest.

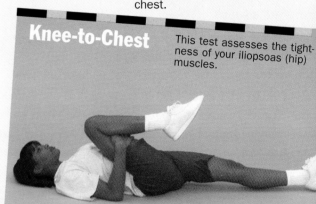

Knee-to-Chest This test assesses the tightness of your iliopsoas (hip) muscles.

Single Leg Lift (Supine) This test assesses the length of your hamstring muscles.

Single Leg Lift
(Prone)

1 Lie facedown on the floor. Lift your straight right leg as high as possible. Hold for a count of 10. Then lower your leg.

2 Repeat using your left leg.

3 Score 1 point if you can lift and hold your right leg 1 foot off the floor and hold for the count. Score 1 point if you can lift your left leg 1 foot off the floor and hold for the count.

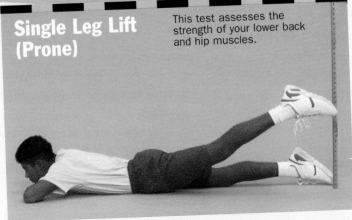

Single Leg Lift (Prone) This test assesses the strength of your lower back and hip muscles.

Curl-Up

1 Lie on your back with your knees bent 90 degrees and your arms extended.

2 Curl up by rolling your head, shoulders, and upper back off the floor. Roll up only until your shoulder blades leave the floor.

3 Score 1 point if you can curl up with your arms held straight in front of you and hold 10 seconds without having to lift your feet off the floor.

4 Score 2 points if you can curl up with your arms across your chest and hold 10 seconds.

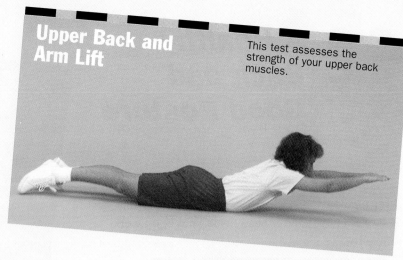

Upper Back and Arm Lift

This test assesses the strength of your upper back muscles.

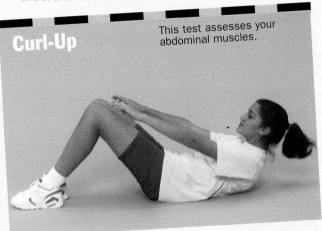

Curl-Up

This test assesses your abdominal muscles.

Upper Back and Arm Lift

1 Lie facedown. Hold your arms straight out in front of your head. Lift your arms and upper body off the floor. Hold for 10 seconds.
Caution: Do not lift your feet off the floor.

2 Score 1 point if you can lift your chin 1 foot off the floor. Score 2 points if you can lift your chin 1 foot off the floor for 10 seconds.

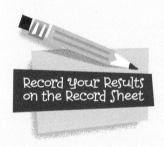

Record your Results on the Record Sheet

Back-to-Wall

1 Stand with your back to a wall so that your heels, buttocks, shoulders, and head are against the wall.

2 Try to press your lower back and neck against the wall without bending your knees or lifting your heels off the floor.

3 Have a partner try to place a hand between your back and the wall.

4 Score 2 points if you can press your back against the wall. Score 1 point if you can press your back against your partner's hand.

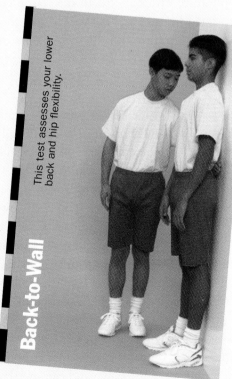

This test assesses your lower back and hip flexibility.

Back-to-Wall

Rating Chart: Healthy Back Test

Rating	Score
Healthy Back	11–12
Average Risk	9–10
Above Average Risk	6–8
High Risk	below 6

5.2

A Healthy Back and Good Posture

Lesson Objectives
After reading this lesson, you should be able to:
1. Explain how good fitness helps your back work efficiently.
2. Describe some common posture problems.
3. List some biomechanical principles that will help you improve posture and avoid back problems.

Lesson Vocabulary
lordosis

Each year as many as 25 million Americans seek a doctor's care for backache. According to some experts, back pain is the leading medical complaint in the United States. Although adults experience most of the back problems, young people do suffer from back pain. Also studies show that back problems often begin much earlier in life. In this lesson you will learn how good fitness helps the back work efficiently. You will also learn how some back problems are related to poor posture.

Back Problems

Backache is considered a hypokinetic condition because weak and short muscles are linked to some types of back problems. Poor posture also is associated with muscles that are not strong or long enough. By building fit muscles to improve your posture, you can help reduce the risk of back pain and look your best. Even if you never experience back pain, a healthy back and good posture are important so that you can function more efficiently in your daily activities.

How does good fitness help the back operate efficiently? Your body parts are balanced like blocks on your legs. Your chest hangs from your spine and is balanced over your pelvis. Your head sits on top of your spine, balanced over the other blocks in the stack. Since your spine is flexible and can move back and forth, the pull of your muscles keeps your body parts balanced. You might recall from the discussion of bio-mechanical principles in Chapter 2 that if your muscles on one side are weak and long, while your muscles on the opposite side are strong and short, your body parts are pulled off balance.

One back problem that often occurs among teens is **lordosis,** which is too much arch in the lower back. Lordosis, also called swayback, results when the abdominal muscles are weak and the iliopsoas muscles are too strong and too short. Lordosis is a problem that can lead to backache.

Even people who are relatively fit in other areas can lack fitness in the muscles that are related to back problems. One reason for this lack of fitness is that sports and games often overdevelop some muscles and neglect others. It is not unusual for basketball players, gymnasts, band members, and other active people to have weak back and abdominal muscles and short hamstring and hip-flexor muscles.

Posture Problems

Just as strong, long muscles contribute to a healthy back, they also are important to good posture. You can see some of the common posture problems associated with poor fitness in the picture to the right. You might recognize some of these problems with your own posture or that of others.

Knowing what constitutes good posture helps improve your own posture. Good posture helps you look good, helps prevent back problems, and helps you work and play more efficiently. In Chapter 17 you will get the opportunity to learn more about your posture using the Good Posture Assessment. You will check to see if you have any of the problems shown in the picture.

Back and Posture Improvement and Maintenance

Recall the Healthy Back Test you did in the Self-Assessment earlier in this chapter. How did you do? If you didn't do well, avoid exercises that require you to arch your back or to lift inefficiently with your back muscles. Instead, use the back exercises in the Activity for this chapter to help correct or prevent back problems. Since back problems are often related to poor posture, some exercises for improving posture have also been included. Also, these biomechanical principles will help you improve your posture and avoid back problems:

• **Use the large muscles of the body when lifting.** Let the strong leg muscles, not the relatively weak back muscles, do the work.

• **When lifting, keep your weight (hips) low.** Squatting with the back straight and the hips tucked helps keep weight low and makes lifting safer.

• **Divide a load to make it easier to carry.** For example, carrying two small suitcases, one in each hand, is easier than carrying one larger suitcase with one hand. A backpack is an efficient way to carry books. If you must carry your books in your arms, carry some in each arm. If you do carry your books in one arm, change arms from time to time.

• **Avoid twisting while lifting.** If you have to turn while lifting, change the position of your feet. It is especially important to avoid twisting your spine as you are straightening or bending it.

• **Push or pull heavy objects rather than lift them.** Heavy lifting can cause injury. Pushing or pulling an object is more efficient than lifting it.

• **Avoid a bent over position when sitting, standing, or lifting.** The levers of your body, such as your spine, do not work efficiently when you are bent over. When sitting in a chair, sit back in the seat and lean against the backrest. Do not work for long periods of time in a bent over position.

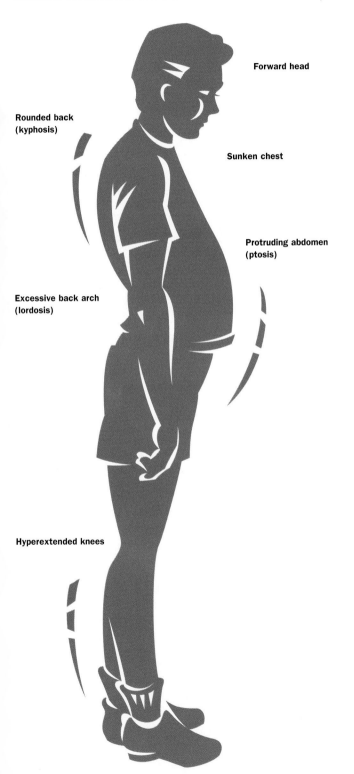

Forward head

Rounded back (kyphosis)

Sunken chest

Protruding abdomen (ptosis)

Excessive back arch (lordosis)

Hyperextended knees

Posture problems

Lesson Review
1. How does good fitness help the back operate efficiently?
2. What are some common posture problems?
3. List some biomechanical principles that will help you improve posture and avoid back problems.

Activity 5
Exercises for Good Posture and Back Care

Safety Tips

As you do these exercises, move only as far as the directions specify.

You now know the importance of strong back muscles and good posture. These exercises will help strengthen the muscles which support your back and improve your posture. You might want to include some of these exercises in your lifetime physical activity program.

Curl-Up

See page 32 for directions for the curl-up. Complete up to 10 repetitions.

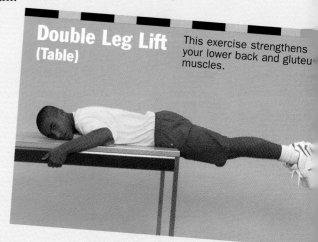

Double Leg Lift (Table) This exercise strengthens your lower back and gluteu muscles.

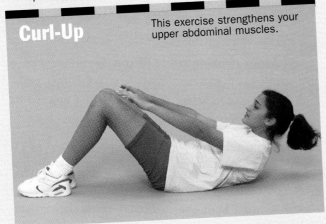

Curl-Up This exercise strengthens your upper abdominal muscles.

Record your Results on the Record Sheet

Double Leg Lift (Table)

1 Lie facedown on a table or bench with a partner holding your upper body. If you have no partner, grasp under the edge of a table.

2 Lift your legs until your legs are even with the top of the table. **Caution: Do not lift any higher. You might lift one leg at a time until you are able to lift both legs at once.**

3 Lower to the beginning position. Repeat up to 10 repetitions.

Trunk Lift (Table)

1 Lie facedown on your back on a table or bench with a partner holding your legs. Your upper body should hang over the edge.

2 Lift your upper body until it is even with the edge of the table. **Caution: Do not lift any higher.**

3 Lower to the beginning position. Repeat up to 10 times.

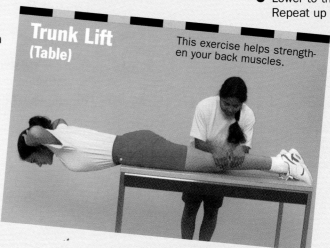

Trunk Lift (Table) This exercise helps strengthen your back muscles.

Reverse Curl

See page 32 for directions for doing the reverse curl. Complete up to 10 repetitions.

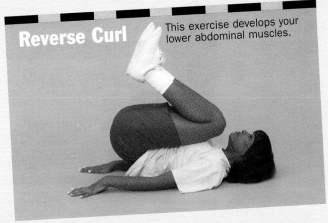

Reverse Curl

This exercise develops your lower abdominal muscles.

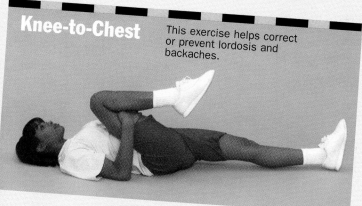

Knee-to-Chest

This exercise helps correct or prevent lordosis and backaches.

Knee-to-Chest

1 Lie on your back. Bend your right knee to your chest.

2 Grasp your thigh under the knee with your arms. Pull it down tight against your chest. Keep your left leg flat on the floor.

3 Return to the beginning position. Repeat with your left leg.

4 Pull both thighs to your chest and hug them. Repeat the exercise up to 10 times.

Arm and Leg Lift

This exercise helps prevent rounded shoulders, sunken chest, and rounded upper back.

1 Lie face down with your arms stretched in front of you.

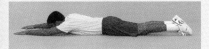

2 Raise your right arm; then lower it. Raise your left arm; then lower it. Finally raise both arms and then lower them.

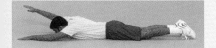

Single Leg Hang

1 Lie on your back on a table. Bend knees to your chest.

2 Grasp your right leg under your knee with your arms. Lower your left leg so that your thigh remains on the table while your knee and the rest of your leg hang over the edge of the table. Have a partner push your left leg down if it comes up. Hold this position for several seconds.

3 Return to the beginning position. Repeat switching leg positions. Repeat 10 times with each leg.

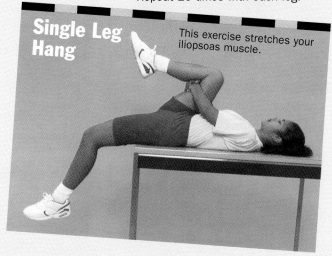

Single Leg Hang

This exercise stretches your iliopsoas muscle.

3 Raise your right leg; then lower it. Raise your left leg and then lower it.

4 Raise your right arm and right leg; then lower them. Repeat with your left arm and left leg.

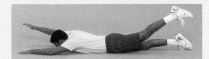

5 Raise your left arm and your right leg; then lower them. Raise your right arm and left leg; then lower them.

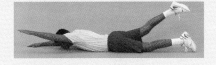

6 Repeat all the steps up to 5 times.
Caution: Do not arch your back.

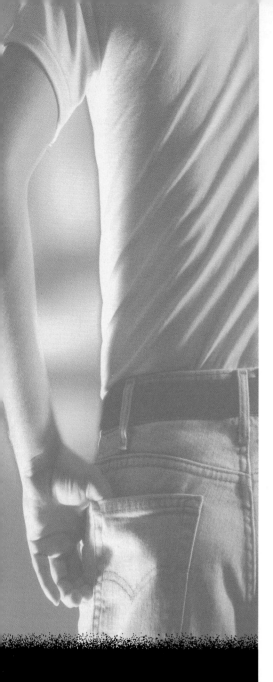

5 Chapter Review

Reviewing Concepts and Vocabulary

Copy the number of each statement on a sheet of paper. Next to each number, write the word or words that correctly complete the sentence.

1. If a person exercises when ill, he or she might be showing a symptom of _____.

2. A stroke causes damage to the _____.

3. During a heart attack, the blood supply to the heart is _____.

4. _____ results when uncontrollable cells invade normal cells and interfere with normal cell function.

5. Any condition caused by doing too much exercise is called a _____.

Number your paper. Next to each number, choose the letter of the best answer.

Column I	Column II
6. osteoporosis	a. having a high percentage of body fat
7. atherosclerosis	b. the body cannot regulate blood sugar level
8. hypertension	c. bones deteriorate and become weak
9. obesity	d. substances build up inside artery walls
10. diabetes	e. blood pressure is consistently higher than normal

On your paper, write a short answer for each statement or question.

11. What are some benefits of physical activity that contribute to positive health?

12. How can exercising when you are young help prevent osteoporosis as you get older?

13. Explain why some sports enthusiasts who are relatively fit, such as basketball players, might lack the types of fitness related to back problems.

14. What are some things you can do to avoid back problems?

15. Why is hypertension considered a primary risk factor?

Thinking Critically

Write a paragraph to answer the following question.

Why is inactivity a primary risk factor for many cardiovascular diseases?

Project

A recent study showed that approximately one-fourth of those who are 18 years and older do not participate in regular leisure time physical activity. What percentage of students your age participate in leisure time physical activity? Conduct a survey to find out. You might also poll those who respond to your survey to find out why they do or do not exercise.

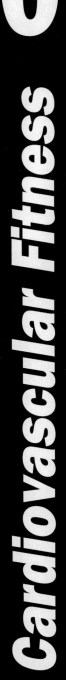

In This Chapter

6

Cardiovascular Fitness

Jump-Rope and Stretch Workout

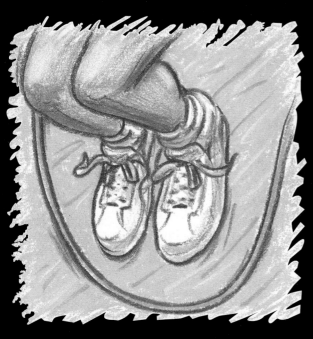

Regular physical activity strengthens your heart and improves other parts of your cardiovascular system. Jump rope is an activity that can be performed by most people to improve cardiovascular fitness. The stretching exercises improve the flexibility of your muscles and joints.

Refer to your instruction sheet to see how to do the Jump-Rope and Stretch Workout. This workout includes only basic jump-rope skills, but you may want to add other, more difficult skills as your ability improves. The stretching exercises require a partner.

Jog Step
Back Saver Toe Touch
Left-Right Swing
Wring the Dish Towel
Two-Foot Balance
Posture Stretch
Two-Foot Hop
Two-Ankle Wrap
Front-Back Jump
Mirror Side Stretch

Lesson 6.1 Activity and Cardiovascular Fitness

Lesson Objectives

After reading this lesson, you should be able to:
1. Describe the benefits of cardiovascular fitness to health and wellness.
2. Explain the relationship between physical activity and good cardiovascular fitness.
3. Describe and demonstrate some methods you can use to assess your cardiovascular fitness.
4. Determine how much cardiovascular fitness is enough.

Lesson Vocabulary

cardiovascular system, respiratory system, cholesterol, lipoprotein, low-density lipoprotein, high-density lipoprotein, vein

The girl in the picture at one time thought she would never be able to run a mile. Now she can. If you are inactive like this girl used to be, consider increasing your physical activity. When you do regular physical activity, you improve your cardiovascular fitness—fitness of the heart, lungs, blood, and blood vessels. Of the eleven parts of fitness, cardiovascular fitness is the

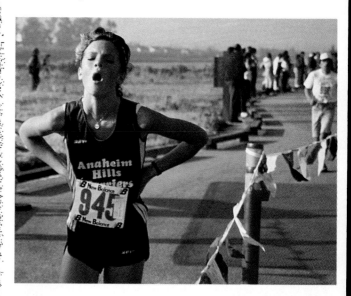

Running is one activity that can improve your cardiovascular fitness.

most important because those who have it receive many health and wellness benefits, including a chance for a longer life. The chart above lists some benefits of cardiovascular fitness. In addition, the activity that you do to improve your cardiovascular fitness will make you look better too!

In this lesson you will learn how proper exercise improves cardiovascular fitness. You will also learn how to assess your own cardiovascular fitness.

Benefits of Physical Activity and Cardiovascular Fitness

Looking good is important to most people, and you most likely are one of them. Doing regular physical activity can help you look better by controlling your weight, building muscle, and developing good posture. In addition, regular exercise produces changes in body organs such as making your heart muscle stronger and your blood vessels healthier. These changes result in improved cardiovascular fitness and wellness, as well as a reduction in risk of hypokinetic diseases.

Regular physical activity benefits two vital body systems. Your **cardiovascular system** includes your heart, blood vessels, and your blood. Your **respiratory system** includes your lungs and the air passages that bring air, including oxygen, from outside the body into the lungs. In your lungs oxygen enters your blood while carbon dioxide is eliminated. The cardiovascular and respiratory systems work together to bring your

body cells the materials they need to function and to rid the cells of wastes. Exercise helps these systems function more effectively (with the most benefits possible) and efficiently (with the least amount of effort).

Heart Because your heart is a muscle, it benefits from exercise and activities such as jogging, swimming, or long-distance hiking. Your heart acts as a pump to supply blood to your body cells. When you do vigorous physical activity, your muscle cells need more oxygen and they produce more waste products. Your heart must pump more blood to supply the increased amount of oxygen and to remove the wastes. If your heart isn't able to pump enough blood, the ability of your muscles to contract will be reduced and they will become fatigued more quickly.

Obviously, your heart's ability to pump blood is very important when doing physical activity, especially for an extended length of time. Your heart has two ways to get more blood to your muscles—by beating faster or by sending more blood with each beat.

You might recall from the Self-Assessment in Chapter 1 that your resting heart rate is the number of heartbeats per minute when you are relatively inactive. A person who does regular physical activity might have a resting heart rate of 55 to 60 beats per minute, while a person who does not exercise regularly might have a resting heart rate of 70 or more beats per minute. A very fit person's heart beats approximately 9.5 million times *less* each year than that of the average person. As you can see in the picture, a fit person's heart works more efficiently by pumping more blood with fewer beats.

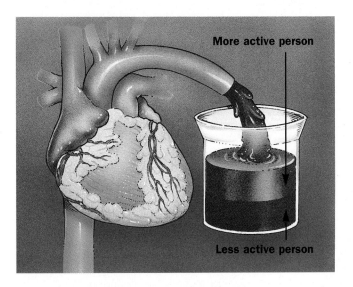

A fit heart pumps more blood with each beat.

Arteries Recall from Chapter 5 that your arteries carry blood away from your heart to other parts of your body. Blood is forced through your arteries by the beating of your heart. A strong heart and healthy lungs are not very helpful if your arteries are not clear and open. You know that fatty deposits on the inner walls of an artery lead to atherosclerosis. An extreme case of atherosclerosis can totally block the blood flow in an artery. Also, the hardened deposits allow blood clots to form, severely blocking blood flow. In either case, the heart muscle does not get enough oxygen and a heart attack occurs.

Blood Although your body needs a certain amount of fat, excessive amounts trigger formation of the fatty deposits along artery walls. **Cholesterol**, a fattylike substance found in meats, dairy products, and egg yolks, can be dangerous because high levels can build in your body without you noticing it.

Regular physical activity helps improve your cardiovascular fitness by reducing LDL (bad cholesterol) levels and increasing HDL (good cholesterol) levels. Also, exercise can help prevent blood clots from forming by reducing the amount of fibrin in the blood. Fibrin is a substance involved in making blood clot. High amounts of fibrin might contribute to the development of atherosclerosis.

Regular physical activity has other cardiovascular benefits. How do the drawings of the two hearts on this page differ? Note that the one on the left has a richer network of blood vessels. Scientists have found that people who exercise regularly develop more branching of the arteries in the heart. The importance of a richer network of blood vessels can be shown in this example. After astronaut Ed White died in a fire in 1967 while training for a mission, an autopsy was performed. Doctors found that one of the major arteries in his heart was completely blocked due to atherosclerosis. Because of all the physical training astronauts do, scientists think

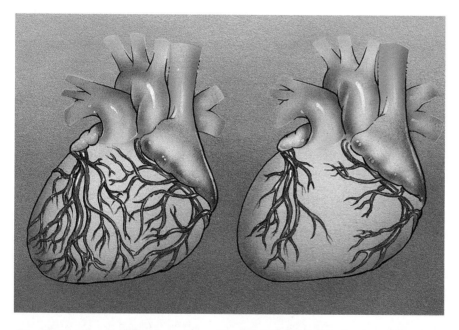

The richer network of blood vessels on the heart to the left is due to regular exercise.

Cholesterol is carried through the bloodstream by particles called **lipoproteins**. One kind, **low-density lipoprotein (LDL)**, is often referred to as "bad cholesterol" because LDLs carry cholesterol which is most likely to stay in the body and contribute to atherosclerosis. Another kind, **high-density lipoprotein (HDL)** is often referred to as "good cholesterol"; HDLs carry excess bad cholesterol out of the bloodstream and into the liver for elimination from the body. Therefore, HDLs appear to help prevent atherosclerosis.

White's body had developed an extra branching of arteries in his heart muscle. Therefore, he didn't die of a heart attack when a main artery was blocked. White had been able to continue a high level of physical fitness training without signs of heart trouble.

Veins Your **veins** carry blood filled with waste products from the muscle cells back to the heart. One-way valves in your veins keep the blood from flowing backward. Your muscles squeeze the veins to pump the blood back to your heart. Regular cardiovascular exercise helps make your muscles squeeze your veins efficiently. A lack of physical activity can cause the valves, especially those in the legs, to stop working efficiently. Proper circulation in your legs is then reduced.

Nerves of Your Heart Your heart muscle is not like your arm and leg muscles. When your arm and leg muscles contract, nerves in the muscles are responding to a message sent by the conscious part of your brain. In contrast, your heart is not controlled voluntarily; it beats regularly without you telling it to do so. Regular cardiovascular exercise can influence your nervous system to slow down your heart rate. As a result your heart works more efficiently because each heartbeat supplies more blood and oxygen to your body than if you did not exercise. In addition, a person with a slower heart rate can function more effectively during an emergency or vigorous physical activity.

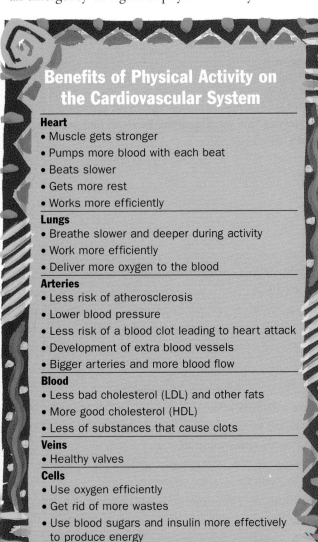

Benefits of Physical Activity on the Cardiovascular System

Heart
• Muscle gets stronger
• Pumps more blood with each beat
• Beats slower
• Gets more rest
• Works more efficiently

Lungs
• Breathe slower and deeper during activity
• Work more efficiently
• Deliver more oxygen to the blood

Arteries
• Less risk of atherosclerosis
• Lower blood pressure
• Less risk of a blood clot leading to heart attack
• Development of extra blood vessels
• Bigger arteries and more blood flow

Blood
• Less bad cholesterol (LDL) and other fats
• More good cholesterol (HDL)
• Less of substances that cause clots

Veins
• Healthy valves

Cells
• Use oxygen efficiently
• Get rid of more wastes
• Use blood sugars and insulin more effectively to produce energy

Muscle Cells For you to be able to do physical activity for a long time without getting tired, your muscle cells must function efficiently and effectively. Regular physical activity helps cells use oxygen and get rid of waste materials effectively. Physical activity also helps the muscle cells use blood sugar, with the aid of the hormone insulin, to produce energy. This is important to good cardiovascular health.

The chart summarizes some of the changes that physical activity produces in your body. These changes account for improvements in cardiovascular fitness.

Cardiovascular Assessment

You might be curious about your cardiovascular fitness—how good is it? Special tests can assess your cardiovascular fitness. The Maximal Oxygen Uptake test is considered the best test of cardiovascular fitness. It is done in a laboratory using special equipment, including a gas meter and a treadmill or a stationary bicycle. Another type of lab test of cardiovascular fitness is the graded exercise test, sometimes called the exercise stress test. This test also requires a treadmill or stationary bicycle and a special heart rate monitor.

Self-Assessment The tests described above are often quite expensive because of the need for special equipment and fitness experts. For this reason several self-assessments have been developed to allow you to conveniently assess your own cardiovascular fitness with a minimum of equipment and expense. You will get an opportunity to try several self-assessments in this class.

Interpreting Self-Assessment Results It is wise to do more than one self-assessment for cardiovascular fitness. Self-assessments are not as accurate as laboratory tests of fitness. However, they do give a good estimate of fitness level. Each assessment has its own strengths and weaknesses. For example, the results of the PACER (Chapter 3) and One-Mile Run (this chapter) are influenced by your motivation; if you don't try very hard, you won't get an accurate score. The Walking Test (Chapter 16) is a good indicator of fitness for most people but is not best for assessing high-level fitness. The Step Test (this chapter) uses heart rate; therefore, motivation does not influence the results as much as in some other assessments. But results on the Step Test can be distorted if you've done other exercise that might elevate the heart rate before doing the assessment. The test also can be influenced

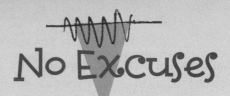

No Excuses

Finding Social Support

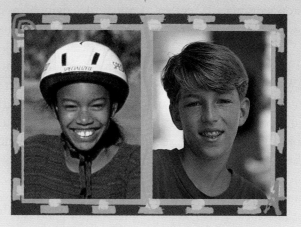

Social support is when members of your family or your friends encourage your physical activities or participate with you. You are more likely to begin or continue an activity if the people you associate with also do it.

Shannon's family has always enjoyed riding bikes. As a toddler, she would ride in the child's seat behind her mother. Every evening the family would ride through the neighborhood. By the time she was in school, Shannon had her own two-wheeler. Now as a teenager, Shannon still loves to ride. Because of school activities, she can't always ride with her family. Shannon wants to continue riding, but she doesn't want to do it alone.

Jim's family never has been very active. Most of his friends tend to watch TV, play video games, or just "hang out" rather than do anything active. Sometimes, Jim watches when a group of his classmates plays a quick game of volleyball after school. They often invite him to join the game. He has been tempted to join, but he has hesitated because he's not friends with any of the players. He knows that he has enjoyed whatever activities he's tried in the past, even though he never continued them for very long.

Both Shannon and Jim need social support. Shannon needs it to continue an activity she already enjoys. Jim needs support to begin an activity and then to continue to reinforce participation in it.

For Discussion

Who might Shannon ask to go riding with her? What could Jim do to become involved in physical activity? What groups of people provide the social support a person receives? Fill out the questionnaire to find out what social support you have.

by emotional factors that cause the heart rate to be higher than normal. Finally, your results may vary depending on when you do an assessment.

Since you may get different ratings on different tests of cardiovascular fitness, consider the strengths and weaknesses of each test when making decisions about which score is most indicative of your fitness.

How Much Cardiovascular Fitness is Enough?

To get the health and wellness benefits associated with cardiovascular fitness, you should achieve the good fitness zone in the rating charts that accompany each Self-Assessment in this book. It is important to know that there are benefits associated with moving out of the low fitness zone. Risk of hypokinetic diseases is greatest for those in the low fitness zone. Since cardio-

vascular fitness is a requirement for high-level performance in many sports, if you aspire to be an athlete you may want to train harder than most people to achieve the high performance zone. Achieving this level isn't necessary to get most of the health and wellness benefits, and it may be difficult for some people.

Lesson Review

1. What are some benefits of cardiovascular fitness to health and wellness?

2. What is the relationship between physical activity and cardiovascular fitness?

3. What are some methods for assessing cardiovascular fitness and how are they performed?

4. How much cardiovascular fitness is enough?

Self-Assessment 6
Cardiovascular Fitness

As you learned in the previous lesson, several tests of cardiovascular fitness can be done in physical-fitness laboratories by trained technicians. But if you want a quicker, easier, and less expensive test, try the Step Test or the One-Mile Run. You might do either of these assessments to see how fit you are. After you have done regular exercise over a period of time, test yourself again to see how much you have improved.

Step Test

1 Use a 12-inch high bench. Step up with your right foot. Step up with your left foot.

2 Step down with your right foot. Step down with your left foot. Repeat this 4-count (up, up, down, down). Step 24 times each minute for 3 minutes.

3 Immediately after stepping for 3 minutes, sit and use the procedure you learned in the Self-Assessment in Chapter 1 to count your own pulse. Begin counting within 5 seconds. Count for 1 minute.

4 Record your results on your worksheet. Check your cardiovascular rating and write it on your record sheet.
Caution: You should only do this test once in class unless your instructor tells you to do otherwise.

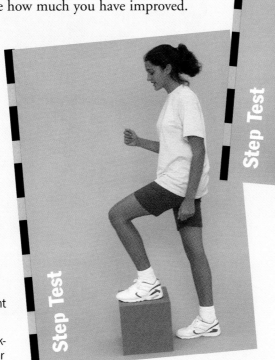

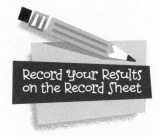

Record your Results on the Record Sheet

Rating Chart: Step Test (beats per minute)*

	13-years old or below		14 to 16-years old		17-years old or above	
	males	**females**	**males**	**females**	**males**	**females**
High Performance	90 or less	100 or less	85 or less	95 or less	80 or less	90 or less
Good Fitness	91–98	101–110	86–95	96–105	81–90	91–100
Marginal Fitness	99–120	111–130	96–115	106–125	91–110	101–120
Low Fitness	above 120	above 130	above 115	above 125	above 110	above 120

* Those who cannot step for 3 minutes receive a low fitness rating.

One-Mile Run

The one-mile run is an alternate test of cardiovascular fitness that you might use. Remember that this test is for your own information. It is not a race. Your goal is a good fitness rating. Once you achieve this rating, a faster time does not necessarily improve your health. However, it might help you perform better in a sport or other activity.

1 Run or jog for 1 mile in the shortest possible time. Try to set a pace that you can keep up for the full mile. A steady pace is best. If you start too fast and then have to slow down at the end, you will probably not be able to run for the entire distance.

2 Your score is the amount of time it takes you to run the mile. Record this score on your record sheet.

3 Find your rating on the cardiovascular fitness rating chart below and write it on your record sheet.

Safety Tips

Exercise several days a week for several weeks before you do this activity.

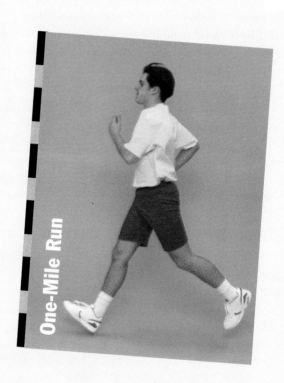

One-Mile Run

One-Mile Run (time in minutes and seconds)

	13-years old or below		14-years old		15-years old		16-years old or above	
	males	females	males	females	males	females	males	females
High Performance	7:30 or less	9:00 or less	7:00 or less	8:30 or less	7:00 or less	8:00 or less	7:00 or less	8:00 or l
Good Fitness	7:31–9:00	9:01–10:30	7:01–8:30	8:31–10:00	7:01–8:00	8:01–9:30	7:01–7:45	8:01–9:0
Marginal Fitness	9:01–10:00	10:31–11:30	8:31–9:30	10:01–11:00	8:01–9:00	9:31–10:30	7:46–8:30	9:01–10
Low Fitness	over 10:00	over 11:30	over 9:30	over 11:00	over 9:00	over 10:30	over 8:30	over 10:0

6.2 Lesson Activity for Health and Wellness

Lesson Objectives
After reading this lesson, you should be able to:
1. Identify areas of the Physical Activity Pyramid that are especially good for building cardiovascular fitness.
2. Explain how to count Calories or your heart rate to determine how much physical activity you need.
3. Explain the difference between aerobic activity and anaerobic activity.

Lesson Vocabulary
aerobic activity, anaerobic activity

You now know that physical activity is important to your cardiovascular fitness. But how do you choose the right kind and amount of activities? In this lesson you will learn how to combine activities from the Physical Activity Pyramid to build cardiovascular fitness. You will also learn how to determine how much activity you need.

The Physical Activity Pyramid and Cardiovascular Fitness

For total physical fitness and for optimal health and wellness benefits, it's important to select activities from all parts of the Physical Activity Pyramid. In this lesson we will focus on Lifestyle Physical Activity, Aerobic Activity, and Active Sport because these activities build cardiovascular fitness and its associated health and wellness benefits.

Lifestyle Physical Activity Not so many years ago lifestyle physical activity was the primary form of activity for most Americans. Farmers did all kinds of physical activity as did people who were required to do physical tasks at work. Now fewer and fewer people do significant physical activity as part of their work. Also electrical appliances and devices have reduced the amount of physical activity done at home.

Though most of us do less of it, lifestyle physical activity is a good way of doing regular activity that can produce cardiovascular benefits as well as contribute to other health and wellness benefits. This type of activity is at the bottom of the Physical Activity Pyramid because it is activity that all people are encouraged to do everyday, or at least most days of the week. In other words, all people are encouraged to do lifestyle physical activities such as mowing the lawn, walking to school or work, walking up stairs instead of riding an elevator, and even doing physical tasks at home such as vacuuming. Activities from this level of the pyramid can be combined with those from other parts of the pyramid to provide a total physical activity program. High school students in particular need more intensity than activities at this level can provide.

Aerobic Activity The term *aerobic* means "with oxygen." **Aerobic activity** is activity that is steady enough to allow the heart to supply all the oxygen your muscles need. Actually, most activities in the Physical Activity Pyramid can be considered aerobic. However, aerobic activity is usually described as "large muscle activities that are sustained for relatively long periods of time." Examples include walking, biking, jogging, cross-country skiing, and aerobic dance. *Aerobic activity* in this book refers to this kind of activity.

Aerobic activity is especially important to building cardiovascular fitness and promoting good health and wellness. Although some people

Physical Activity Pyramid

Rest or Inactivity
watching TV
reading

Exercise for Flexibility
stretching

Exercise for Strength & Muscular Endurance
weight training
calisthenics

Aerobic Activity
aerobics
jogging
biking

Active Sport
tennis
basketball
racquetball

Lifestyle Physical Activity
walk rather than ride
climb the stairs
do yard work

can get enough lifestyle physical activity to enjoy adequate fitness and wellness benefits, for most people additional aerobic exercise is strongly recommended.

Active Sport Active sports such as basketball, racquetball, and even golf can contribute to a total program for improving cardiovascular fitness and reaping health and wellness benefits. When activities such as these are done intensely enough to expend relatively large numbers of Calories or to increase the heart rate for a period of time, they are especially effective. Research has shown that people who play active sports throughout life are likely to have good health and wellness and, therefore, a reduced risk of early death.

The way you do an activity, including sports, has much to do with the benefits you receive from it. For example, golf is most beneficial when you walk and carry or pull your own clubs. Riding a cart limits the benefits you gain from the activity.

How Much Cardiovascular Activity Is Enough?

In 1995 the Centers for Disease Control and Prevention issued national guidelines for physical activity: "Every American should accumulate 30 minutes or more of moderate intensity physical activity on most, preferably all, days of the week." This amount of activity is the minimum each person should do to get health and wellness benefits and to achieve at least adequate cardiovascular fitness.

For teenagers there are two basic guidelines concerning how much activity is enough. These guidelines are presented in the following sections with information that will help you know if you have done enough physical activity to meet them.

Counting Physical Activity Calories The first national guideline indicates that teenagers should "be physically active daily, or nearly every day, as part of play, games, sports, work, transportation, recreation, physical education, or planned exercise . . ." As you can see, this guideline allows you to choose from any of the activities in the pyramid. Even activities for strength, muscular endurance, and flexibility can contribute to meeting this guideline.

Experts have shown that even modest amounts of activity are better than no activity at all. One way to determine if you do enough of these activities would be to count physical activity Calories. Notice in the

Physical Activity Threshold and Target Zones

Threshold of Training		
	Counting Calories	**Counting Heart Rate**
Frequency	5 days a week	3 days a week
Intensity	200 Calories a day or 1000 to 1400 Calories a week	50% of heart rate range 60% of maximum heart rate
Time	Activity can be accumulated during the day in periods of 5 minutes or longer	20 continuous minutes

Target Fitness Zone		
	Counting Calories	**Counting Heart Rate**
Frequency	5 to 7 days a week	3 to 6 days a week
Intensity	200 to 500 a day or 1000 to 3500 Calories a week	50-85% of heart rate range 60-90% of maximum heart rate
Time	Activity can be accumulated during the day in periods of 5 minutes or longer	20-60 continuous minutes

chart above that the FIT formula for Calorie counting suggests that, as a minimum (threshold), you should expend at least 200 Calories a day in physical activity. This would amount to 1000 to 1400 Calories expended each week based on 5 to 7 active days a week. Some people will expend these Calories in lifestyle activities such as walking to school or mowing the lawn. Others will expend them in aerobic exercises or in active sports or other activities in the pyramid. Most of us will choose physical activities from all areas of the pyramid.

For optimal benefits to health and wellness (target zone), 2000 to 3500 Calories per week should be expended in activities from the Physical Activity Pyramid. Over time, people who expend an appropriate number of Calories in physical activity will be able to move out of the low or marginal fitness categories and reach the good fitness zone. You can use the chart in the Activity at the end of this chapter to determine the number of Calories expended in several physical activities. A more complete list of energy expenditures is included in Chapter 7, page 97.

Counting Heart Rate The second national guideline suggests teenagers ". . . should engage in three or more sessions per week of activities that last 20 or more minutes at a time and that require moderate to vigorous levels of exertion." To meet this guideline you can use the FIT formula for heart rate shown in the chart.

Your heart rate must be elevated above the threshold of training heart rate and into the target fitness zone for cardiovascular fitness. At a minimum you must be active three times a week for 20 minutes each time. For best results you should be active five or six days a week for up to 60 minutes per day. Experts have learned that you need one or two days of rest from this type of higher intensity physical activity. If you exercise more often, you risk getting injured.

Heart rate counting activity produces health and wellness benefits, although most experts would encourage you to do lifestyle activity in addition to high heart rate activity. Heart rate counting activity is especially effective in producing cardiovascular fitness improvements such as those needed for participation in varsity sports or other activities requiring fitness in the high performance zone. You can quickly see the advantages of both Calorie counting and heart rate counting by reading the chart below.

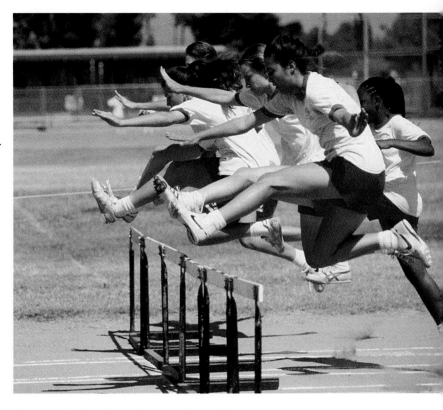

Fast running is a form of anaerobic activity.

Anaerobic Physical Activity The girls in the picture above are doing **anaerobic activity**—activity done in short bursts. Anaerobic activities include sprinting, swimming very fast, and bursts of activity in sports such as football. When you do anaerobic activity, your body cannot supply blood and oxygen to the muscles as fast as the muscles use it. Without oxygen, you can't exercise very long. You need frequent rests

during anaerobic activity to "catch your breath." Anaerobic fitness is important to being a good sports performer, but anaerobic activities are not included in the pyramid as a type of activity that provides significant health and wellness benefits.

If you are interested in anaerobic activity, you should participate three to six days a week. The intensity of your activity should be at the upper level of the target zone since your exercise bouts are short. Keep your heart rate high for 10 to 40 seconds followed by walking or slow jogging. This slow pace should last three times the length of the exercise. Alternate fast and slow exercise bouts. The total exercise time should be at least 15 minutes. Consult your teacher or a coach for more information on this type of activity.

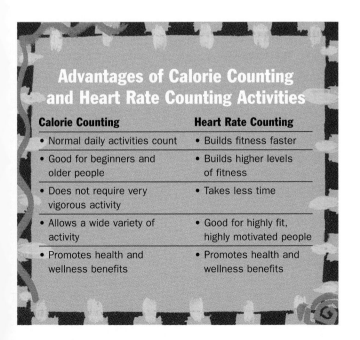

Advantages of Calorie Counting and Heart Rate Counting Activities

Calorie Counting	Heart Rate Counting
• Normal daily activities count	• Builds fitness faster
• Good for beginners and older people	• Builds higher levels of fitness
• Does not require very vigorous activity	• Takes less time
• Allows a wide variety of activity	• Good for highly fit, highly motivated people
• Promotes health and wellness benefits	• Promotes health and wellness benefits

Lesson Review
1. How can you select activities from the Physical Activity Pyramid that build cardiovascular fitness?
2. Explain how to count Calories to determine how much physical activity you need. How would you use your heart rate instead of counting Calories?
3. What is the difference between aerobic activity and anaerobic activity?

Activity 6
Cardiovascular Fitness: How Much Activity Is Enough?

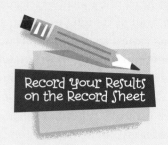
Record Your Results on the Record Sheet

Part 1: Calculating Target Heart Rate Zone

Recall that one way to determine if you have enough activity is to be sure that you are exercising in your target heart rate zone. In the first chapter you learned how to count heart rate and how to use a chart to see if you were elevating your heart rate high enough to get fitness benefits from exercise. The target heart rate chart you used was based on a "typical" person your age. As you grow older, you need to be able to calculate your own target heart rate at any age. Two methods to determine your target heart rate zone are explained below. Use your record sheet to calculate your target heart rate zone using both methods.

Heart Rate Range Method

1 Begin by estimating your maximal heart rate, the highest heart rate you attain in very vigorous activity. To do this, subtract your age from 220. In the example at the right you can see that the maximal rate for a 30-year-old person would be 190.

2 Next determine your heart rate range by subtracting your resting heart rate from your maximal heart rate. The resting heart rate in the example is 70 and the heart rate range is 120.

3 To calculate your threshold heart rate, multiply your heart rate range by 50%. Then add your resting heart rate. In the example the threshold would be 130.

4 Calculate your target ceiling heart rate by repeating Steps 1–3, but in Step 3 multiply by 85%, not 50%.

5 Your target heart rate zone will be between the values you calculate for your threshold heart rate and your ceiling heart rate. In the example the person has a target heart rate zone between 130 and 172.

Example: Heart Rate Range
(for a 30-year-old person with a resting heart rate of 70)

Threshold Heart Rate

Step 1	220	
	– 30	(age)
	190	(maximal heart rate)
Step 2	– 70	(resting heart rate)
	120	(heart rate range)
Step 3	x .50	(threshold percent)
	60	
	+ 70	(resting heart rate)
	130	(threshold heart rate)

Target Ceiling Rate

Step 1	220	
	– 30	(age)
	190	(maximal heart rate)
Step 2	– 70	(resting heart rate)
	120	(heart rate range)
Step 3	x .85	(target ceiling percent)
	102	
	+ 70	(resting heart rate)
	172	(target ceiling rate)

Target Heart Rate Zone

130–172 beats per minute

Percent of Maximal Heart Rate Method

1 Estimate your maximal heart rate by subtracting your age from 220.

2 To find your threshold heart rate, multiply this number by 50%.

3 To calculate your target ceiling rate, repeat Steps 1 and 2, but in Step 2 multiply by 85%.

4 Your target heart rate zone will be between the values you calculated for your threshold heart rate and your ceiling heart rate.

Note: New American College of Sports Medicine Guidelines suggest that very low fit people or those who are totally sedentary should use 40% rather than 50% as the threshold value.

Part 2: Walking and Jogging

When using the heart rate counting method for determining how much activity you need, it is important to be able to continue to exercise in your target heart rate zone. In this part of the activity you will walk and jog in your target heart rate zone.

Walking

1 Walk briskly for 5 minutes.

2 At the end of your walk, immediately count your one-minute heart rate. Record your heart rate on your record sheet.

3 Determine if your heart rate reached your heart rate threshold of training (lower limit of your target heart rate zone). You can use the zone you calculated using either method in Part 1.

4 Check to see that your heart rate did not exceed your target ceiling heart rate (the upper limit of your target heart rate zone).

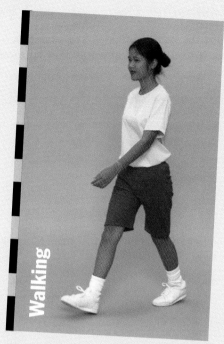

Walking

Jogging

1 Jog at a steady pace for 5 minutes.

2 At the end of your jog, immediately count your one-minute heart rate. Record your heart rate on your record sheet.

3 Determine if your heart rate reached your heart rate threshold of training (lower limit of your target heart rate zone). You can use the zone you calculated using either method in Part 1.

4 Check to see that your heart rate did not exceed your target ceiling heart rate (the upper limit of your target heart rate zone).

Part 3: Exercise to Expend 200 Calories

You know that you should expend at least 200 Calories a day. In this part of the activity you can see how much activity is required to expend 200 Calories.

1 Use the Energy Expenditure chart below to determine how many Calories you used during your 5-minute walk and the 5-minute jog. Record this information on your record sheet.

2 Use the remainder of the class in an attempt to expend a total of 200 Calories. You may choose from any of the activities in the Energy Expenditure chart below. Be sure to use the Calories expended in the walk and jog you did in Part 2.

3 Count your heart rate at least 2 times in this part of the activity to see if you are in your target heart rate zone.

Energy Expenditure

	Calories Used (per minute)					
Activity	**Weight (in pounds):** less than 100	101–125	126–150	151–175	176–200	201–225
Walking	2.3	2.9	3.5	4.1	4.7	5.2
Walking (brisk pace)	3.4	4.3	5.3	6.2	7.1	8.0
Fitness Calisthenics	3.3	4.2	5.1	6.0	6.9	7.8
Badminton	3.7	4.7	5.7	6.7	7.7	8.7
Volleyball	3.8	4.8	5.8	6.8	7.8	8.8
Basketball (half court)	3.3	4.2	5.1	6.0	6.9	7.8
Jogging (12-minute mile)	7.1	9.0	10.8	12.6	14.5	16.4

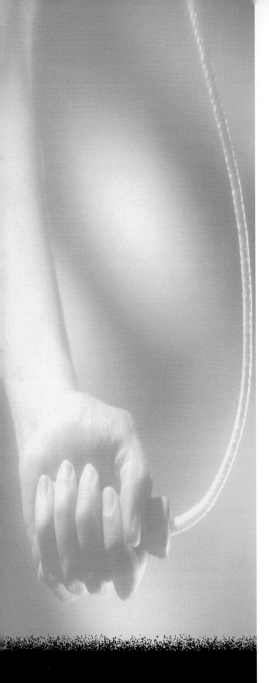

6 Chapter Review

Reviewing Concepts and Vocabulary

Copy the number of each statement on a sheet of paper. Next to each number, write the word or words that correctly complete the sentence.

1. Vessels that carry blood to the heart are called _____.

2. Walking, jogging, and bicycling are examples of _____ activity.

3. The body system that includes your heart, blood vessels, and blood is the _____.

4. Carriers of cholesterol and other fats in the blood are called _____.

5. The body system that includes your lungs and air passages is the _____.

Number your paper. Next to each number, choose the letter of the best answer.

Column I	Column II
6. aerobic activity	a. fattylike substance in the blood
7. cholesterol	b. heart can supply necessary oxygen to muscles
8. high-density lipoprotein	c. bad cholesterol
9. low-density lipoprotein	d. heart cannot supply necessary oxygen to muscles
10. anaerobic activity	e. carries cholesterol out of the blood-stream

On your paper, write a short answer for each statement or question.

11. How can you use the Calorie counting method to determine how much physical activity you need?

12. Explain how cardiovascular fitness helps your cardiovascular system work more efficiently and helps prevent cardiovascular diseases.

13. Explain why cholesterol can be dangerous to your health

14. Activities from which areas of the Physical Activity Pyramid are best for building cardiovascular fitness?

15. Why should you do more than one self-assessment for determining cardiovascular fitness?

Thinking Critically

Write a paragraph to answer the following question.

You decide that you need to develop a program to improve your cardiovascular fitness. What are some lifetime changes that you should incorporate into your program? Explain.

Project

Investigate the amount of cholesterol in your favorite foods. Use package labels and reference books to find the amounts. Develop a list of substitute foods you might use in place of those foods you currently use that are high in cholesterol.

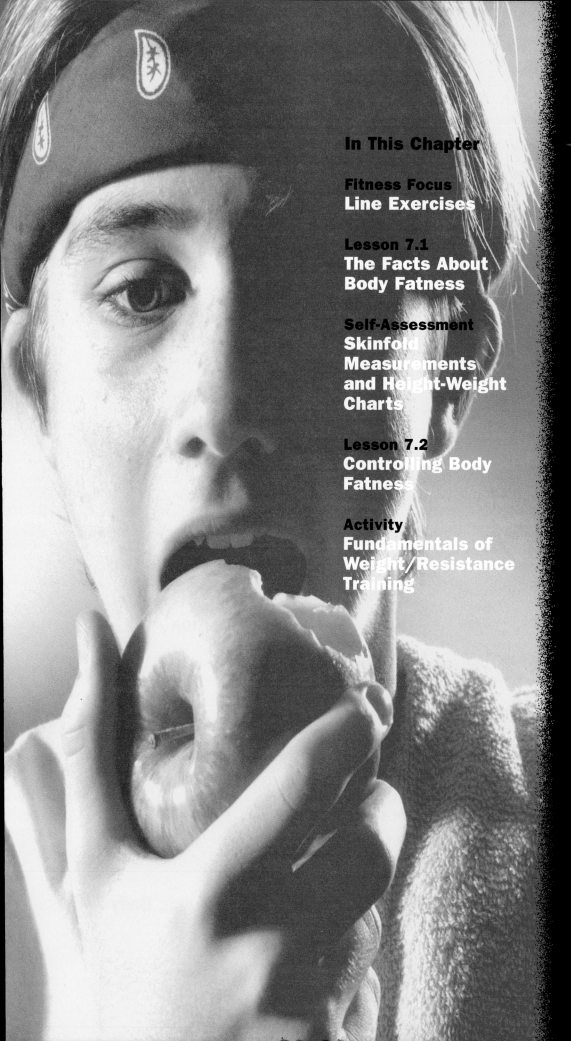

7

Physical Activity and
Fat Control

Line Exercises

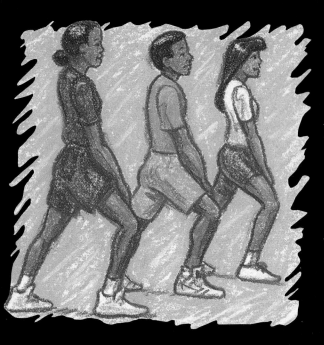

Line exercise is a good type of physical activity for expending Calories. For this reason, it is particularly good for controlling body fatness and building cardiovascular fitness. Line exercises can be done individually or in a group. Music adds to the enjoyment of line exercises. Advantages of this type of physical activity include:
• It can be done in a relatively small space.
• It is fun and easy to learn.
• It is aerobic, so it produces many health and wellness benefits.
• You can create your own routines.
See your instruction sheet to learn more about line exercises.

Routine 1:	Routine 2:
Step Touch	Grapevine
Double Step Touch	Hitch Hiker
Forward Walk	The Point
Backward Walk	Backward Walk
Grapevine	Rocker Step
Slap, Step, and Turn	Hop Turn

7.1
Lesson

The Facts About Body Fatness

Lesson Objectives
After reading this lesson, you should be able to:
1. Describe a good level of body fat for health.
2. Explain how the level of body fat is related to good health.
3. Explain how body fatness can be assessed.

Lesson Vocabulary
body composition, basal metabolism, underfat, overfat, essential body fat, anorexia nervosa, anorexia athletica, bulimia, underwater weighing, skinfolds, caliper

Body fatness is a part of health-related physical fitness. Body fatness refers to the percentage of your total body that is comprised of fat tissue. For good health, it is important to have optimal amounts of body fat. In this lesson you will learn what level of body fat is best for you, how body fatness affects your health, and how to assess your body fatness.

Body Composition
Together, all the tissues that make up your body are called your **body composition.** For a typical 150-pound person, 15 percent to 25 percent of the body composition is fat and 75 percent to 85 percent is lean body tissue. Lean tissue includes muscles, bones, skin, and body organs such as the heart, liver, kidneys, and lungs.

People who do regular physical activity typically have a larger percentage of lean body weight, especially from muscle and bone, and less body fat than those who do not do such activity. Having a relatively low percentage of your total body weight as fat is desirable. However, for good health, it is important that your body composition include some body fat.

Factors Influencing Body Fatness
In Chapter 1, you learned about some of the factors that influence physical fitness. Many factors also influence body fatness.

Heredity You inherit your body type from your parents. Some people are born with a tendency to be lean, muscular, or fat. Inherited tendencies make keeping body fat levels in the good fitness zone easy for some people, but difficult for others. You need to consider heredity when you are determining your goals for body fatness.

Metabolism Your **basal metabolism** is the amount of energy your body uses just to keep you living. This energy is measured in units called Calories. Your basal metabolism does not include the Calories you burn in work, recreation, studying, or even sitting and watching television. Some people have a higher basal metabolism than others. This means that their bodies, at complete rest, burn more Calories than the bodies of those with low metabolism. People with a high metabolism can consume more Calories than others can without increasing the level of body fatness.

Metabolism is affected by heredity, age, and maturation. Most young people have a high metabolism

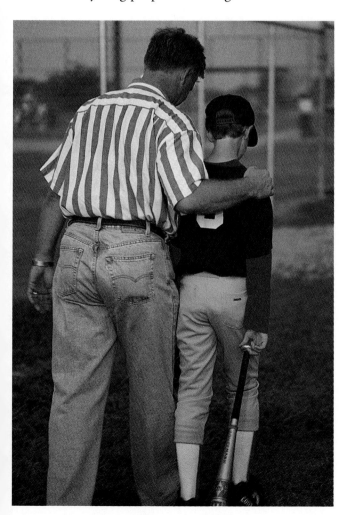

Age, heredity, and maturation affect metabolism.

because their bodies are growing and building muscle. As you grow older, your rate of metabolism becomes slower. Then most people need to reduce the number of Calories in the diet to avoid gaining fat. How might the rates of metabolism of the people in the picture be likely to differ?

Maturation As you grow older and the hormone levels in the body begin to change, levels of body fatness also change. During the teen years, female hormones cause girls to develop more body fatness than boys. Because of male hormones, teenage boys have greater muscle development than girls.

Early Fatness Children who are too fat develop extra fat cells that make it more difficult to control fatness levels later in life. Keeping body fatness levels within the good fitness zone during the childhood and teen years will help keep body fat levels in check throughout life.

Diet The amount of energy in foods is measured in Calories. A typical male your age needs to consume about 2,500 to 3,000 Calories a day to maintain an ideal level of body fat. A typical female your age needs about 2,000 to 2,500 Calories a day. Most males need more Calories than females because they are larger and have more muscle mass.

Physical Activity Your body burns Calories for energy. The more vigorous activity you do, the more energy your body uses and the more Calories you need. An inactive person uses less energy each day than an active person and therefore needs to consume fewer Calories.

Body Fatness: How Much is Good?

About one-half of your body fat is located deep within your body. The remaining fat is between your skin and muscles. A fit person has the right amount of body fat — neither too much nor too little.

Weight Versus Fat The terms *underweight* and *overweight* do not provide a great deal of information about fitness or about a person's body composition. *Underweight* and *overweight* refer to how much you weigh compared to others. Muscles weigh more than fat. Thus, you can weigh more than someone else of the same size because you are more muscular and have less body fat than the other person. For example, the runners in the picture have strong muscles. They may weigh more than other people who appear to be the same size. On the other hand, you can weigh less than someone else of the same size because you have smaller bones.

The terms *overfat* and *underfat* are very useful because they describe how much of your total body weight is made up of fat. **Underfat** means having too little body fat; **overfat** means having too much body fat. *Obesity* is a term used to describe people who are very overfat.

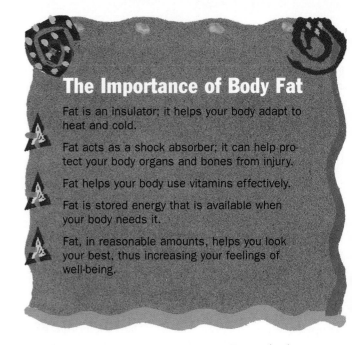

The Importance of Body Fat

- Fat is an insulator; it helps your body adapt to heat and cold.
- Fat acts as a shock absorber; it can help protect your body organs and bones from injury.
- Fat helps your body use vitamins effectively.
- Fat is stored energy that is available when your body needs it.
- Fat, in reasonable amounts, helps you look your best, thus increasing your feelings of well-being.

Body Fat in Females and Males From the late teens on, females generally have a higher percentage of body fatness than do males. Teenage girls should not have less than 11 percent or more than 25 percent body fat. Over 35 percent fat is considered obese for females. Teenage boys should not have less than six percent or more than 20 percent body fat. Over 30 percent is considered obese for males.

Too Little Body Fat

The minimum amount of body fatness is called **essential body fat** because if fat levels in the body drop below this amount, health problems result. The chart on this page shows several reasons why your body needs some body fat.

Being underfat can result in abnormal functioning of various body organs. In fact, exceptionally low body fat levels can result in serious health problems, particularly among teenagers.

Eating Disorders **Anorexia nervosa** is a serious eating disorder. A person who has this disorder severely restricts the amount of food he or she eats in an attempt to be exceptionally underfat. In addition, many persons with anorexia do extensive physical activity to further lower their levels of body fat to extremely dangerous levels.

Anorexia is most common among teenage girls, though it is becoming increasingly common among teenage boys. Anorexics are usually very hard workers and high achievers. They have a distorted view of their bodies and see themselves as being too fat even when they are extremely thin. A fear of maturity, and the

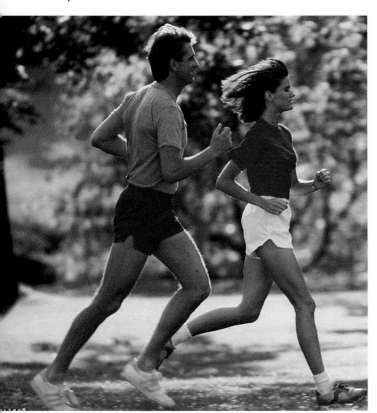

People who are muscular can weigh more than others of the same size because they have more muscle and less body fat.

weight gain associated with adulthood, is a characteristic of persons with this disorder. Anorexics often try to hide their condition by wearing baggy clothing, only pretending to eat, and exercising in private. Anorexia is a life-threatening condition, and those who have the condition need immediate professional help.

Anorexia athletica has many symptoms that are similar to those of anorexia nervosa. It is most common among athletes involved in sports such as gymnastics, wrestling, and cheerleading in which a low body weight is desirable. This condition can lead to anorexia nervosa. The disorder is thought to be related to the pressure to maintain a low weight and an excessive preoccupation with dieting and exercising for weight loss.

Bulimia is an eating disorder in which a person does binge eating, or eats very large amounts of food within a short period of time. Bingeing is followed by purging. Techniques of purging include vomiting and the use of laxatives to rid the body of food and prevent its digestion. Bulimia can result in loss of teeth, gum diseases, severe digestive problems, and other significant health problems.

Identifying the symptoms of eating disorders early is extremely important. Conditions associated with an excessive desire to lose fat and maintain very low body fat levels can be serious health problems.

Overfatness, Health, and Wellness

Having too much fat can be unhealthful. Scientists report that persons who are overfat have a higher risk of heart disease, high blood pressure, diabetes, and other diseases. Being overfat also reduces a person's chances of successful surgery. In addition, an overfat person tires more quickly and easily than a lean person. For this reason, an overfat person might be less efficient in work and recreation.

Body Fat Assessment

You might wonder how to assess body fatness and make determinations about how much you should weigh. There are several ways to make such assessments.

Underwater Weighing The best way to assess your body fat level is by using **underwater weighing**. With this technique, you are immersed in a tank of water and then weighed. Lean people weigh more under water; they sink. People with more fat weigh less under water; they float.

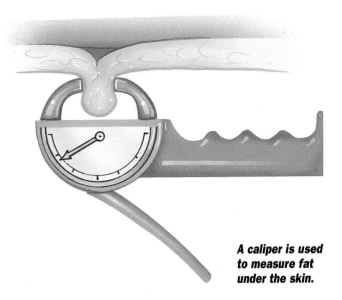

A caliper is used to measure fat under the skin.

Measurements of your lung capacity are also taken because the amount of air in your lungs influences your weight. A formula is applied to your underwater weight and lung capacity to scientifically determine your body fatness. Underwater weighing is accurate, but this procedure requires time, is expensive, and must be done by an expert.

Skinfold Measurements Your body fatness can also be determined by measuring the thickness of **skinfolds,** the fat under the skin. Look at the picture illustrating the measurement of a skinfold. A special instrument called a **caliper** is used to measure skinfold thickness. You will learn to do skinfold measurements in the Self-Assessment feature in this chapter.

Body Measurements You can also use body measurements to estimate your percentage of body fat. One procedure uses weight and waist measures for males and height and hip measurements for females. This method is less accurate than skinfold measures.

Body Mass Index You learned about the body mass index in Chapter 4. This index is a better indicator of fat than height and weight alone, but it does not give as accurate an assessment of body fatness as underwater weighing or skinfold measurements.

Height-Weight Charts A common method of assessing body weight is through the use of height-weight tables. The tables, shown in the Self-Assessment on page 95, list normal weight ranges for people according to age, height, and sex. Note that this procedure

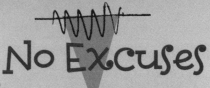

No Excuses

Eliminating Irrational Beliefs

People make decisions based on what they believe to be true. However, what they believe is not always true. Some "facts" that people believe about physical activity are actually irrational beliefs. Despite evidence that shows that certain beliefs are not based on facts, some people continue to hold to their beliefs. These irrational beliefs can keep people from participating in physical activities.

The last thing Melissa wanted to do was go on a bike ride, but Ako kept bugging her to go. Her stomach was already grumbling, and dinner was still two hours away. She explained. "I'm trying to lose weight. If I go riding, I'll eat twice as much at dinner. Then how am I going to lose this fat?"

"Melissa, if you want to lose weight, exercise will help your body use up more Calories."

"I know exercise uses up Calories! That's why riding a bike would make me hungrier. Then I'd probably eat lots more Calories than I used up riding my bike. I

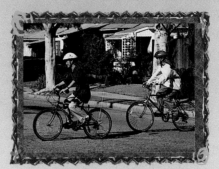

think I'll just watch TV."

Ako wasn't ready to give up. "Just ride with me once," she suggested. "I bet you'll eat less than if you just watched TV."

"Is that true? I'll eat less?"

Ako felt sure Melissa wouldn't eat more because she exercised.

"Well, let's find out," Melissa said. "Where's my bike?"

For Discussion

What is an irrational belief? What irrational beliefs did Melissa have? What are some ways that Melissa could find out whether exercise increases the appetite? What are some other irrational beliefs about exercising and losing weight? Why do you think people have such beliefs? Fill out the questionnaire to see whether you have any irrational beliefs that you should check out.

does not assess body fatness. It can mistakenly classify a thin, muscular person as overweight or mistakenly classify an overfat person who has little muscle as within a normal weight range. These tables are convenient, but should not be the only source of information about body composition. You will use height-weight charts in the Self-Assessment feature on page 95 of this chapter.

Waist-to-Hip Ratio Evidence indicates that people with a very large waist compared to hip size tend to have more fat inside the body and may be at risk for health problems. You can measure the circumference of your hips and waist and calculate a ratio. It is a useful indicator of health risk that can be used throughout life. You can learn more about waist-to-hip ratio in Chapter 15.

Other Measurements X rays, computers, and other machines have been developed to test body fatness. Many are expensive and require trained people to do the assessment. Others are unreliable. The methods listed above are ones that are easiest to do and give you reasonably good measures of body fatness and normal body weight levels.

Lesson Review
1. Describe a good level of body fat.
2. Explain how the level of body fat is related to good health.
3. Name three methods of assessing body fat, and explain the accuracy of each.

Skinfold Measurements and Height-Weight Charts

One way to estimate your body fat percentage is to use skinfold measures. You can assess your body weight using height-weight charts. When you do this assessment, keep the following points in mind:

• Your fitness scores are your personal information and should be kept confidential.

• Be sensitive to the feelings of others when body fatness measurements are being taken. Taking the measurements privately may be appropriate.

• You can use your results to help build a fitness profile.

Part I: Skinfold Measurements

Skinfold measurements can be used to estimate body fat percentage and target weight. For teenagers, upper arm (triceps) and calf measurements provide a good estimate of body fatness. Work with a partner to take each other's measurements. Write your results on your record sheet.

• Triceps skinfold: Pick up a skinfold on the middle of the back of the right arm, halfway between the elbow and the shoulder. The arm should hang loose and relaxed at the side.

• Calf skinfold: Stand up and place your right foot on a chair. Pick up a skinfold on the side of your right calf half way between your shin and the back of your calf, where the calf is largest.

1 Use your left thumb and index finger to pick up the skinfold. Do not pinch or squeeze the skinfold.

2 Hold the skinfold with your left hand while you pick up and use the caliper with the right hand to get a reading.

3 Place the caliper over the skinfold about one-half inch below your finger and thumb. Hold the caliper on the skinfold for three seconds, and then note the measurement. Read the caliper measurement to the nearest one-half millimeter (mm), if possible.

4 Have your partner take three measurements each for the triceps and the calf skinfolds. Use the middle of the three measures as your score. For example, an 8, 9, and 10 give a score of 9. If your three measurements differ by more than 2 mm, take a second, or even third set of measurements. Do the same measures on your partner.

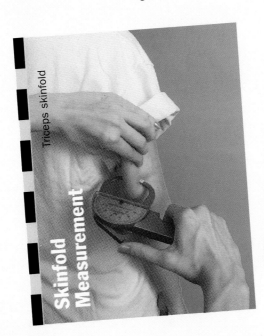

Triceps skinfold / Skinfold Measurement

Calf skinfold / Skinfold Measurement

5 Add the triceps and calf scores. Use the table below, Skinfold Measurements and Body Fat Percentages, to estimate your body-fat percentage. Use a ruler to connect your sum of skinfolds with the percent fat figure. For example, if you are a male and your skinfolds' sum is 27 mm, then your body fat percentage is approximately 22%. Then look at the rating chart at the right to determine your fitness rating for body fatness.

6 Next, look at the Target Body Weight Tables on your worksheet. Find the row showing your body weight and the column with your estimated sum of skinfolds. Your target weight is where the columns intersect. If your skinfolds' sum is less than 27 mm for females and 22 mm for males, you are already at or below your target weight. The target is meant to give you an idea of a weight that will put you in the good fitness zone for body fatness. People should determine their own targets based on the factors that influence body fatness discussed earlier in this chapter.

Rating Chart: Body Fatness

Fitness Rating	% fat	% fat
	males	females
Too Little Fat	less than 6	less than 12
High Performance	6–9.9	12–14.9
Good	10–19.9	15–24.9
Marginal	20–24.9	25–29.9
Too Much Fat	25 or more	30 or more

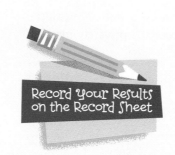

Record your Results on the Record Sheet

Skinfold Measurements and Body Fat Percentages (sum of triceps plus calf skinfolds)

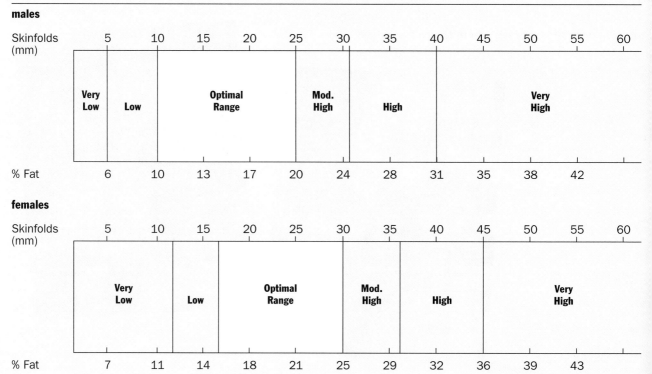

males

Skinfolds (mm): 5 10 15 20 25 30 35 40 45 50 55 60

Very Low | Low | Optimal Range | Mod. High | High | Very High

% Fat: 6 10 13 17 20 24 28 31 35 38 42

females

Skinfolds (mm): 5 10 15 20 25 30 35 40 45 50 55 60

Very Low | Low | Optimal Range | Mod. High | High | Very High

% Fat: 7 11 14 18 21 25 29 32 36 39 43

Part 2: Height-Weight Charts

You can also use height-weight charts to estimate the weight range that is appropriate for you.

1 Remove your shoes.

2 Take your own height and weight measures or ask a partner to help you.

3 Look at the Normal Weight Ranges table on this page to determine the normal weight range for a person your sex, age, and height.

4 Record your height, weight, and normal weight range on the record sheet. Compare your target weight from skinfolds and your normal weight range. Then answer the questions on your record sheet.

Note: As you learned on page 90, people who build muscle in exercise tend to be high in weight. Fit active people may exceed normal weight ranges.

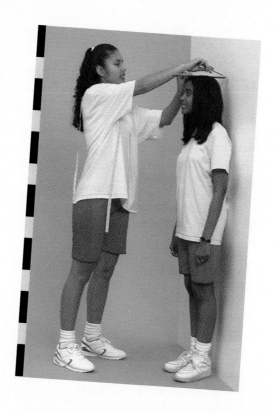

Normal Weight Ranges

males Height feet	inches	Age 13-14	15-16	17-20	females Height feet	inches	Age 13-14	15-16	17-20
4	6	69-72			4	6	73-76		
4	7	73-76			4	7	76-79		
4	8	78-81			4	8	79-82		
4	9	82-85	82-85		4	9	86-89	91-94	
4	10	87-90	87-90		4	10	91-94	98-101	99-102
4	11	88-91	88-91		4	11	96-99	102-105	104-107
5	0	89-92	97-100	101-104	5	0	104-107	106-109	109-112
5	1	97-100	101-104	106-109	5	1	105-108	109-112	113-116
5	2	100-103	106-109	114-117	5	2	106-109	112-115	116-119
5	3	106-109	111-114	121-124	5	3	110-113	115-118	120-123
5	4	113-116	115-118	124-127	5	4	115-118	120-123	125-128
5	5	116-119	120-123	129-132	5	5	119-122	124-127	129-132
5	6	120-123	126-129	134-137	5	6	126-129	128-131	134-137
5	7	126-129	132-135	137-140	5	7	127-130	131-134	137-140
5	8	130-133	135-138	140-143	5	8	128-131	135-138	143-146
5	9	135-138	139-142	147-150	5	9	129-132	137-140	148-151
5	10	141-144	142-145	149-152	5	10	130-133	139-142	153-156
5	11	146-149	149-152	152-155	5	11		142-145	158-161
6	0	151-154	152-155	156-159	6	0		146-149	163-166
6	1		158-161	162-165					
6	2		160-163	167-170					
6	3			177-180					
	and over								

7.2 *Controlling Body Fatness*

A major health goal is to help Americans achieve and maintain acceptable levels of body fatness throughout life. In this lesson, you will learn the FIT formula for fat control and appropriate activities for gaining weight and losing body fatness.

Balancing Calories

Balancing Calorie intake and expenditure affects body fat levels. The foods you eat contain Calories that your body uses for energy. Since fat is stored energy (stored Calories), one way to lose fat is to take in fewer Calories than your body needs or uses. A pound of fat contains 3,500 Calories. Therefore, you can lose a pound of fat by eating 3,500 Calories less than you normally do in a given time or by burning 3,500 Calories more than normal by doing physical activity.

Eating foods that provide more Calories than your body uses will cause you to gain weight. Therefore, you can gain a pound of fat by eating 3,500 Calories more than you usually do within a given time.

The FIT Formula

Both diet and physical activity play an important role in maintaining a good level of body fatness. Because both diet and physical activity are important for fat control, each has a fitness target zone, shown in the chart below.

Gaining Weight

Combining proper physical activity and diet is the best weight gain method. Strength/muscular endurance exercises can help you gain weight. Resistance exercise, which helps build muscle, is especially effective since muscle weighs more than fat.

Remember that physical activity burns Calories. Therefore, when you are active, you need to increase your intake of Calories in order to gain weight. You will learn in Chapter 17 that you do not need to eat special diets or take protein supplements to gain weight. You need only eat a well-balanced diet that contains an increased number of Calories.

Fitness Target Zones for Fat Control

	Diet	Physical Activity
Frequency	• Eat 3 regular meals daily or 4 or 5 small meals. Regular, controlled eating is best for losing fat. Skipping meals and snacking is usually not effective.	• Participate in physical activity daily. Regular physical activity is best for losing fat. Short or irregular physical activity does little for controlling body fat.
Intensity	• To lose a pound of fat, you must eat 3,500 Calories less than normal.	• To lose a pound of fat, you must use 3,500 Calories more than normal.
	• To gain a pound of fat, you must eat 3,500 Calories more than normal.	• To gain a pound of fat, you must use 3,500 Calories less than normal.
	• To maintain your weight, you must keep the number of Calories you eat the same.	• To maintain your weight, you must keep your level of physical activity the same.
Time	Neither diet nor physical activity results in quick fat loss. Medical experts recommend that a person lose no more than 1 or 2 pounds of weight per week without medical supervision. Both diet and physical activity can be used to safely lose 1 or 2 pounds per week.	

Energy Expenditure

Activity	Weight: 100 lbs.	120 lbs.	150 lbs.	180 lbs.	200 lbs.
		Calories Used (per hour)			
Backpacking/Hiking	307	348	410	472	513
Badminton	255	289	340	391	425
Baseball	210	238	280	322	350
Basketball (half court)	225	225	300	345	375
Bicycling (normal speed)	157	178	210	242	263
Bowling	155	176	208	240	261
Canoeing (4 mph)	276	344	414	504	558
Circuit Training	247	280	330	380	413
Dance, Ballet/Modern	240	300	360	432	480
Dance, Aerobic	315	357	420	483	525
Dance, Social	174	222	264	318	348
Fitness Calisthenics	232	263	310	357	388
Football	225	255	300	345	375
Golf (walking)	187	212	250	288	313
Gymnastics	232	263	310	357	388
Horseback Riding	180	204	240	276	300
Interval Training	487	552	650	748	833
Jogging (5½ mph)	487	552	650	748	833
Judo/Karate	232	263	310	357	388
Racquetball/Handball	450	510	600	690	750
Rope Jumping (continuous)	525	595	700	805	875
Running (10 mph)	625	765	900	1035	1125
Skating, Ice/Roller	262	297	350	403	438
Skiing, Cross-Country	525	595	700	805	875
Skiing, Downhill	450	510	600	690	750
Soccer	405	459	540	575	621
Softball (fast pitch)	210	238	280	322	350
Swimming (slow laps)	240	272	320	368	400
Swimming (fast laps)	420	530	630	768	846
Tennis	315	357	420	483	525
Vollyball	262	297	350	403	483
Walking	204	258	318	372	426
Weight Training	352	399	470	541	558

Physical Activity and Calories

Every physical activity burns Calories. You might wonder how many Calories are burned by different activities.

The Energy Expenditure table shows the approximate number of Calories burned per hour during vigorous recreational activities. Find the weight value nearest your own weight. Add five percent to the number of Calories for each 10 pounds you weigh above the listed weight value. Or, subtract five percent from the number of Calories for each 10 pounds you weigh below the listed weight value. Use this table to determine which physical activities are best for burning Calories. Then see which activities appeal to you.

Physical Activity and Fat Loss

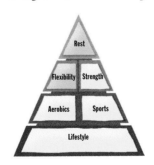

A combination of physical activity and eating fewer Calories is the best way to lose fat. Research shows that a person who reduces Calorie intake without increasing activity will lose both fat and muscle tissue. A person who increases physical activity and reduces Calorie consumption loses mostly body fat. Notice that physical activities from most levels of the Physical Activity Pyramid shown here are appropriate for controlling body fatness.

Have you Heard?

If you maintain your normal intake of Calories and increase your activity by playing one-half hour of tennis daily, you will lose 16 pounds in a year. If you briskly walk 15 minutes a day instead of watching TV, you will lose five to six pounds in a year.

Lifestyle Activities Lifestyle physical activities are especially effective in long-term fat control. Studies indicate that lifestyle activities are just as effective as organized sports and games for losing fat, and more effective for permanent fat loss.

Aerobic Activities Aerobic activities are effective for fat loss. You can do them for relatively long periods of time, burning many Calories.

Active Sports More vigorous activities, such as sports, can be effective for expending Calories.

However, they are often quite vigorous and you may not be able to continue them for long periods of time. Participation in sports is more sporadic than participation in lifestyle activities.

Strength/Muscular Endurance Exercises
Remember that these exercises can help you gain weight by building muscle tissue. However, these exercises, combined with the proper diet, also can contribute to fat loss since they do burn Calories.

Myths About Fat Loss

Some people have some incorrect ideas about physical activity and fat loss. Read the table below to identify some mistaken ideas and learn some facts about losing body fat.

No matter what your body is like now, regular physical activity and the proper diet will help you control body fatness. When you are fit, you look better, feel better, and have fewer health problems than people who are overfat and unfit.

Lesson Review
1. Explain how to use the FIT Formula to control the level of body fatness.
2. How can physical activity help you maintain a good level of body fatness?

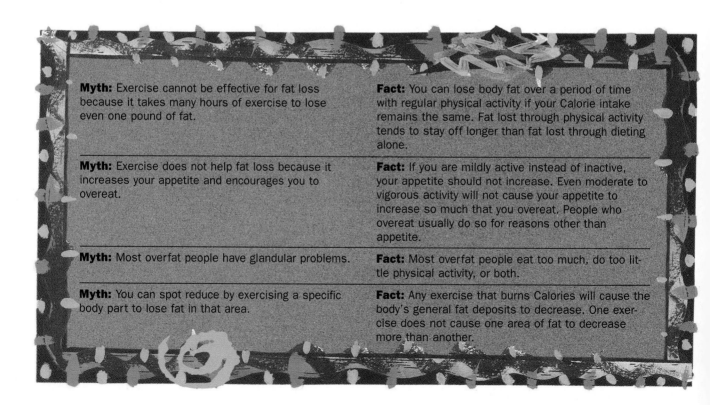

Myth: Exercise cannot be effective for fat loss because it takes many hours of exercise to lose even one pound of fat.	**Fact:** You can lose body fat over a period of time with regular physical activity if your Calorie intake remains the same. Fat lost through physical activity tends to stay off longer than fat lost through dieting alone.
Myth: Exercise does not help fat loss because it increases your appetite and encourages you to overeat.	**Fact:** If you are mildly active instead of inactive, your appetite should not increase. Even moderate to vigorous activity will not cause your appetite to increase so much that you overeat. People who overeat usually do so for reasons other than appetite.
Myth: Most overfat people have glandular problems.	**Fact:** Most overfat people eat too much, do too little physical activity, or both.
Myth: You can spot reduce by exercising a specific body part to lose fat in that area.	**Fact:** Any exercise that burns Calories will cause the body's general fat deposits to decrease. One exercise does not cause one area of fat to decrease more than another.

Activity 7
Fundamentals of Weight/Resistance Training

Although cardiovascular exercises are essential for improving body composition, training for muscular strength and endurance can significantly decrease your percentage of body fat, as well as increase your lean body mass. It firms muscles so that you look trim and fit.

Training for muscular strength and endurance is done through resistance training, that is, working your body's muscles against a force. This force can be provided by your own body weight, free weights, weight machines, or machines using other kinds of resistance, such as friction. Exercises done on machines are generally safe; but exercises with free weights can be dangerous, both because the weights are heavy and because it's hard to keep your balance and to keep control of the weights you are lifting.

To get you started on improving body composition and to prepare you for lifting heavier weights in Chapters 7 and 8, this activity will introduce you to safe training with free weights. (If you don't have access to free weights, instructions for working the same muscles on machines are also provided.) You will learn correct lifting and spotting techniques. Spotting is providing assistance to a partner by being prepared to catch the weight if the partner loses control of the weight or gets off balance.

Because the potential for injury is great, it is essential that you work through each of the mastery levels listed below. To keep track of your progress, an observer will check off your mastery of correct spotting and lifting techniques as well as your maturity and cooperation in assisting and giving coaching (feedback). Record your results on your record sheet.

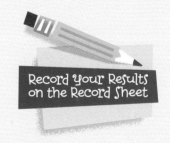

Record Your Results on the Record Sheet

• **Level 1 Mastery: Lifting technique, no weight** Perform each exercise without any weights by using a wand or stick instead of a barbell. Concentrate on correct form (placement of body parts) when you are working. Give useful coaching when you are watching your partners.

• **Level 2 Mastery: Spotting technique, no weight** While your partner performs the lift with the wand, you and another partner practice correct spotting technique. Pay particular attention to your leg and hand positions.

• **Level 3 Mastery: Lifting and Spotting, light weights** Perform each exercise, using very light weights, 5 lifts each. Practice your lifting and spotting techniques, and continue to give each other coaching on both lifting and spotting techniques.

• Warm up and stretch before beginning this activity.

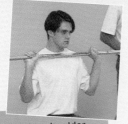

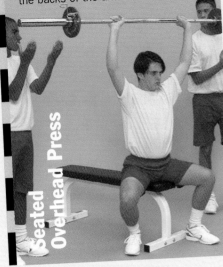

Uses muscles on top of the shoulder, between the shoulder blades, and on the backs of the arms.

Seated Overhead Press

Seated Overhead Press

Weights: Barbell, dumbbells

Spotting: Requires 2 spotters. Spotters stand by lifter's shoulders on either side of bench. Place barbell in lifter's hands, so that bar is across the front of lifter's shoulders and collarbone. Keep your hands palms up under the bar. Be ready to take bar if lifter loses control, especially at top of lift if barbell begins to move backwards or if lifter begins to tremble.

1 Sit on end of the bench in front stride (split-foot) position.

2 Grasp the barbell with your hands facing away from your body, hands slightly wider than your shoulders.

3 Tighten your abdominal, back, and arm muscles. Tip your head back slightly.

4 Push the bar straight up, directly over head, keeping your arms perpendicular. **Caution: Do not let the bar go forward or backward. Do not lock your elbows. Do not arch your back.**

5 Lower the barbell to the starting position. For machine instructions, see page 124.

Half Squat

Weights: Barbell, dumbbells

Spotting: Requires 2 spotters. Spotters stand by lifter's shoulders, one on each side. Place barbell on lifter's shoulders. Keep your hands palms up under the bar. Be ready to take it if lifter loses control.

1 Stand in a side-stride position with your feet a shoulder's distance apart or slightly wider, toes straight ahead or slightly turned out. Keep your head up, and back and abdominal muscles tight. Your back should be as erect as possible, but slightly arched.

2 Hold the barbell across the back of your shoulders at the base of your neck, hands slightly wider than your shoulders, palms facing away from your body. Elbows point toward the floor, and forearms are perpendicular to the floor.

3 Squat until knees are at a right angle. Then rise. When rising, keep the back arched and concentrate on forcing the hips forward. **Caution: Do not round the back. Do not lean too far forward at the hips or let knees get in front of toes. Do not squat too deeply.** To work the same muscles on a machine, do the leg press. Instructions are on page 124.

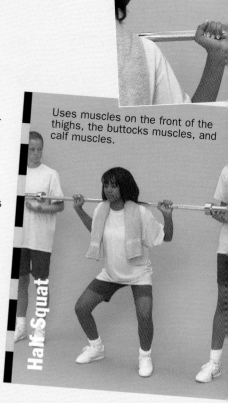

Uses muscles on the front of the thighs, the buttocks muscles, and calf muscles.

Half Squat

Hamstring Curl

Weights: Weighted boot or ankle weight

Spotting: One person can assist lifter to put on the boot or ankle weight.

1 Put the weight on one foot or ankle. Lie face down on a bench, with your knee caps hanging over the edge. Grasp the bench with your hands.

2 Lift the weighted boot by flexing your knee to a right angle. **Caution: Do not lock knees when you extend.**

3 Repeat on the other leg. For machine instructions, see page 124.

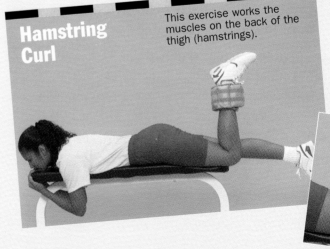

Hamstring Curl

This exercise works the muscles on the back of the thigh (hamstrings).

Biceps Curl

Weights: Barbell, dumbbells

Spotting: Spotters are not required but can place barbell in lifter's palms-up hands.

1. Stand erect, feet in side-stride position. Tighten your abdominal and back muscles.

2. Grasp the bar with palms up, hands slightly wider than your shoulders.

3. Keep your elbows close to your sides and lift the weight by bending your elbows only. Raise the weight to near your chin, then return. **Caution: Do not move other joints, especially in the back.**

4. You can repeat this exercise with your palms down to work the weaker elbow muscles. For machine instructions, see page 125.

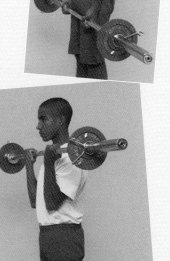

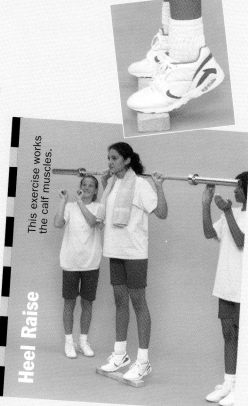

This exercise works the calf muscles.

Heel Raise

Heel Raise

Weights: Barbell, dumbbells

Spotting: Requires 2 spotters. Spotters stand by lifter's shoulders, one on each side. Place barbell on lifter's shoulders, into lifter's palms-up hands.

1. Stand with balls of feet on a 2-inch board, toes turned in slightly.

2. Rise on your toes, then lower to starting position. **Caution: Keep your spine straight.**

3. Advanced lifters may also try toes out and toes straight ahead. For machine instructions, see page 125.

This exercise works muscle on the front of the upper arm (biceps) and other elbow flexor muscles.

Biceps Curl

Bench Press

Weights: Barbell, dumbbells

Spotting: Requires 2 spotters. Spotters stand by lifter's shoulders on either side of bench. Place bar in the palms-down hands of lifter. Keep your hands palms up under bar. Be prepared to take it if lifter loses control.

1. Lie on your back on a bench with your feet on floor, lower back flat. Extend your arms perpendicularly to the floor, into the "up" position.

2. Grasp the bar with a palms-down grip, hands slightly wider than shoulder width, elbows straight, bar approximately over your collar bones. **Caution: Do not lock your elbows.**

3. Lower the bar until it touches your chest, even with a line just below your armpits. When the bar touches your chest, your forearms should be perpendicular to the floor and your elbows should point neither at your feet nor out to the side but halfway in between (45 degrees).

4. Push the bar up to the starting position, arms perpendicular to the floor. The bar follows a slightly curved path. **Caution: Do not bounce the bar off your chest. Do not arch your back or lift your hips. Do keep your arms perpendicular to the floor. If the weight gets in front of or behind your arms, you will lose control and get pinned. For machine instructions, see page 125.**

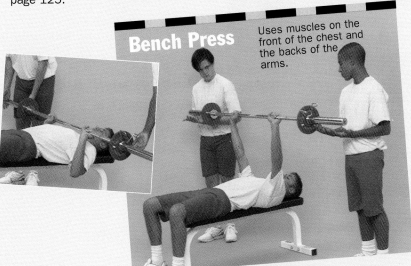

Bench Press

Uses muscles on the front of the chest and the backs of the arms.

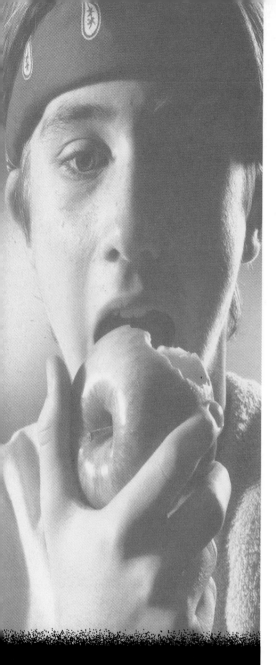

7 Chapter Review

Reviewing Concepts and Vocabulary

Copy the number of each statement on a sheet of paper. Next to each number, write the word or words that correctly completes the sentence.

1. An eating disorder characterized by bingeing and purging is _____.

2. The minimum amount of body fat needed for good health is _____.

3. Your _____ is the amount of energy your body uses at complete rest.

4. A term used to describe a person who is very overfat is _____.

5. People with _____ see themselves as too fat even when they are extremely thin.

6. A technique for assessing body fat levels that involves being weighed under water is _____.

Number your paper. Next to each number, choose the letter of the best answer.

Column I	Column II
7. overfat	a. fat under the skin
8. skinfolds	b. too much body fat
9. anorexia athletica	c. all the tissues that make up your body
10. underfat	d. eating disorder most common among athletes
11. caliper	e. used for skinfold measurements
12. body composition	f. too little body fat

On your paper, write a short answer for each statement or question.

13. Explain why maintaining essential body-fat levels is important for good health.

14. Describe one myth about fat loss and explain how it is incorrect or misleading.

15. Why is a combination of diet and physical activity best for maintaining ideal levels of body fatness?

Thinking Critically

Write a paragraph to answer the following question.

You want to develop your own program for increasing your level of body fatness. How would you use the FIT Formula to help you reach a good level of body fatness?

Project

Keep a record of your Calorie intake and your physical activity for one week. How might you adjust your Calorie intake and your amount of physical activity to better maintain or improve your levels of body fatness? Make a written plan for the following week incorporating changes that might help you reach or maintain ideal levels of body fatness.

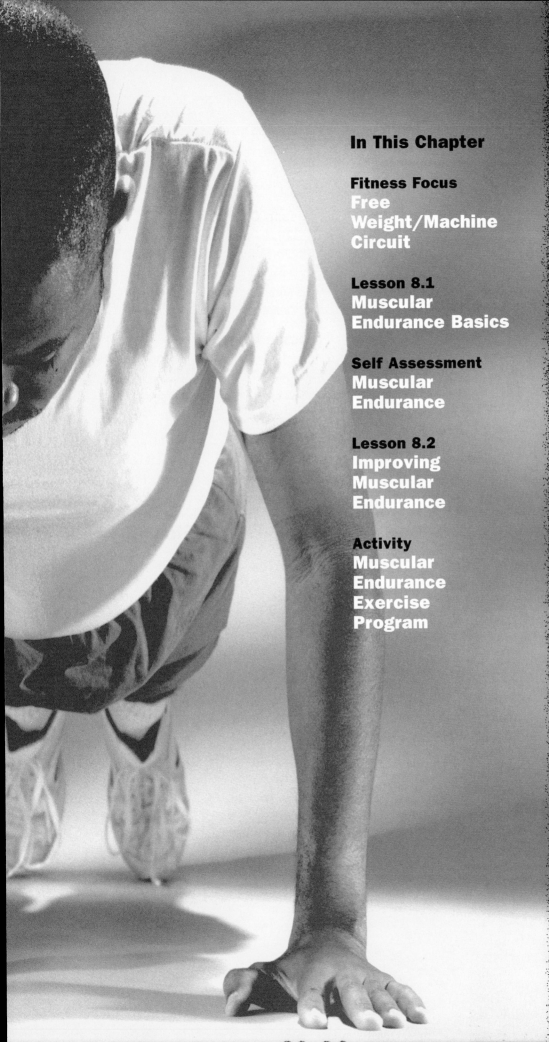

In This Chapter

Muscular Endurance 8

Free Weight/ Machine Circuit

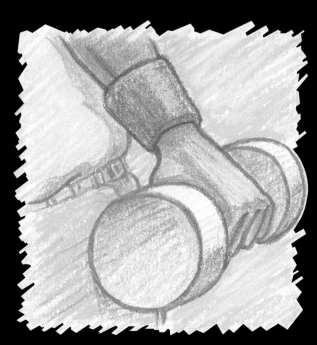

Circuit training is a fun way to add variety to your workouts. This circuit is designed to build muscular endurance. It combines free weights and resistance machines to work different muscle groups at each station. Use this circuit to build endurance by using light weights and many repetitions. Your instruction sheet will explain how to do the exercises in this circuit.

Machine:	Free Weights:
Seated Overhead Press	Sitting Leg Lift
	Lower Leg Lift
Bench Press	Curl-Up (modified)
Trunk Lift (decline)	Kneeling Leg Lift
Leg Press	Side Leg Raise
Hamstring Curl	Heel Raise
Lat Pull-Down	Side Bender
Seated Rowing	

Lesson 8.1

Muscular Endurance Basics

Lesson Objectives
1. Tell the differences among muscular endurance, cardiovascular fitness, and muscular strength.
2. Describe benefits of good muscular endurance.
3. Name and describe the three types of muscles.
4. Explain how muscles make bones move.

Lesson Vocabulary
resistance, skeletal muscles, isotonic contraction, isotonic exercises, isometric contraction, isometric exercises, muscle fibers

In this lesson, you will learn about muscular endurance and how it improves your health and affects your life. Also, the structure of muscles will be described.

Endurance and Strength
Distinguishing among muscular endurance, cardiovascular fitness, and muscular strength can be difficult. In fact, training for any one of the three tends to develop some of the other two. For example, if you swim to increase cardiovascular fitness, you may get an increase in strength as well as muscular endurance.

Muscular Endurance vs. Cardiovascular Fitness
Cardiovascular fitness is the ability of the heart, lungs, and blood vessels to function efficiently during vigorous activity. The rider in the first picture needs good cardiovascular fitness to ride for a long time.

Muscular endurance is the ability to contract muscles many times without tiring or to hold one contraction for a long time. The person in the second picture needs good muscular endurance to carry even lightweight bags a long way.

You can have muscular endurance without cardiovascular fitness, or cardiovascular fitness without muscular endurance. Riding a bicycle especially requires cardiovascular fitness, but requires some muscular endurance as well.

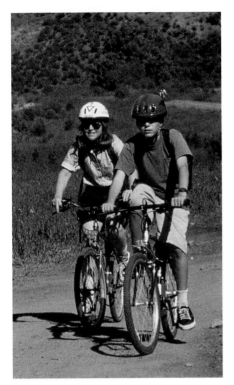

Cardiovascular Fitness

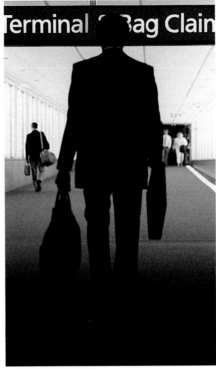

Muscular Endurance

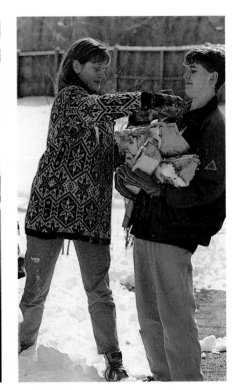

Strength

Muscular Endurance vs. Strength *Strength* indicates the amount of force a muscle can exert. The amount of weight a muscle group can lift one time measures strength. Endurance is measured by how many times a muscle group can repeat an exercise or how long a muscle group can hold a contraction without tiring.

Both muscular endurance and strength are developed by resistance exercises. **Resistance** is a force that acts against your muscles. It is usually measured in terms of pounds. You can lift your own body weight, free weights, or weights in a weight machine. Some machines use other forces, such as hydraulic pressure, air pressure, or friction to provide resistance.

Strength and endurance use resistance in different ways. Strength is developed by doing an exercise only a few times, but with a lot of resistance. The boy holding logs needs strength. Muscular endurance is developed by doing an exercise many times, but with less resistance, such as a light weight.

Strength training tends to increase the size of the muscles as they become stronger. This increase in muscle size is called hypertrophy. Because muscular endurance training uses less weight, endurance training does not cause as much hypertrophy.

The Muscular Endurance-Strength Continuum
Exercises used to develop muscular endurance and strength differ only in the number of repetitions and the amount of resistance. The relationship between endurance and strength can be illustrated by a continuum. The continuum shown below has marks on one edge representing pounds of resistance, and marks on the other edge representing number of repetitions.

The continuum shows the resistance and repetitions that a person might use for a leg press exercise. You can see on the left that an adult might use near maximum resistance (60 pounds) with few repetitions (4) to develop strength. For endurance, a person might use light resistance (20 pounds) with a near maximum number of repetitions (20), as shown on the right.

Using the resistance and the number of repetitions from the middle of the continuum would develop both endurance and strength. This continuum also

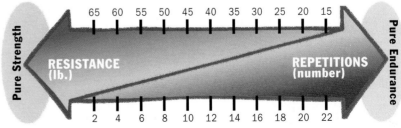

Muscular Endurance - Strength Continuum

shows that usually when you train for strength you will develop some endurance, and when you train for endurance you will develop some strength.

Benefits of Muscular Endurance

Muscular endurance exercise improves appearance, fitness, and physical and mental health. Good muscular endurance enables people to work longer without getting tired. Those with good muscular endurance find it easier to maintain good posture. In addition, they are less likely to have backaches, muscle soreness, and muscle injuries.

Muscular endurance training also increases your lean body mass and decreases fat. This improvement in body composition can help you look and feel better. Muscular endurance developed through physical activity decreases heart rate, helping reduce the risks of cardiovascular disease. Resistance training, whether done for endurance or strength, also strengthens your bones.

The Structure of Muscles

Your body has three types of muscles: smooth, cardiac, and skeletal. Smooth muscles make up the walls of internal organs such as the stomach and blood vessels. Your heart is made of cardiac muscle. Both smooth

and cardiac muscles are classified as involuntary muscles because you cannot consciously control their movements.

Skeletal muscles are attached to bones and make movement possible. These are muscles you use to do physical activity. They are called voluntary muscles because you control them.

As the diagram shows, muscles are attached to bones on either side of a joint. The bones act as levers to which the muscles apply force. An **isotonic contraction** is a muscle contraction that pulls on the bones and produces movement of body parts. **Isotonic exercises** involve isotonic contractions in which body parts move. An **isometric contraction** occurs when muscles contract and pull with equal force in opposite directions so no movement can occur. **Isometric exercises** involve isometric contractions and body parts do not move.

Types of Muscle Fibers

Muscles are made of muscle fibers. **Muscle fibers** are muscle cells, which are long, thin, and cylinder-shaped. The strength and endurance of skeletal muscles depends on whether the muscles are made of slow, fast, or intermediate fibers and how much exercise they get.

Slow-twitch fibers contract at a slow rate. These

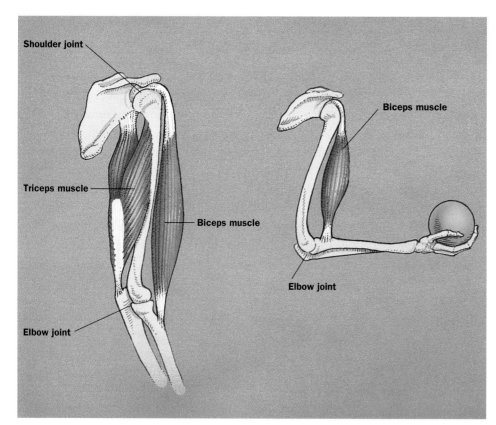

Shoulder joint

Triceps muscle

Biceps muscle

Elbow joint

Biceps muscle

Elbow joint

Muscles apply force to bones.

No Excuses

Thinking Success

An optimist is a person who expects a good or favorable outcome from a situation. This positive thinking is an example of "thinking success." The optimist thinks that he or she can succeed at a specific activity. A person who "thinks success" will more often be successful than a person who has negative thoughts.

Aaron loves baseball. For two years he played on a team that won most of the regular season's games. The team even played in the league's championship game. During that time, Aaron played well at second base and hit a few home runs.

This year Aaron moved up to a new team. Most of the players in the new level were older, bigger, and stronger than he was. During the first game, he was hit by a pitch. He struck out each time he was at bat. In fact, he didn't even hit the ball one time. The coach noticed that Aaron no longer swung at the ball with confidence.

Luckily, the coach knew that Aaron had the physical

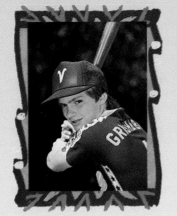

strength and skills needed to hit the ball. He only needed to change the way he was thinking. He wouldn't hit the ball until he thought he could. The coach had Aaron practice drills that he could successfully complete. He taught Aaron to mentally see himself hitting the ball and to say and believe "yes, yes, yes," as he stood waiting for the pitch. He also taught Aaron not to think obsessively about the times he struck out or failed to make a play. "After all," the coach told Aaron, "even the best professionals only get a hit about one out of three tries. The next play is the one to think about." Aaron improved his hitting as he gained confidence.

For Discussion

How did Aaron's negative feelings affect the way he played baseball with the new team? How was he able to change his attitudes to think about success? What are some other ways a person can change negative thoughts into positive ones? Fill out the questionnaire to find out how negative or positive your thoughts are.

fibers have good endurance. They are involved in cardiovascular activities as well. Fast-twitch fibers contract fast. They are the muscle fibers you use for strength activities. Intermediate-twitch fibers have characteristics of both slow- and fast-twitch fibers. They contract fast and have good endurance. You use them for activities that involve both strength and cardiovascular fitness.

The types of fibers in our muscles are determined by our genes; however, we can increase the strength and endurance of our muscles by proper training.

Lesson Review
1. What are the differences among muscular endurance, cardiovascular fitness, and muscular strength?
2. What are the benefits of good muscular endurance?
3. Name and describe the three types of muscles.
4. Explain how muscles make bones move.

Self-Assessment 8
Muscular Endurance

Many tests can help you evaluate your muscular endurance, but the best ones assess your body's large muscles. In this Self-Assessment you will perform some isotonic and some isometric tests. Follow these directions to evaluate your muscular endurance.

• Warm up before doing these assessment activities.

• Write on your record sheet the number of times you complete each test. Check *yes* if you could do the test as long or as many times as indicated. Check *no* if you could not. If you cannot pass all the tests, you need to work on muscular endurance.

• Look up your rating on the rating chart and write your rating on your record sheet.

Rating Chart: Muscular Enduran...

Fitness Rating	Number of Tests Passe...
Good	5
Marginal	3 or 4
Low	less than 3

Side Stand
(isometric)

1 Lie on your side.

2 Use both hands to get your body in position so that it is supported by your left hand and the side of your left foot. Keep your body stiff.

3 Raise your right arm and leg in the air. Hold.

4 Return to starting position and repeat the test on the right side.

Pass (males) = hold position for 30 seconds on each side

Pass (females) = hold position for 20 seconds on each side

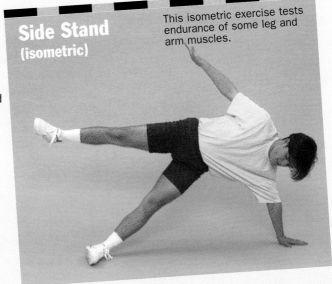

Side Stand (isometric)

This isometric exercise tests endurance of some leg and arm muscles.

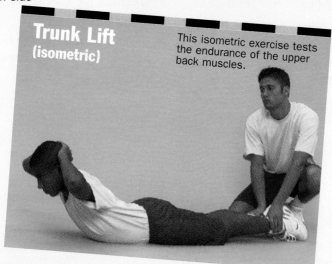

Trunk Lift (isometric)

This isometric exercise tests the endurance of the upper back muscles.

Trunk (Upper Back) Lift (isometric)

1 Lie facedown on the floor. Clasp your hands behind your neck. Have a partner hold your feet down with both hands.

2 Slowly lift your head and chest off the floor no more than 12 inches. Hold.
Caution: It is extremely important not to lift more than 12 inches.

Pass (males) = hold for 30 seconds

Pass (females) = hold for 20 seconds

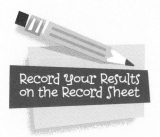

Safety Tips

Avoid arching your lower back repetitively to avoid straining or pulling the muscles in that area.

Sitting Tuck
(isotonic)

1 Sit on the floor with your knees bent and arms outstretched.

2 Lean back and balance on your hips. Keep your knees bent near your chest (feet off the floor).

3 Straighten your knees so the body forms a "V." You may move your arms sideways for balance.

4 Bend your knees to your chest again. Repeat as many times as you can. Count each time you push your legs out.

Pass (males) = 25 times

Pass (females) = 20 times

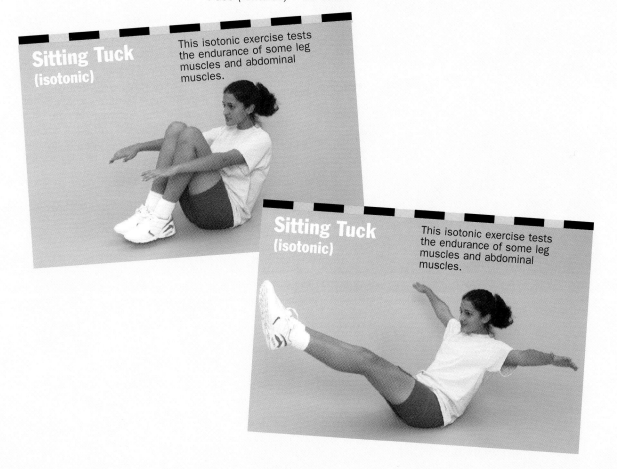

Sitting Tuck (isotonic)
This isotonic exercise tests the endurance of some leg muscles and abdominal muscles.

Sitting Tuck (isotonic)
This isotonic exercise tests the endurance of some leg muscles and abdominal muscles.

Leg Change
(isotonic)

1 Assume a push-up position with weight on your hands and feet.

2 Pull your right knee under your chest, and keep the left leg straight.

3 Change legs by pulling your left leg forward and pushing your right leg back.

4 Continue changing legs. **Caution: Do not let your lower back sag.**

5 Repeat this exercise for 1 minute and count the number of leg changes.

Pass = 25 changes

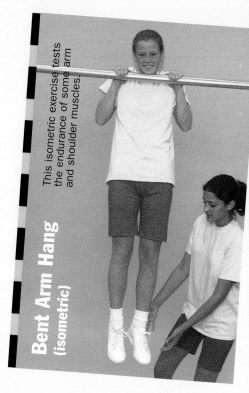

This isometric exercise tests the endurance of some arm and shoulder muscles.

Bent Arm Hang
(isometric)

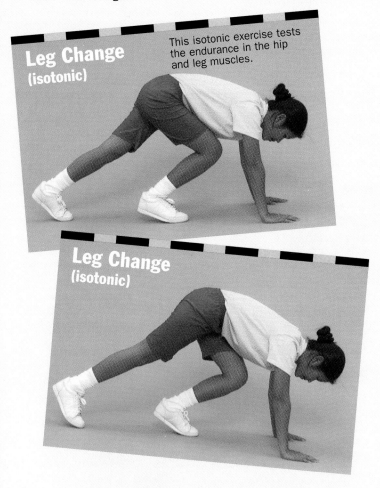

Leg Change
(isotonic)

This isotonic exercise tests the endurance in the hip and leg muscles.

Leg Change
(isotonic)

Bent Arm Hang
(isometric)

1 Hang from the chinning bar with your palms facing away from your body.

2 You may stand on a chair and/or with the help of a partner, lift your chin above the bar.

3 On a signal, the partner lets go or removes the chair. Count the time or duration of the hang. The time begins when the chair is removed and ends when the chin touches or goes below the bar, or the head tilts backward.

Pass (males) = hold for 16 seconds

Pass (females) = hold for 12 seconds

Lesson 8.2 — Improving Muscular Endurance

Lesson Objectives

After reading this lesson, you should be able to:
1. Apply the three fitness principles to muscular endurance training.
2. Describe how the FIT Formula applies to muscular endurance exercise.
3. Give the guidelines for safe and enjoyable muscular endurance exercise.

Lesson Vocabulary

repetitions, sets, calisthenics, resistance training

In this lesson you will learn how to apply the three training principles and the FIT Formula to muscular endurance exercise. You will also learn guidelines for choosing and performing endurance exercises.

The Physical Activity Pyramid

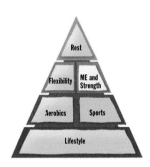

Muscular endurance is essential for health, wellness, and good appearance. Selecting activities from the *Strength and Muscular Endurance* section of the Physical Activity Pyramid will help you improve your muscular endurance and develop overall fitness.

Fitness Principles and Muscular Endurance

You probably will hear the terms *reps* and *sets* in relation to muscular endurance exercises. The diagram on this page can help you understand these terms. **Repetitions,** or reps, are the number of consecutive times you do an exercise. A **set** is one group of repetitions. For example, suppose you do an exercise 11 times, then rest; repeat it 11 times, then rest; and repeat another 11 times. Then you will have completed a total of 3 sets of 11 repetitions each.

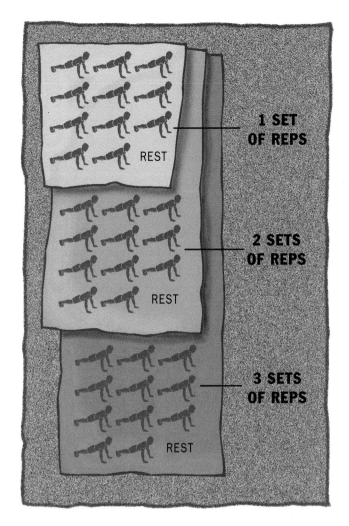

Reps and Sets

Principle of Overload As you learned from the Muscular Endurance-Strength Continuum shown on page 105, muscular endurance is best developed by doing a relatively high number of reps and using low to moderate resistance (load). The overload principle is applied by adjusting the intensity of both reps and load. To get strength, you use 7 to 10 reps lifting relatively heavy weights. To get muscular endurance, you use 11 to 25 reps using lighter weights. You start doing one set and gradually work up until you can do 3 sets. When it becomes easy to do 3 sets, then you apply the Principle of Progression.

Principle of Progression To apply the Principle of Progression, you gradually increase the number of times you do the exercise, and the number of sets that you perform. For example, to build muscular endurance, you might start doing a biceps curl with 10 pounds and lift it 11 reps for 3 sets. Then your goal is to increase the number of reps in each set until you can do 3 sets of 25. When it becomes easy to do 3 sets of 25, increase the weight and start all over again. Continue until you reach your desired level of muscular endurance.

Principle of Specificity Make certain that you exercise each specific group of muscles in your arms, legs, and trunk through their full range of motion. Also consider how you use those muscles in your everyday life and in sports and other physical activities. Design exercises that closely resemble the specific activities for which you will need endurance. For example, if you play the piano, do exercises that develop endurance in the muscles that help you hold an erect sitting position and that help you use your arms and fingers for long periods.

The FIT Formula for Muscular Endurance

The frequency, intensity, and time recommended for your target zone are shown in the table below. You may either do calisthenics, in which you lift the weight of your body parts, or work against the resistance of weights or machines. These kinds of exercises involve isotonic muscle contractions. Notice that the FIT table shown below is divided into two sections—one section for isotonic exercises and the other for isometric exercises.

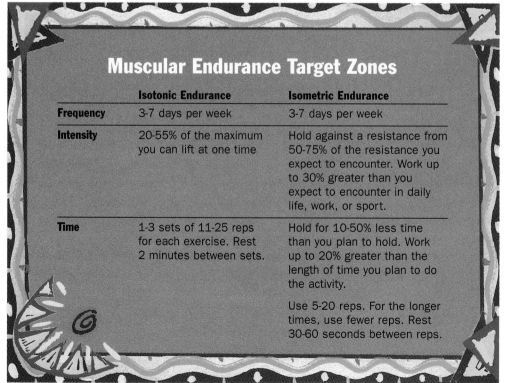

Have you Heard?

Good muscular endurance is best achieved by doing multiple sets rather than doing one set of repetitions to exhaustion.

Training Programs for Muscular Endurance

Muscular endurance programs include: calisthenics, resistance training, circuit resistance training, isometric training, and other physical activities.

Exercises that use all or part of your body weight as the resistance are called **calisthenics.** You can do calisthenics anywhere with little or no special equipment. Calisthenic exercises appear in the Self-Assessment and Activity in this chapter and in Chapters 4 and 5.

Resistance training involves using resistance, in the form of free weights or machines to develop muscular endurance or strength. In the next chapter, you will study the use of weights and machines for strength development. These exercises are equally effective for muscle endurance if you use less weight, more repetitions, and the muscular endurance FIT Formula and target zones.

A circuit can be designed to develop muscular endurance, such as the circuit in this chapter's Fitness Focus. Circuit resistance training can be designed around a resistance machine or perhaps a combination of calisthenics, free weights, and machine stations. Usually the circuit is repeated several times.

Isometric exercises help build muscular endurance in those muscles that you use isometrically in your daily

Muscular Endurance Target Zones

	Isotonic Endurance	Isometric Endurance
Frequency	3-7 days per week	3-7 days per week
Intensity	20-55% of the maximum you can lift at one time	Hold against a resistance from 50-75% of the resistance you expect to encounter. Work up to 30% greater than you expect to encounter in daily life, work, or sport.
Time	1-3 sets of 11-25 reps for each exercise. Rest 2 minutes between sets.	Hold for 10-50% less time than you plan to hold. Work up to 20% greater than the length of time you plan to do the activity. Use 5-20 reps. For the longer times, use fewer reps. Rest 30-60 seconds between reps.

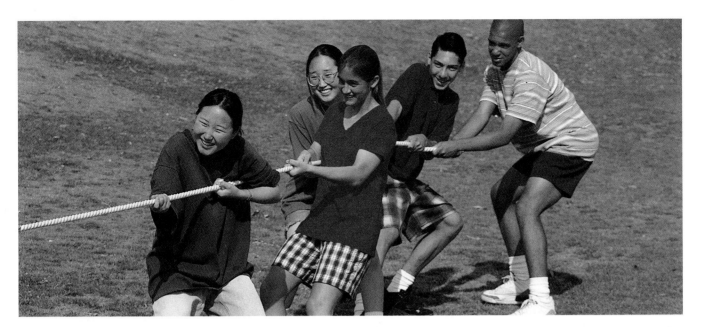

Tug-of-war is an example of an activity that builds muscular endurance.

routines. Your postural muscles, especially the abdominal muscles, need a lot of this kind of training. Chapter 17 includes some sample isometric exercises.

Many activities such as jogging, swimming, and aerobics that are used for cardiovascular fitness can also help develop muscular endurance. Repetitive sports skills, such as practicing your tennis swing or throwing a baseball, are specific endurance exercises. Many enjoyable sports and games, such as the tug-of-war shown above, can be used to develop endurance.

Guidelines for Muscular Endurance Exercise

To avoid injury and increase your enjoyment of the activities, you should follow these guidelines when exercising for muscular endurance.

• Always warm up and stretch gently before exercising.

• Breathe normally. Holding your breath may cause an abdominal hernia or cause you to black out.

• Start with low intensity exercises and progress slowly. Too many reps and sets too soon will cause muscular soreness and slow your progress.

• Use good body mechanics and correct technique. To work a specific set of muscles, the movement must be done exactly right or you may actually be working the wrong set of muscles or straining other body parts.

• Take your time and work rhythmically.

• Always move through a full range of motion so you don't lose your flexibility. (See Chapter 10 for more on flexibility and range of motion.)

• Avoid working the same muscles in two consecutive exercises.

• Exercise each specific muscle group. If there is a muscle you do not know how to isolate, ask your instructor about it. Most people tend to exercise their chest muscles (pectorals), biceps, and other muscles on the front of the body, while neglecting the muscles on the back. Include exercises for the triceps on the backs of your arms, the hamstrings on the backs of your legs, and the muscles between your shoulder blades.

• Vary your exercise routine to avoid boredom. There are many ways to exercise the same muscles effectively.

Lesson Review
1. How do the three fitness principles apply to muscular endurance training?
2. How does the FIT Formula apply to muscular endurance exercise?
3. Give the guidelines for safe and enjoyable muscular endurance exercise.

Activity 8
Muscular Endurance Exercise Program

This activity shows you some calisthenics that you can use to build muscular endurance. It includes only eight groups of muscles, and for most teens will be only light to moderate in intensity. When you design your own program, you can choose the intensity and exercises that are best for you. While performing these exercises, keep these points in mind.

• Learn how to do each exercise correctly.

• Do the exercises in the order and with the number of repetitions listed in the table.

• If you cannot complete an exercise as many times as directed, just do as many as you can.

• Your instructor will tell you when to start and stop the exercise. Between exercises, walk or jog if you finish before others in your group.

• For each exercise, write on your record sheet the number of repetitions you were able to complete in the one minute time allowed (up to 25 reps). If more than one set is completed, record the number of sets as well as reps per set.

• After you have been exercising for a few weeks, add one or two sets to your workout. Then do the warm-up only before the first set and the cool-down only after the last set.

Safety Tips

In some exercises, such as the curl-up, the feet should not be anchored. When doing the Trunk Lift you can anchor the feet as long as you limit your lift to about 12 inches

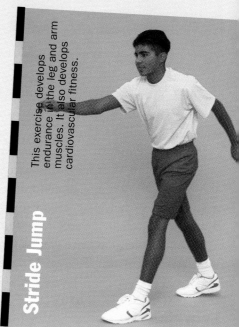

This exercise develops endurance in the leg and arm muscles. It also develops cardiovascular fitness.

Stride Jump

Stride Jump

1 Stand with your left leg forward and right leg back. Hold your right arm shoulder high straight in front of your body and your left arm straight behind you.

2 Jump, moving your right foot forward and left foot back. As your feet change places, your arms switch position. Keep feet 18-24 inches apart.

3 Continue jumping, alternating feet and arms. Count 1 each time the left foot moves forward.

Sample Muscular Endurance Exercise Program

Exercise	Length of time or number of reps
Warm-Up and Stretch	Use the warm-up in Chapter 1 (3 minutes)
1. Stride Jump	1 every 3 seconds for 1 minute = 20 reps
2. Side Leg Raise (right leg)	1 every 3 seconds for 1 minute = 20 reps
3. Side Leg Raise (left leg)	1 every 3 seconds for 1 minute = 20 reps
4. Bridging	1 every 3 seconds for 1 minute = 20 reps
5. Trunk (Upper Back) Lift	1 every 3 seconds for 1 minute = 20 reps
6. Push-Up or Modification	1 every 4 seconds for 1 minute = 15 reps
7. Prone Arm Lift	1 every 3 seconds for 1 minute = 20 reps
8. High Knee Jog	Right foot down every 3 seconds for 1 minute = 20 reps
9. Curl-Up with Twist	1 every 3 seconds for 1 minute = 20 reps
Cool-Down and Stretch	Same as warm-up (3 minutes)

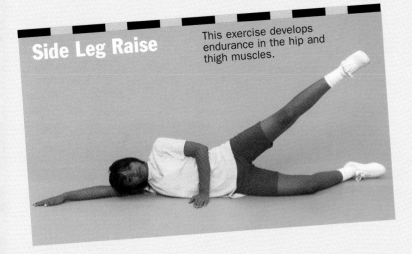

Side Leg Raise

This exercise develops endurance in the hip and thigh muscles.

Side Leg Raise

1 Lie on your right side. Use your arms for balance.

2 Lift top (left) leg 45 degrees. Keep your knee cap pointing forward and ankle pointing toward ceiling. If the leg is allowed to rotate so knee points upward, you will work the wrong muscles.

3 Lower your leg. Repeat the movement. An ankle weight could be used to increase intensity.

4 Roll over and repeat exercise with right leg.

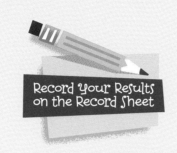

Record Your Results on the Record Sheet

Trunk (Upper Back) Lift

1 Lie facedown with your hands clasped behind your neck.

2 Pull your shoulder blades together, raise your elbows off the floor, then lift your head and chest off the floor. Arch the upper back until your breastbone (sternum) clears the floor. You may need to hook your feet under a bar or have someone hold your feet down. **Caution: Do not lift your chin more than 12 inches off the floor.**

3 Lower your trunk and repeat.

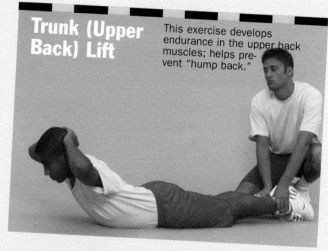

Trunk (Upper Back) Lift

This exercise develops endurance in the upper back muscles; helps prevent "hump back."

Bridging

1 Lie on your back with your knees bent and feet close to buttocks.

2 Contract the buttocks muscles. Lift the buttocks and lower back off the floor until there is no bend at the hip joint. **Caution: Do not let the lower back arch.**

3 Lower the hips to the floor and repeat.

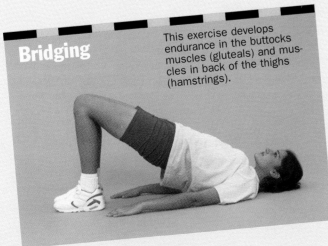

Bridging

This exercise develops endurance in the buttocks muscles (gluteals) and muscles in back of the thighs (hamstrings).

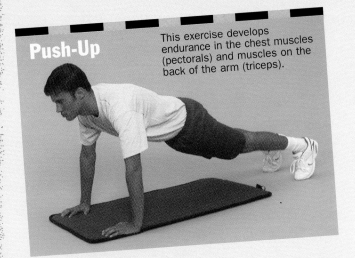

Push-Up

This exercise develops endurance in the chest muscles (pectorals) and muscles on the back of the arm (triceps).

Push-Up

1 Lie facedown with your hands placed under your shoulders.

2 Push up, keeping your body rigid, until your arms are straight and you are in a lean-rest position on hands and toes.

3 Keep the body rigid and lower until your chest touches the floor. **Caution: Do not allow the hips to sag and do not bend at the hips more than 5 degrees.**

Half Push-Up

1 If you cannot complete 20 reps of the push-up, try this version. Lie facedown with your hands placed under your shoulders.

2 Push up only until your upper arms are parallel with the floor and the elbows are bent approximately at a right angle.

3 Keep the body rigid and lower until your chest touches the floor. **Caution: Do not allow the hips to sag and do not bend at the hips more than 5 degrees.**

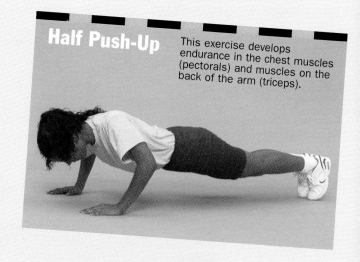

Half Push-Up

This exercise develops endurance in the chest muscles (pectorals) and muscles on the back of the arm (triceps).

Knee Push-Up

1 If you cannot complete 20 reps of the half push-up, try this version. Lie facedown with your hands placed under your shoulders.

2 Push up, keeping your body rigid, until your arms are straight, but keep your knees on the floor.

3 Keep the body rigid and lower until your chest touches the floor. **Caution: Do not allow the hips to sag and do not bend at the hips more than 5 degrees.**

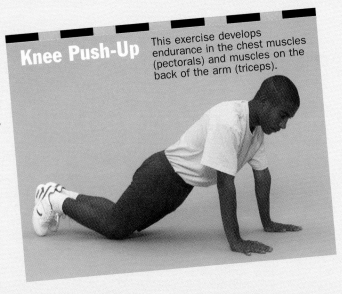

Knee Push-Up

This exercise develops endurance in the chest muscles (pectorals) and muscles on the back of the arm (triceps).

High Knee Jog

1 Jog in place. Try to lift your knees so that your upper leg is parallel with the floor.

2 Count 1 each time the right foot touches the floor. Try to do 1 to 2 jog steps per second.

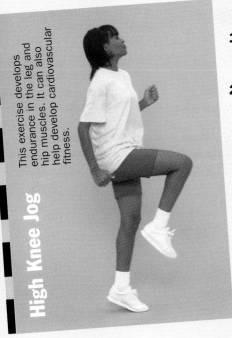

This exercise develops endurance in the leg and hip muscles. It can also help develop cardiovascular fitness.

High Knee Jog

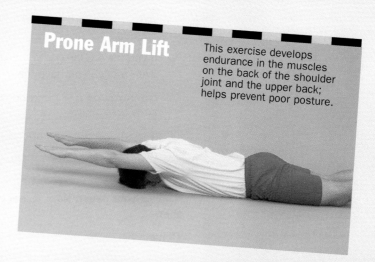

Prone Arm Lift

This exercise develops endurance in the muscles on the back of the shoulder joint and the upper back; helps prevent poor posture.

Prone Arm Lift

1 Lie facedown on the floor with your arms extended and held against your ears.

2 Keep your forehead and chest on the floor and lift your arms so the hands are 6 inches off the floor.

3 Lower your arms and then repeat. Keep your arms touching your ears and your elbows straight.

Curl-Up with Twist

1 Lie on your back with your knees bent to about a right angle (90 degrees), feet flat on the floor. Extend your arms down along your sides.

2 Flatten your lower back to the floor. Tuck your chin and lift your head. Then raise your shoulder blades, twisting to the left and reaching with both arms outside your left leg. Curl-up until both shoulder blades are off the floor.

3 Curl-down to the starting position and repeat, twisting to the right. Continue alternating right and left twists.
Caution: Always flatten your lower back and tuck your chin as you curl up and curl down. Do not let anyone hold your feet.

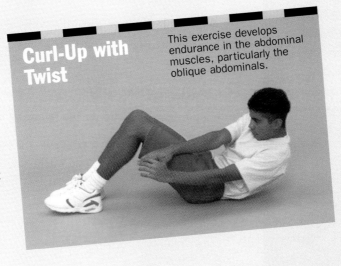

Curl-Up with Twist

This exercise develops endurance in the abdominal muscles, particularly the oblique abdominals.

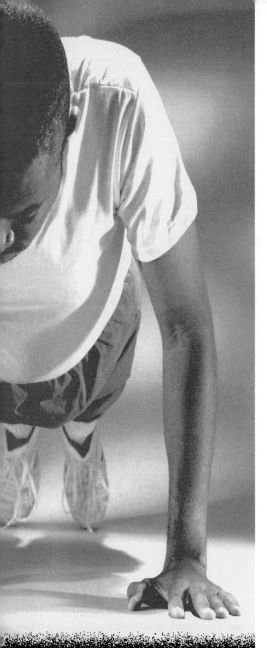

8 ▶ Chapter Review

Reviewing Concepts and Vocabulary

Copy the number of each statement on a sheet of paper. Next to each number, write the word or words that correctly completes the sentence.

1. _____, a force that acts against your muscles, is often measured in pounds.

2. If you have poor _____ your leg muscles might get tired when you run, even though you have the _____ to keep going.

3. When you do _____, body parts move; but when you do _____, no body parts move.

4. A _____ consists of one group of _____.

5. When you do _____, you use your body weight as the resistance.

Number your paper. Next to each number, choose the letter of the best answer.

Column I	Column II
6. strength	a. muscle contractions that pull with equal force in opposite directions so no movement can occur
7. isotonic contraction	b. muscle cells
8. muscle fibers	c. muscles contractions that pull on the bones and produce movement
9. skeletal muscles	d. the amount of force a muscle can exert
10. isometric contraction	e. muscles attached to bones

On your paper, write a short answer for each statement or question.

11. How do muscles make bones move?

12. How many days a week should you train for muscular endurance?

13. Why is it important to do muscular endurance exercises exactly right?

14. What kinds of physical activities can you do to build muscular endurance?

15. Why should you start with low intensity exercises for muscular endurance?

Thinking Critically

Write a paragraph to answer the following question.

Suppose you want to plan a program of physical activity to increase your muscular endurance. What activities would you choose? How would your program affect other areas of your health-related fitness? Explain how it might help reduce your risk of disease or physical disorders.

Project

Over the years, many people have performed feats of muscular endurance. Find out what some of those feats are, who performed them, and how they trained for these feats.

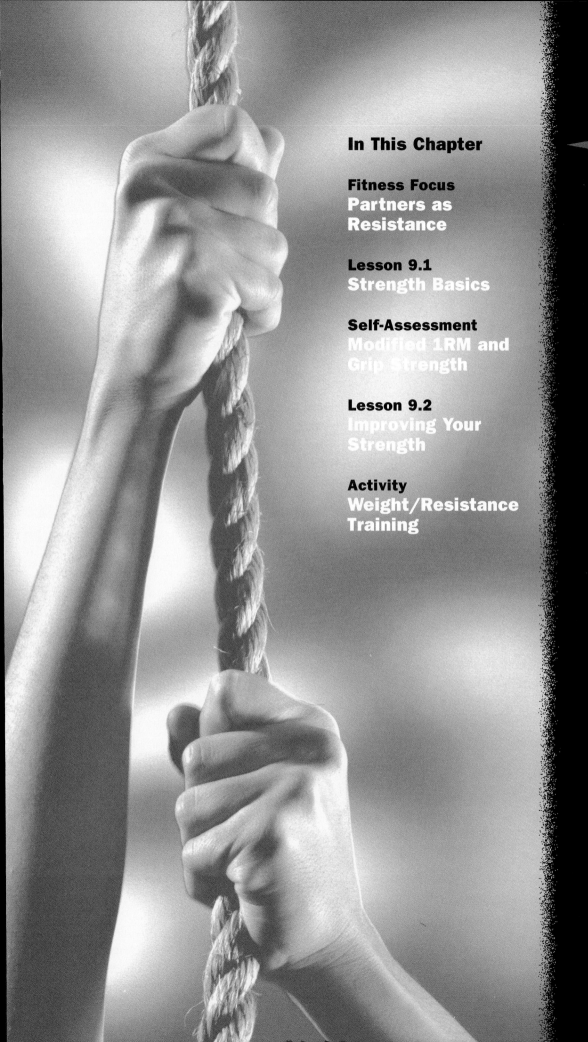

Strength

9

Partners as Resistance

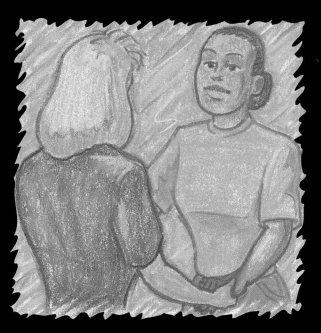

To build strength and muscular endurance, you have to work your muscles against a resistance. Resistance can be provided by free weights, machines, or your own body weight. But in these exercises, you are going to use a partner's body weight as resistance. Choose a partner who is about your height and weight, then try these exercises. A word of caution: To avoid injuring each other, be gentle when you provide resistance or try to move your partner's body parts. A description of the exercises is on your instruction sheet.

Shoulder Moves
Elbow, Flex and Extend
Neck, Flex and Extend
Knee Flex
Hip Moves
Shoulder Rotation
Hand Tussle
Noses

Lesson 9.1 ## Strength Basics

Lesson Objectives
After reading this lesson, you should be able to:
1. Describe health and wellness benefits of strength.
2. Describe some myths about strength and tell why they are wrong.
3. Explain why preteens and teens must take special care when strength training.

Lesson Vocabulary
muscle-bound, anabolic steroids, 1RM

In this lesson you will learn about the benefits of strength, some common misconceptions about strength training, and some special considerations for preteens and teens. You will also learn how to assess your strength.

Health and Wellness Benefits
Strength is the amount of force a muscle can exert. Strong muscles help you jump, lift, push, and do other activities. If your muscles regularly work against heavy loads, they will stay strong. If you do not use your muscles, they become weak.

Strength enables you to work and play with less fatigue. Muscular strength can help prevent some health problems. For example, strong abdominal muscles can reduce the risk of backache. Exercises for muscle strength also strengthen bones, making them less likely to fracture or become porous.

Strong muscles are necessary for certain sports and exercises. Strength can help prevent muscle injuries and muscle soreness. Strong muscles help you withstand vigorous activity.

Strong muscles give your body a firm appearance. Muscles also burn more Calories than fat does. Strong muscles help you maintain good posture.

Strength for Preteens and Teens
In young people between the ages of about 11 and 18, the bones are rapidly growing at the growth centers. The diagram on the next page shows the location of a growth center in a bone. These growth

centers are soft cartilage and can be easily injured. For example, if a heavy weight is lifted, the force can cause the part of the bone above the growth center to slide past the part of the bone below it. The result could be a broken bone or damage to the growth center. By age 19 or 20, the soft growth cartilage turns to bone and is no longer as easily injured.

To avoid injury, preteens and teenagers should use a strength training program especially designed for their age group. Adult training programs should *not* be used. Your teacher can give you an appropriate and safe training program. The teacher should be available while you are training to check your form and guide you. Follow the techniques for lifting and spotting described in the Activity for Chapter 7 and the guidelines in Chapters 8 and 9 to avoid injury.

Knob of Bone (epiphysis)

Growth Center (epiphyseal growth plate)

Shaft of Bone (diaphysis)

Arm bone

Anabolic Steroids

Anabolic steroids are synthetic drugs that resemble the male hormone testosterone. For certain diseases, doctors prescribe these drugs in small doses. However, some people illegally buy and use anabolic steroids to increase muscle size and strength. Not only are anabolic steroids *illegal* to use without a doctor's prescription, they are also extremely dangerous. The chart at the right lists some of the harmful effects of steroids. The use of anabolic steroids is prohibited by the United States Olympic Committee and by most other athletic associations.

Teenagers are at high risk for harm from steroids because their bodies are still growing. Anabolic steroids can damage the growth centers of bones, causing the long bones of the body to stop growing. This can prevent a person from growing to his or her full height. Many side-effects, such as hair loss, acne, and deepening voice and dark facial hair growth in women, do not go away when the drug is stopped.

Have you Heard?

Adolescents' muscles can be stronger than their bones. Teens have been known to break their own bones by moving in ways that involve strong muscle contractions. Lifting weights that are too heavy or trying to lift heavy weights with quick contractions can cause such problems. A common injury is the separation of the end of the bone from the shaft at the growth cartilage.

Myths and Misconceptions

The amount of strength you need to stay healthy and to do what you want depends upon your own personal needs and interests. For example, people who have jobs requiring a lot of lifting need more strength than people who work at a desk. Some people think that only males need to be concerned about their strength. This notion is false. Both males and females need strength to be healthy, to avoid injury, to look good, and to save themselves or others in an emergency.

Some women fear that strength training will cause their bodies to look masculine. However, the hormones in females' bodies prevent them from developing large, bulky muscles even when they exercise regularly.

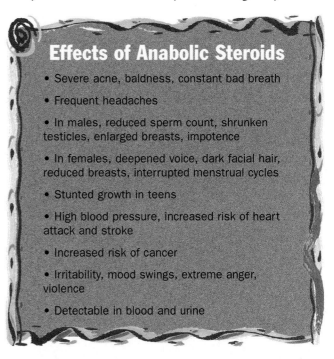

Effects of Anabolic Steroids

- Severe acne, baldness, constant bad breath
- Frequent headaches
- In males, reduced sperm count, shrunken testicles, enlarged breasts, impotence
- In females, deepened voice, dark facial hair, reduced breasts, interrupted menstrual cycles
- Stunted growth in teens
- High blood pressure, increased risk of heart attack and stroke
- Increased risk of cancer
- Irritability, mood swings, extreme anger, violence
- Detectable in blood and urine

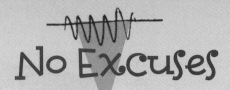

No Excuses

Building Knowledge

A misconception is a belief based on incorrect or misunderstood information or lack of facts. The best way to counter a misconception is to increase knowledge so that you can interpret facts correctly.

Mary Lou had tried several exercise programs, but did not find one she felt would meet her goal of attaining strength and firm muscles. She never even considered weight training because she believed she would develop big, bulky muscles.

One day Mary Lou's physical education teacher took her class to the weight room. There, she explained how to use the free weights and machines for the best benefit. Over the next several weeks, the class practiced the correct use of the weight training equipment. As a class assignment, Mary Lou's physical education teacher had each member of the class find one newspaper or magazine article on weight training and write a report on it. Mary Lou learned that muscles will not become bulky if weight training is done properly.

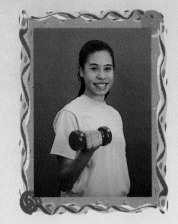

Mary Lou realized that the correct weight training program would give her exactly what she was looking for. Now she works out with weights three days each week. The knowledge Mary Lou gained about weight training has dispelled her original misconceptions.

Now Mary Lou is trying to help others change their irrational beliefs about weight training. When friends ask her why she's trying to build big muscles, she tells them, "If strength and firm muscles are what you're after, you should give weight training a try."

For Discussion
What misconception did Mary Lou have? How was she able to build knowledge to dispel her misconception? What are some other misconceptions people have about physical activity? Fill out the questionnaire to find out about your knowledge regarding physical activity and how you use it to make decisions about being active.

Women and girls who perform strength exercises do develop strong muscles. Both men and women look more attractive with strong muscles because they are more likely to have good posture and firm bodies.

Muscle-Bound Body Some people think that strength training will cause them to be **muscle-bound,** that is, to have tight, bulky muscles that prevent them from moving freely. It is not strength training, but rather incorrect strength training, that causes inflexibility. Failure to stretch or training muscles only on one side of a joint are two examples of incorrect training that can cause a muscle-bound condition. Another example of incorrect training is failure to move your joints through their full range of motion when you lift weights or do other resistance exercises. For example, your elbow joint can bend to allow your hand to reach

your shoulder and to let your arm straighten completely. When you do a biceps curl with weights, bring the weight all the way to the shoulder then straighten the elbow each time you lower the weight. *Caution:* Do not bend your elbow or any other joint backward beyond a full range of motion. You can damage the joint if you move it in a way it was not designed to move.

Lesson Review
1. How does strength contribute to your health and wellness?
2. Describe some myths about strength and tell why they are wrong.
3. Why must preteens and teens take special care when strength training?

Self-Assessment 9
Modified 1RM and Grip Strength

Part 1: Estimating Your 1RM

1RM means one repetition maximum. It represents the maximum amount of weight a group of muscles can lift at one time. As you have learned, it is dangerous for teens to lift maximum weights. Therefore, this assessment has been modified to allow you to lift less than maximum weights, then use a table to determine your 1RM. The results you get will enable you to safely determine the amount of weight to use in your strength training.

The modified 1RM can be done with free weights or machines. The table lists the muscle groups and the free weight or machine exercise to perform to determine your 1RM. Instructions for the free weight exercises are in the Chapter 7 Activity, pages 99 to 101. The instructions for the machine exercises follow. The exercises on the weight machines are very similar to those done with the free weights.

Do the exercises in the order listed in the table. The exercises were selected so that most of the major muscle groups are used and you do not use the same muscles consecutively. Additional weight training exercises appear in the Chapter 11 Activity.

Follow these directions for each exercise.

• Choose a weight that you think you can lift 5 to 10 times but is too heavy for you to lift more than 10 times.

• Using correct technique, lift the weight as many times as you possibly can. Count the number of lifts and write the number on your record sheet.

• If you were able to do more than 10 lifts, wait until another day before you try a heavier weight for that exercise. Go to the next muscle group exercise.

• If you can tell that you will not be able to lift the weight at least 5 times, stop and choose a lighter weight.

• If you were able to do 5 to 10 lifts and no more, then refer to the 1RM table on page 126. Find the weight you lifted in the left-hand column. Now find the number of reps you did in the top row. Your 1RM score is the number in the box where the horizontal weight row and the vertical rep column intersect. Write this number on your record sheet.

Safety Tips

• When doing strength training exercises, 7 to 10 reps are recommended for teens over the age of 13. However, doing 5 to 6 reps is acceptable for this assessment as long as you do this number of reps just for self-assessment and only occasionally.

• Follow the resistance training guidelines on page 130.

Resistance Exercises by Muscle Group

Muscle group	Free Weight	Machine
Hamstrings	Hamstring Curl	Hamstring Curl
Deltoids, upper back muscles, triceps	Seated Overhead Press	Seated Overhead Press
Quadriceps, gluteals, calf	Half Squat	Leg Press
Biceps, elbow flexors	Biceps Curl	Biceps Curl
Calf	Heel Raise	Heel Raise
Pectorals and triceps	Bench Press	Bench Press

Hamstring Curl

1 Lie facedown on the bench with the kneecaps extending over the edge of the bench. Hook your heels under the cylindrical pads. Grasp the handles on the bench.

2 Bend your knees so that you lift the cylindrical pads. Bend the knees through their full range of motion. The pads will almost touch your buttocks at the top of the lift.

3 Lower to the starting position. **Caution: Do not lock the knees when putting your heels under the pads. If necessary, have a partner lift the pads so you can avoid this.**

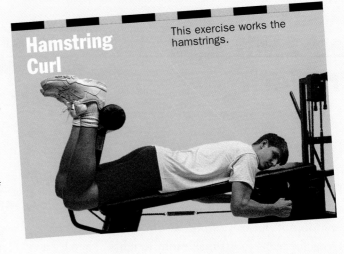

Hamstring Curl

This exercise works the hamstrings.

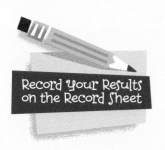

Record Your Results on the Record Sheet

Seated Overhead Press

1 Sit on the stool with the handles even with your shoulders. Grasp the handles with palms facing away from you. Tighten your abdominal muscles.

2 Push upward on the handles, extending your arms until the elbows are straight. **Caution: Do not arch your back. Do not lock your elbows.**

3 Lower to the starting position.

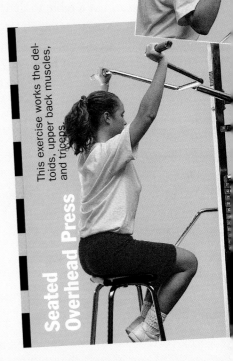

This exercise works the deltoids, upper back muscles, and triceps.

Seated Overhead Press

Leg Press

1 Adjust the seat distance for leg length comfort. The closer the seat, the greater the range for working and the greater the intensity. Sit with your feet resting on the pedal.

2 Push the pedal until your legs are straight. **Caution: Do not lock your knees.**

3 To work your calf muscles, point your toes to push farther. Remember not to lock your knees.

4 Slowly return to your starting position.

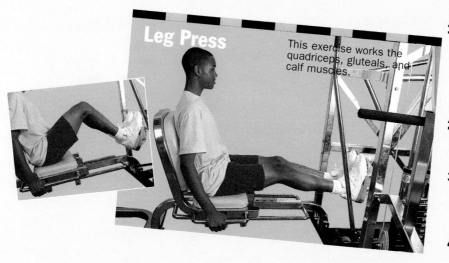

Leg Press

This exercise works the quadriceps, gluteals, and calf muscles.

Biceps Curl

1 Stand in front of the station and grasp the handle of the low pulley, palms up. Tighten your abdominals and buttocks muscles (gluteals).

2 Pull the handle from thigh level to chest level. Bend your elbows, but keep them close to your sides.
Caution: Do not move other body parts.

3 Return to the starting position.

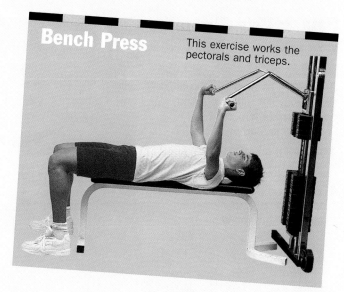

Bench Press

This exercise works the pectorals and triceps.

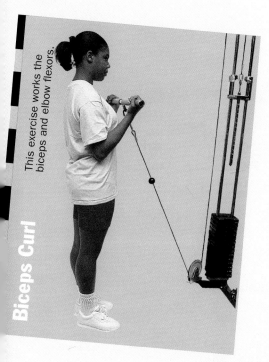

This exercise works the biceps and elbow flexors.

Biceps Curl

Bench Press

1 Lie on your back on the bench with your feet flat on the floor. Grasp the handles with your palms facing away from your body. Flatten your back.

2 Push upward on the handles, extending your arms completely.
Caution: Do not lock your elbows. Do not arch your back.

3 Return to the starting position.

Heel Raise

1 Place a 2-inch thick board on the floor. Stand with the balls of your feet on the board and the handles even with your shoulders.

2 Grasp the handles with your palms facing away from your body. Keep your hands and arms stationary during the lift.

3 Rise on the balls of your feet, and then lower to the starting position.

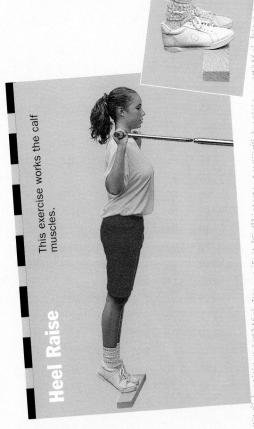

This exercise works the calf muscles.

Heel Raise

Part 2: Grip Strength

1 Adjust the dynamometer to fit your hand size.

2 Squeeze as hard as possible. You may not touch your body with your arm or hand, but you may bend or extend the elbow.

3 Record the best of two scores for each hand.

4 Write your scores on the record sheet and add them together. Look up your rating on the Grip Strength Rating table and then record it.

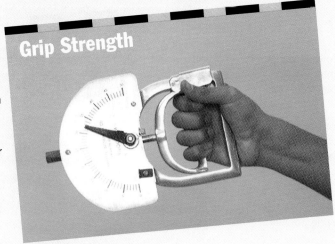

Rating Chart: Grip Strength

	Below 15 years old		15–17 years old		18 years old and above	
	males	**females**	**males**	**females**	**males**	**females**
Good Fitness	191 or more	121 or more	226 or more	136 or more	253 or more	156 or more
Marginal Fitness	158-190	99-120	191-225	114-135	209-252	116-155
Low Fitness	157 or less	98 or less	190 or less	113 or less	208 or less	115 or less

Predicted 1RM Based on Reps-to-Fatigue

Wt	Repetitions						Wt	Repetitions					
	5	**6**	**7**	**8**	**9**	**10**		**5**	**6**	**7**	**8**	**9**	**10**
30	34	35	36	37	38	39	**145**	163	168	174	180	186	193
35	40	41	42	43	44	45	**150**	169	174	180	186	193	200
40	46	47	49	50	51	53	**155**	174	180	186	192	199	207
50	56	58	60	62	64	67	**160**	180	186	192	199	206	213
55	62	64	66	68	71	73	**165**	186	192	198	205	212	220
60	67	70	72	74	77	80	**170**	191	197	204	211	219	227
65	73	75	78	81	84	87	**175**	197	203	210	217	225	233
70	79	81	84	87	90	93	**180**	202	209	216	223	231	240
75	84	87	90	93	96	100	**185**	208	215	222	230	238	247
80	90	93	96	99	103	107	**190**	214	221	228	236	244	253
85	96	99	102	106	109	113	**195**	219	226	234	242	251	260
90	101	105	108	112	116	120	**200**	225	232	240	248	257	267
95	107	110	114	118	122	127	**205**	231	238	246	254	264	273
100	112	116	120	124	129	133	**210**	236	244	252	261	270	280
105	118	122	126	130	135	140	**215**	242	250	258	267	276	287
110	124	128	132	137	141	147	**220**	247	255	264	273	283	293
115	129	134	138	143	148	153	**225**	253	261	270	279	289	300
120	135	139	144	149	154	160	**230**	259	267	276	286	296	307
125	141	145	150	155	161	167	**235**	264	273	282	292	302	313
130	146	151	158	161	167	173	**240**	270	279	288	298	309	320
135	152	157	162	168	174	180	**245**	276	285	294	304	315	327
140	157	163	168	174	180	187	**250**	281	290	300	310	321	333

9.2 Lesson — Improving Your Strength

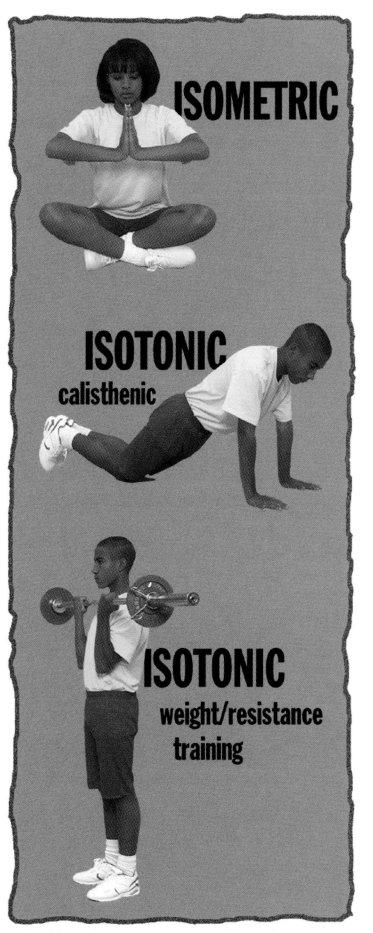

ISOMETRIC

ISOTONIC
calisthenic

ISOTONIC
weight/resistance training

Strength Exercises

Lesson Objectives
After reading this lesson, you should be able to:
1. Name and describe the types of exercises you can do to improve your strength.
2. Describe progressive resistance exercise and why it is important.
3. List the guidelines for resistance training.

Lesson Vocabulary
weight training, progressive resistance exercise

In this lesson you will learn how to include strength training in your total fitness program. You will find out about the types of exercises that improve strength. You also will learn about guidelines to keep you safe while improving strength.

The Physical Activity Pyramid and Strength

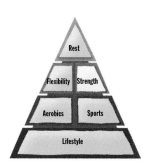

Strength is an important part of the Physical Activity Pyramid, shown at the left. Several types of exercises can help you improve your muscular strength. Some are shown in pictures on this page. These exercises involve the exertion of near maximal muscular force against a resistance.

Isometric Exercises In isometric exercises, also called static exercises, muscles contract but the body parts do not move. You will have the opportunity to try many isometrics in the Activity for Chapter 17.

Isotonic Exercises Isotonic exercises, also called dynamic exercises, are those in which the muscles contract and body parts move. There are several types of isotonic exercises used for strength development: isokinetics, plyometrics, calisthenics, and weight training.

- **Isokinetic Exercise** Isokinetic exercises are done with a special apparatus such as the Exergenie or machines such as the Cybex. These devices control the speed of movement of a body part so that it remains constant, even when you try to move faster. These machines also provide a constant force throughout the range of motion. They are often used in rehabilitation and can be regulated to predetermined speeds.

- **Plyometrics** These exercises are used by athletes to train for the development of power. Power is the rapid application of strength. Plyometric exercises involve a quick stretch followed by a strong muscle contraction. A common drill to develop power in the legs is a series of consecutive hops or jumps. As a general rule, plyometrics are *not* recommended for preteens and teens. They can place a great deal of stress on the tendons.

- **Calisthenics** These exercises are done using your body weight as resistance. Calisthenics include exercises such as push-ups, pull-ups, trunk curls, and squats. You have used this type of exercise in the Self-Assessments in Chapters 2, 3, and 4 and in your endurance workout in Chapter 8.

- **Weight/Resistance Training** Weight training involves the lifting of weights to build strength or endurance. The weights can be free weights or those on weight machines, or homemade weights such as plastic bottles filled with water or sand. Because the weights are often made of iron, this kind of exercise is usually called "pumping iron." Many machines use forces other than weight to provide resistance. For example, some machines use hydraulic pressure, air pressure, or friction to provide resistance.

The terms *resistance training* and *resistance machines* are used to describe strength training, unless the use of weights is specifically intended. *Resistance* includes all types of resistance including weights. The table compares the advantages and disadvantages of resistance machines and free weights.

Resistance Machines vs. Free Weights

	Resistance Machines	Free Weights
Safety	• Safer because weights cannot fall on the lifter. • Less need for a spotter.	• Greater chance of injury from falling weights. • Spotter required to help you because it's easy to lose control of the weights.
Cost	• Very expensive to own. • If you don't own the machines, you must join a club to use them.	• Inexpensive
Versatility	• Can easily isolate a particular muscle group to work.	• Requires more balance, coordination, and concentration. • You use more muscles and the movements are more like moving heavy loads in daily life.
Convenience	• Requires a lot of floor space. • You must go to where they are.	• Takes up little space. • Some weights are small enough to be carried around. • Can easily scatter and get lost or stolen.

Types of Weight Training

There are different forms of weight training. Some are just for athletes who compete.

- **Weight Training** This non-competitive form of exercise is done to improve muscular strength and endurance. Participants exercise against resistance for about 3 to 25 repetitions. They usually use a load between 50% and 80% of the maximum weight they can lift, so it is called "sub-maximal" resistance.

- **Circuit Weight Training** This is the same as weight training except that it is usually used to develop aerobic endurance as well as strength and muscular endurance. Circuit Training was described in Chapter 8. Sample circuits are included in Chapters 8 and 15.

- **Weight Lifting** This is an Olympic sport involving the use of free weights. The athletes try to lift a maximum load. There are only two exercises: the *snatch* and the *clean and jerk*.

- **Power Lifting** This is another competitive sport using free weights. The athletes try to make one maximal lift. There are only three exercises: the *bench press, squat,* and *deadlift.*

- **Body Building** This sport can also be done for competition. The athletes are primarily concerned about the appearance of their bodies. They are judged based on how large and well defined their muscles are. They train with more repetitions than weight lifters and power lifters.

Progressive Resistance Exercise

When you do an exercise with a weight or other resistance to improve strength, your muscles get stronger and you soon feel that the exercise is easy. You will not get any stronger unless you increase the amount of resistance you use in the exercise. The gradual increase of resistance used in strength training exercises is called **progressive resistance exercise** or PRE. There is general agreement among researchers that PRE is the best way to develop strength.

Fitness Principles and Strength

The three basic fitness principles can be applied to strength exercises. You have read about these principles—overload, progression, and specificity—in previous chapters.

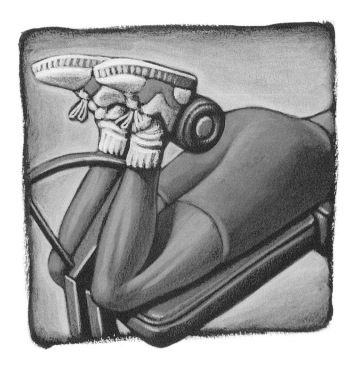

Doing an exercise involving knee flexion to strengthen the hamstring muscles illustrates the principle of specificity.

Principle of Overload A muscle must contract harder than normal to become stronger. In other words, the muscles must work against a greater load than they normally have in regular daily activity. Experts say a muscle must be contracted to at least 60% of its maximum to increase strength. If a muscle is worked against less than normal resistance, it will weaken. If a muscle is always worked against the same amount of resistance, it will maintain the same strength because over time muscles adapt to the stress put upon them.

Principle of Progression Overload gradually—increase the load over a period of time—to get the best improvement in muscle strength. You can injure yourself if you try to lift too much weight too soon. Also, lifting too much weight will not result in as much strength gain as would occur if you progressed gradually. To progress, you must continue increasing the resistance until you are as strong as you want to be. The concept of progressive resistance exercise is based on the principles of overload and progression.

Principle of Specificity You must exercise the specific muscles you wish to develop. If you wish to strengthen the muscles on the back of the thigh, you must specifically overload the particular group of muscles called the hamstrings, by doing an exercise such as the one shown above involving flexion of the knee.

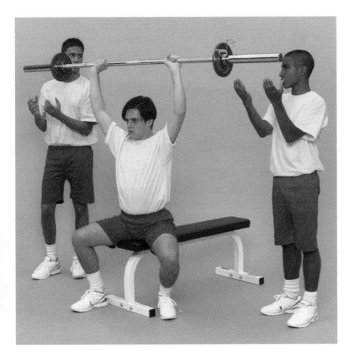

The principle of progression: To improve muscle strength, increase the load gradually over a period of time.

Fitness Target Zones for Strength

	Isotonic	Isometric
Frequency	Non-consecutive days, at least 2-3 days a week.	Every other day and at least 2-3 days a week.
Intensity	*Teens:* 60 to 75% of 1RM for 7-10 reps *Adults:* 75 to 90% of 1RM 4 to 8 reps	Contract the muscles as tightly as possible for the required length of time.
Time	*Teens:* 7-10 repetitions per set for 3 sets. *Adults:* 4-8 reps per set for 3 sets.	Hold the contraction for 7-10 seconds. Rest 30 seconds. This is one set. Do two more sets.

Note: Children 13 years of age and younger should do no fewer than 8 reps.

The principle of specificity also means that you should do some strength exercises that resemble the movement that you want to eventually use. For example, to strengthen the arm, a baseball pitcher might make a pitching motion against an elastic band.

The Fit Formula and Strength

The table shows the amount of exercise needed to improve muscle strength. Notice that you should not do your strength training on consecutive days. Your muscles need time to recover and grow.

To improve strength, adults need to use a resistance of 75% to 90% of their maximum. Teens should use 60% to 75% of their maximum. For some people, lifting parts of the body, such as the arms and legs, is enough. For others, lifting the entire body as in a push-up, might be necessary. Stronger people may need to lift extra weight to overload the muscles enough to develop strength. If you do isometric exercises, contract your muscles as hard as you can for each exercise.

The isotonic strength training programs for teens in this book use 7-10 reps. As an adult, when your skeleton has matured and your bones have stopped growing, you will use fewer reps and more resistance.

Resistance Training Guidelines

You can safely participate in resistance training and see much improvement in your strength and physique. Here are some safety guidelines especially for teens to keep in mind:

• Do not hold your breath when you lift. This can cause you to "black out." Some resistance trainers recommend exhaling on the lift and inhaling on the return movement.

• Always be sure to use spotters whenever you are working with free weights.

• Avoid maximal lifts.

• Avoid overhead lifts with free weights; if possible, use machines for these.

• Be sure to learn to use proper form. Avoid positions that cause the lower back to arch or the wrists to bend backward.

• Avoid jumping (plyometric) machines and machines that do not fit you (most of these are made for adults).

• Avoid fast, sudden, power moves such as those used in plyometric training. Make sure that you use sensible, safe, slow, nonexplosive movements.

• Never use weights carelessly.

• Concentrate on your technique and on what you are doing.

• Use resistance (weight) that you can lift 7 to 10 reps. Your muscles may be strong enough to lift more, but your bones are not!

• Never compete when you do strength training. For example, do not have a contest to see who can lift the most weight. Genetic differences largely determine how strong a person can be. You need only be concerned with trying to improve your strength and enjoying the exercise.

• Consider other forms of resistance such as calisthenics, elastic bands, or isometrics.

Lesson Review
1. What types of exercises can you do to improve your strength?
2. What is progressive resistance exercise and why is it important?
3. List six guidelines that teens should follow for resistance training.

Activity 9
Weight/Resistance Training

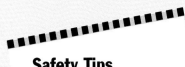

Safety Tips

• Make all moves slowly.

• Exhale on the lift; inhale on the return to starting position. Don't hold your breath.

• Handle all weights with care and awareness of the potential for serious injury.

In this activity, you will use your 1RM values from the Self-Assessment to determine the amount of weight you should be able to lift 7 times, your 7 RM. You may do this activity on free weights or machines.

If you do the exercises with free weights, follow the order in the table on page 123 and the instructions for each exercise in the Chapter 7 Activity, pages 99 to 101. If you do the exercises on machines, follow the order in the table on page 123 and the instructions for each exercise in the Chapter 9 Self-Assessment, pages 123 to 125.

Follow these general directions.

• Determine your 7RM by multiplying your 1RM for each activity by the appropriate percentage for your age. See the table to determine your percentage. Write your 7RMs for each exercise on your record sheet.

• Warm-up and stretch.

• At each station, select the weight nearest your 7RM for that exercise. Do 7 repetitions. If you are unable to complete 7 reps, make a note of it on your record sheet and use a lower weight next time.

• Your machine partner will assist by changing weights and coaching you on technique. The free weight partners will help you change weights, spot for you on the lifts, and coach you on technique.

• Exchange places with your partner(s). Continue this procedure at each station, rotating in the order they are listed or in the order prescribed by your instructor.

• When you and your partner(s) have completed the stations, you have completed one set. Continue rotating for 2 more sets (a total of 3 sets). If instructed to do so, change from machine to free weights or vice versa for the second set.

• Cool down and stretch.

• After some experience, these exercises will feel easier. Then increase the reps until you can do 10. When 10 reps feels easy, increase the weight and drop back to 7 reps.

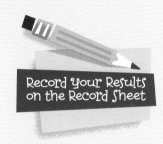

Record Your Results on the Record Sheet

7RM

Age	Percentage
13	60%
14	65%
15	75%
16	75%

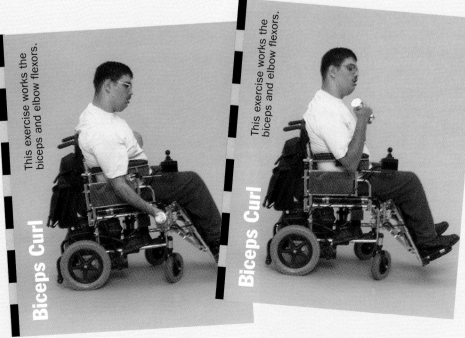

This exercise works the biceps and elbow flexors.

Biceps Curl

This exercise works the biceps and elbow flexors.

Biceps Curl

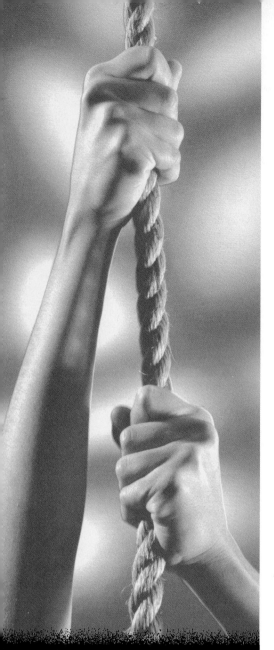

9 Chapter Review

Reviewing Concepts and Vocabulary

Copy the number of each statement on a sheet of paper. Next to each number, write the word or words that correctly completes the sentence.

1. _____ is the amount of force a muscle can exert.

2. The place in your bones where growth is rapidly occurring is called the _____.

3. _____ are drugs that are similar to the male hormone testosterone, but are illegal and dangerous to use to build strength.

4. A person can become _____ if he or she does strength training improperly by developing some muscles while ignoring others.

5. When you do calisthenics to develop strength, you use your body weight as the _____.

Number your paper. Next to each number, choose the letter of the best answer.

Column I	Column II
6. weight training	a. the maximum amount of weight a group of muscles can lift one time
7. progressive resistance exercise	b. rapid application of strength
8. power	c. the lifting of weights to build strength or endurance
9. 1RM	d. the gradual increase of weight used in strength training

On your paper, write a short answer for each statement or question.

10. How do strong muscles help you look better and prevent health problems?

11. Why can't preteens and teens do the same strength training programs that adults do?

12. Why should you assess your strength before you start a strength training program?

13. Why should you gradually increase the amount of weight you use?

14. How often should you do your strength training program?

15. Why is it dangerous to hold your breath when you lift weights?

Thinking Critically

Write a paragraph to answer the following question.

Your friend Derrick is excited about an article he read in a muscle magazine. He tells you that he's going to take some steroids to make his muscles big and strong. What would you tell your friend? What would you recommend he do to strengthen his muscles safely?

Project

Find out about rules and laws governing the use of anabolic steroids. What is the policy in your school regarding the consequences for those found using these drugs? What local and state laws apply to use of anabolic steroids?

10

Flexibility

Cooperative Games

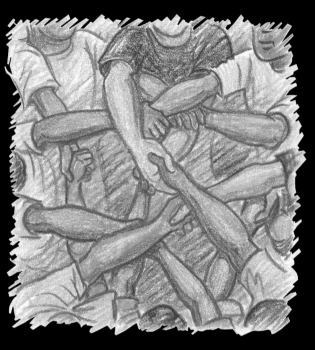

Strangely enough, the concept of cooperative games grew out the Vietnam War experience in the 1970s. Cooperative games are the opposite of war and competition. In these games, you have fun by playing for all you are worth, and everyone wins by cooperating with each other. Even when games are arranged so that teams compete, the winning is not important. Sometimes members of the opposite team have been known to change sides and try to help the losing team! The fun is in the play, not in the winning. Follow the directions on your instruction sheet to play some of the following games and see how much fun you can have. Then you can try to make up your own cooperative game!

Human Knots
Catch the Dragon's Tail
Stand-Up
Blanket Ball Volleyball
Triangle Tag
Earth Ball

10.1 Nature and Purpose of Flexibility

Lesson

Lesson Objectives
After reading this lesson, you should be able to:
1. Describe the characteristics of flexibility.
2. Explain how you benefit from good flexibility.
3. Explain why it is important to balance strength and flexibility exercises.
4. Explain how the fitness principles of overload, progression, and specificity apply to flexibility.

Lesson Vocabulary
range of motion, hypermobility, arthritis, laxity

In this lesson, you will learn about the importance of being flexible and how to improve flexibility by applying fitness principles. You will also learn to evaluate flexibility in some of your own joints.

What Is Flexibility?
Flexibility is the ability to move your joints through a full range of motion. A joint is a place in the body where bones come together. The best known joints include the ankles, knees, and hips in the legs; the knuckles, wrist, elbows, and shoulders in the arms; and the joints between the vertebrae in the spine. Some joints such as the knees and elbows work like a hinge, permitting movement in only two directions. Other joints such as the hip and shoulder work like a ball and socket, allowing movement in all directions. **Range of motion** is the amount of movement you can make in a joint.

Benefits of Good Flexibility
Improved Function Everyone needs a minimum amount of flexibility to maintain health and mobility. Some people need additional flexibility. For example, dancers and gymnasts must be very flexible to perform their routines. Plumbers, painters, and dentists often need to bend and stretch. Some musicians need very flexible fingers and wrists.

Flexibility is important to many athletes because it allows a greater backswing in throwing and striking movements. A long backswing enables a faster forward swing. In the case of weight lifting, shot put, and some other sports, the greater backward movement is believed to allow a faster "snap back" of the muscle on the forward movement, producing more power.

Improved Health and Wellness Stretching exercises can help prevent injury and muscle soreness and have a beneficial effect on a number of conditions. For example, musicians who are flexible are less likely to have pain in the joints they use. Stretching exercises can often alleviate menstrual cramps in women. Stretching exercises can prevent or provide relief from leg cramps and shin splints, pains in the front of the shins caused by overuse. Stretching short muscles helps improve posture. Good posture helps prevent or relieve back pain and reduces fatigue. A stretch can help your muscles relax. In Chapter 18 you will learn how stretching exercises can help relieve stress.

Characteristics of Flexibility

Body Build and Flexibility Some people will not be able to score as well on flexibility tests as others no matter how much they stretch. Anatomical differences in our bodies help determine what we can and cannot do. Rather than comparing your scores on fitness tests with those of others, compare your scores with your own previous scores and seek to improve.

Can short people touch their toes more easily than tall people? No, a shorter person does tend to have relatively short legs and trunk, but also tends to have short arms (although there are exceptions). In contrast, a tall person tends to have longer legs and trunk, as well as longer arms.

Generally, females tend to be more flexible than males. Also, young people tend to be more flexible than older people. However, flexibility exercises can help you maintain flexibility throughout your life.

Hypermobility Some people are unusually flexible in certain joints, and people often refer to them as being "double jointed." This condition is called **hypermobility**, the ability to extend the knee, elbow, thumb, or wrist joint past a straight line, as if the joint could bend backwards. Hypermobility is usually an inherited trait and tends to be more common in some races and ethnic groups. Some people who have hypermobile

joints are prone to joint injuries and may be more likely to develop **arthritis**, a disease in which the joints become inflamed. For the most part, however, those with hypermobile joints do not have problems, other than a slight disadvantage in some sports. For example, when doing the push-up exercise, the elbows of a hypermobile person might easily lock when the arms straighten. Then it is difficult to unlock the elbows to begin the downward movement.

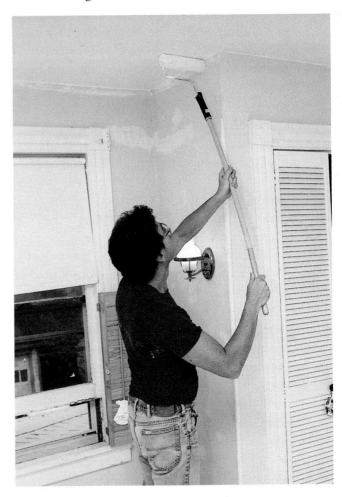

Flexibility can help a person paint hard-to-reach places.

Joint Laxity When a joint allows the bones to move in ways other than intended, it is sometimes described as looseness, or **laxity**. Laxity occurs when the ligaments around the joint are overstretched, most likely from injury or incorrect exercise. If laxity occurs in a knee joint, it may lead to knee sprains and torn cartilage or a dislocated knee cap. Ligaments cannot be strengthened by doing exercises. However, strengthening the muscles around the joint can help reduce looseness.

Balancing Strength and Flexibility

Strength and flexibility exercises should go together. Everyone needs strong muscles, but as you learned earlier, exclusive use of strength exercises can lead to a loss of normal range of motion and a condition sometimes called "muscle-bound." On the other hand, if you only do flexibility exercises, then your joints may become susceptible to injury because strong muscles are needed to reinforce the ligaments that hold the bones together.

A balanced exercise program includes both strength and flexibility exercises for all your muscles so that they can apply equal force on all sides of a joint. People commonly use the muscles (flexor) on the front of the body a great deal because many daily activities emphasize the use of those muscles. For example, the majority of people have strong biceps (on the front of the arm), pectoral muscles (on the front of the chest), and quadriceps muscles (on the front of the thigh). The pull of these strong muscles results in the body hunching forward. To avoid becoming permanently hunched over, you need to make certain that these strong, short muscles on the front of the body get stretched. At the same time, you must strengthen the weak, long, relatively unused muscles on the back of the body. The table shows the muscles most in need of flexibility exercises in most people.

Are there muscles that don't need stretching? For most people, there probably are. For example, most people eventually begin to develop a hunched over posture often called "humpback." Since the upper back muscles become overstretched in people with this postural problem, they should avoid further stretching of those muscles. Another example might be the abdominal muscles. If you neglect to keep these important muscles strong, they begin to sag and the abdomen protrudes, leading to poor posture. Most people do *not* need to stretch the abdominal muscles.

Muscles That Need the Most Stretching

Muscle	Reason
Chest muscles	To prevent poor posture
Front of shoulders	To prevent poor posture
Front of hip joint	To prevent swayback posture, backache, or a pulled muscle
Back of thigh (hamstrings)	To prevent swayback posture, backache, or a pulled muscle
Inside of thigh	To prevent back, leg, and foot strain
Calf muscles	To avoid soreness and Achilles tendon injuries, which may occur from running and jumping
Lower back	To prevent soreness, pain, and back injuries

Each person must evaluate his or her own needs to avoid stretching already overstretched muscles and avoid strengthening muscles that are already so strong that they are out of balance with their opposite muscles. Keeping muscles on opposites sides of a joint in balance helps them pull with equal force in all directions. Such a balance helps align your body parts properly, so that your posture is good.

Fitness Principles and Flexibility

The principles of overload, progression, and specificity apply to flexibility, just as they apply to the other components of health-related fitness.

Principle of Overload You need to stretch your muscles longer than normal to increase your flexibility. To stretch a muscle, you need to lengthen it more than you do in your daily activities. To achieve this kind of stretch, you usually need a force greater than your own opposing muscles. For example, if you want to stretch your chest muscles, you cannot get an overload just by pulling your arms back and holding them in that position. You need additional force, such as your own body weight when you put your arms on either side of a door frame and lean forward. You can use another body part, a partner, or a weight to assist in the stretch. Be sure to give feedback when a partner helps you stretch so that she or he can apply the proper amount of force!

No Excuses

Building Intrinsic Motivation

Some people need to be rewarded by others to stay physically active. When they are no longer rewarded, they use it as an excuse to stop being active. They have extrinsic motivation—motivation given by others. People who have intrinsic motivation are self-motivated—they are active because they want to be. The more intrinsic rewards you get from physical activity, the more likely you are to remain active.

James pulled on his track shirt and stuffed his jeans and T-shirt into his locker. "I can't wait for track season to be over," he told Leon. "If the coach makes us do sprints again today, I'm going to pretend I sprained my ankle or something."

"I like sprints," Leon said as he tied the laces on his running shoes. "You get to see what you can do when you go all out."

"I'm already 'all out'—all out of here as soon as possible! If I weren't going to get a letter jacket at the end of track this year, I'd quit now."

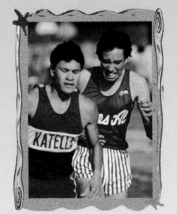

"What about next year? Are you going out for track again?" Leon asked.

"Nah. I can barely beat you and Angelo now in the 400. If I can't run faster than you two, how am I going to place in meets with other schools? I'm slowing down. It's time to quit while I'm ahead."

"Why don't you try out for something different next year? I'm thinking about soccer," Leon said. "I figure all this running would help me there. And it would motivate me to jog all summer to keep in shape"

"Yeah, maybe I'll try out for the soccer team, too. If I jogged with you this summer, maybe I'd stay motivated."

For Discussion

How does James show that he's extrinsically motivated? How does Leon show that he is intrinsically motivated? What could James do to become more intrinsically motivated? Fill in the questionnaire to evaluate your own motivation to be physically active.

Principle of Progression You need to gradually increase the intensity of exercise. Intensity can be increased by stretching farther as you gain flexibility. Up to a point, you may also progress by gradually increasing the amount of time you hold the stretch or the number of repetitions. Eventually you will achieve your flexibility goals. Then you need to maintain the flexibility you have achieved.

Principle of Specificity Flexibility exercises improve only the specific muscles at the specific joints that you stretch. To develop overall flexibility, you must stretch all of your body's muscles that need stretching.

Maintaining Flexibility Once you have reached an acceptable level of flexibility for your muscles, you must continue to move all of your joints and muscles

through this new and improved range of motion on a regular basis. If you do not use the range of motion you have available in a joint, the muscles will begin to shorten again and you will lose that flexibility.

Lesson Review
1. What are the characteristics of flexibility?
2. How do you benefit from good flexibility?
3. Why is it important to balance strength and flexibility exercises?
4. How do the fitness principles of overload, progression, and specificity apply to flexibility?

Arm, Leg, and Trunk Flexibility

Safety Tips

Warm up before taking a flexibility test. Warm muscles are less likely to be injured and will stretch farther.

This Self-Assessment helps you evaluate the flexibility of some of your muscles and joints. Follow these general directions for the following tests.

• Perform each exercise as described and illustrated here.

• Stretch and hold the position for 2 seconds while a partner checks your performance.

• Use the Record Sheet to help you score this test. Record only the first trial. You are expected to do these tests in class only once, unless your instructor tells you otherwise. You will want to retest yourself periodically, so there is space on the record sheet to write the results of your retests in the future.

Arm Lift

1 Lie facedown. Hold a ruler or stick in both hands. Keep fists tight, palms facing down.

2 Raise your arms and the stick as high as possible. Keep your forehead on the floor and your arms and wrists straight.

3 Hold this position while your partner checks the height of the stick with a ruler.

4 Record 1 check mark in the correct column.

Pass = 10 inches or more

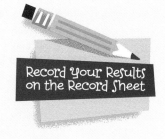

Record Your Results on the Record Sheet

Rating Chart: Flexibility

Fitness Rating	Score
Good	8–10
Marginal	5–7
Low	0–4

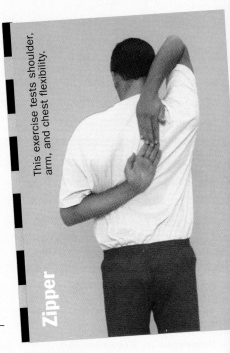

This exercise tests shoulder, arm, and chest flexibility.

Zipper

Zipper

1 Reach your right arm and hand over your right shoulder and down your spine, as if you were pulling up a zipper.

2 Hold this position while you reach your left arm and hand behind your back and up the spine to try to touch or overlap the fingers of your right hand.

3 Hold while your partner checks.

4 Repeat, reaching your left arm over your shoulder.

5 Record 1 check mark for each side.

Pass = touch or overlap fingers

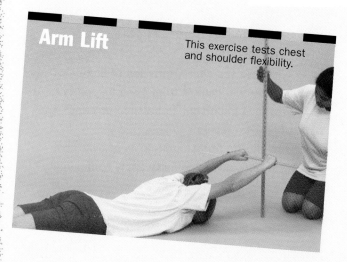

Arm Lift

This exercise tests chest and shoulder flexibility.

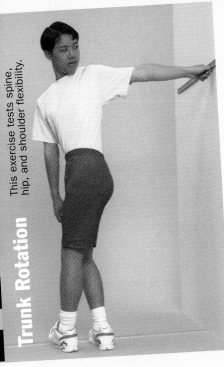

This exercise tests spine, hip, and shoulder flexibility.

Trunk Rotation

Wrap Around

1 Raise your right arm and reach behind your head. Try to touch the left corner of your mouth. You may turn your head and neck to the left.

2 Hold while your partner checks.

3 Repeat with your left arm.

4 Record 1 check mark for each side.

Pass = touching corner of mouth

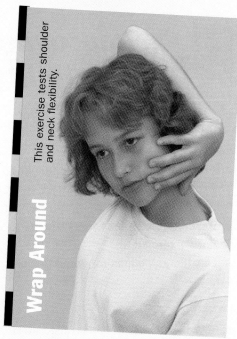

This exercise tests shoulder and neck flexibility.

Wrap Around

Trunk Rotation

1 Stand with your toes on the designated line. Your right shoulder should be an arm's length (fist closed) from the wall, and directly on a line with the target spot.

2 Drop your right arm and extend your left arm to your side at shoulder height. Make a fist, palm down.

3 Without moving your feet, rotate your trunk to the left as far as possible. Your knees may bend slightly to permit more turn, but don't move your feet. Try to touch the target spot or beyond with a palm-down fist.

4 Hold while your partner checks.

5 Repeat, rotating to the right.

6 Record 1 check mark for each side.

Pass = touch center of target or beyond

Knee-to-Chest

1 Lie on back. Extend left leg. Bring right knee to chest. Place hands on back of right thigh. Pull knee down tight to your chest.

2 Keep your left leg straight and both the leg and lower back flat on the floor.

3 Hold. Your partner checks that your knee is on your chest and uses a ruler to measure the distance that your left calf is from the floor.

4 Record score. Repeat with your left knee. Record 1 check mark for each side.

Pass = calf one inch or less from floor

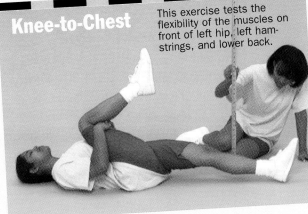

Knee-to-Chest

This exercise tests the flexibility of the muscles on front of left hip, left hamstrings, and lower back.

Ankle Flex

1 Sit erect on the floor with your legs straight and together. You may lean backward slightly on your hands if necessary.

2 Flex your ankles by pulling your toes toward your shins as far as possible.

3 Hold this position while your partner checks the angle that the soles of your feet make with the floor. The partner will align a T-square or a book with the floor, and see whether the soles are at least perpendicular to the floor.

4 Record 1 check mark in the correct column.

Pass = soles angled 90° or more

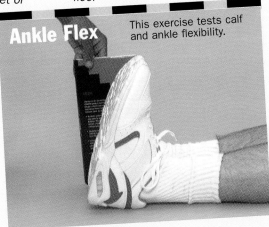

Ankle Flex

This exercise tests calf and ankle flexibility.

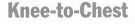

10.2 Improving Flexibility
Lesson

Lesson Objectives
After reading this lesson, you should be able to:
1. Explain the differences among static stretching, PNF stretching, and ballistic stretching.
2. Describe the fitness target zones for static and ballistic exercise.
3. List the guidelines for doing flexibility exercises safely.

Lesson Vocabulary
range of motion (ROM) exercise, stretching exercise, static stretching, PNF stretching, ballistic stretching

In this lesson, you will learn about the types of exercise used for flexibility. In addition, you will see how to apply the FIT principle to maintain or build flexibility. Finally, you will learn safety guidelines and try some stretching exercises for different muscle groups.

The Physical Activity Pyramid

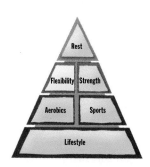

Flexibility in the joints of the body is essential for good health as well as for efficient, effective functioning. Selecting activities from the Flexibility Fitness section of the Physical Activity Pyramid will help you improve your flexibility and develop overall fitness.

Types of Flexibility Exercises

Jogging, swimming, and other activities and sports help improve your cardiovascular fitness, strength, and muscular endurance. However, to improve flexibility, you must perform specific exercises to maintain and improve the range of motion in your joints. Properly selected exercises can improve your flexibility and provide many other benefits such as helping to relieve muscle cramps. There are two main types of flexibility exercises: range of motion and stretching.

Range of Motion (ROM) Exercise The term **range of motion exercise,** usually called ROM exercise, refers to flexibility exercises that are used to maintain the range of motion already present in your joints. ROM exercises are probably the best type of flexibility exercise to use in a warm-up routine. Some experts think that when you stretch your muscles farther than their present range during the warm-up, the muscles are more likely to be injured in the workout or sport that follows.

If you are as flexible as you need to be, then you should move your body to maintain that flexibility. Without attempting to stretch muscles any farther, it is wise to move all of the joints through their complete range of motion at least three times a week. For example, if your self-assessment scores are in the good zone where you wish to be, then you should regularly exercise to maintain that amount of flexibility.

Stretching Exercise Whereas a ROM exercise maintains your current level of flexibility, a **stretching exercise** works to increase your range of motion by stretching farther than your current range of motion. There are three types of stretching exercises: static, PNF, and ballistic.

Static stretching is stretching slowly as far as you can without pain, until you feel a sense of "pulling" or "tenseness," then holding the stretch for several seconds. Done correctly, static stretching increases your flexibility and can help you relax. Static stretching exercises are safer than ballistic exercises because you are less likely to stretch too far and injure yourself. Static stretching can be especially beneficial for people who have bad backs, previous muscle or joint injuries, or arthritis. Even athletes should perform static stretches at the beginning and end of their exercise programs to warm up and cool down. By themselves, static stretches might not build enough flexibility for an athlete, so athletes may need to add PNF and/or ballistic stretches.

PNF (proprioceptive neuromuscular facilitation) is a stretching technique used by physical and occupational therapists. It has recently become popular among athletes. **PNF stretching** is a variation of static stretching that is more effective for improving flexibility. A PNF stretch involves using the body's reflexes to relax the muscle before you stretch it, so that you can stretch it farther. Some variations of PNF require a partner to assist you, but there is one form that is easy for you to use with or without a partner. It is called CRAC (contract-relax-antagonist-contract). After you contract a muscle that you want to stretch, the muscle automatically relaxes. Contracting the opposing muscles during the stretch also makes the muscle you are stretching relax. CRAC does both of these. Some samples of CRAC are included in the Activity at the end of this chapter.

Ballistic stretching is a series of quick but gentle bouncing or bobbing-type motions that are not held for a long time. If you are active in sports, part of your exercise program should include movements that are used in your sports. If you move or stretch muscles quickly in a sport (for example, fast throwing or sprinting), then some of your flexibility exercises should resemble the sport's movement. Although ballistic stretching might be more effective than static stretching, you must be careful to stretch gently. Stretching too quickly or overstretching can cause injury.

Some teachers and coaches have been opposed to all ballistic stretching because of the possibility of overstretching if it is not done carefully. Actually, studies show that ballistic stretching does not cause as much muscular soreness as static stretching. If you are an athlete and wish to achieve a high performance level of flexibility, you may wish to apply the principle of specificity by using a ballistic stretching exercise that closely mimics the backswing so common to sports. An example of this is seen at baseball games when the batter takes a few easy swings with a weighted bat or does trunk twists with a bounce in each direction before getting in the batters box. Another example is the track athlete who stretches the Achilles tendon with a few gentle bounces on the heels.

The Fit Formula for Flexibility

To improve the flexibility of your joints and increase the length of your muscles, you must exercise in the fitness target zone for flexibility. Flexibility has two different target zones: one for static exercise and one for ballistic exercise.

Scientists are not sure about the best length of time to hold a stretch or the ideal number of repetitions, but studies on animals suggest that four repetitions are enough. The FIT chart above is a good guideline to follow.

Guidelines for Flexibility Exercises

To get the most benefit and the most enjoyment from your exercise program, it is important to perform the exercises correctly and observe certain cautions to avoid injury. Before you begin stretching, keep these

Fitness Target Zones for Flexibility

	Static/PNF	Ballistic
Frequency	• Stretch each muscle group daily, if possible, but at least 3 days a week. ROM before and stretch after workouts.	• *Caution:* Before doing ballistic stretching, read about ballistic stretching on page 141 and the guidelines on pages 141-142. • Stretch each muscle group daily, if possible, but at least 3 days a week.
Intensity	• The muscle must be stretched beyond its normal length. • You must have a partner or equipment, or you can use your own body weight to provide an overload.	• The muscle must be stretched beyond its normal length. • Use slow, *gentle* bounces or bobs, using the motion of your body part to stretch the specific muscle. *Caution:* No stretch should cause pain, especially sharp pain. Be especially careful when doing ballistic stretching.
Time	• Hold each stretch for 10 to 30 seconds. Rest for 10 seconds. • Stretch each muscle group. Start with 1 set of 1 rep and progress to 3 to 4 sets, 1 rep each.	• Bounce against the muscle slowly and gently 10 to 15 times. Rest for 10 seconds. • Stretch each muscle group. Start with 1 set of 10 to 15 reps, and progress to 3 sets.

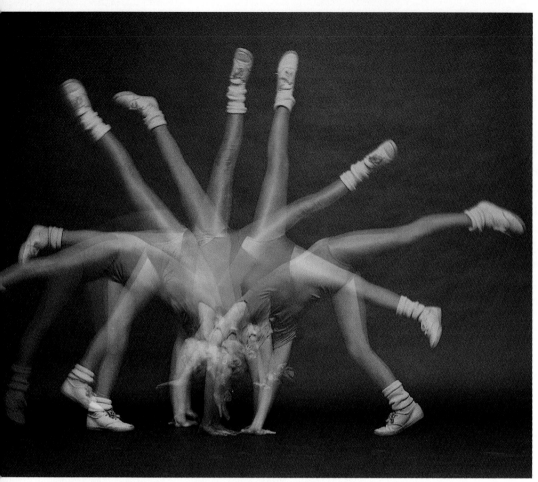

Flexibility is essential for a dance routine such as this one.

• As you learned in Chapter 2, some popular exercises should be avoided because they can cause injury. Avoid the following: rolling the head and neck in a full circle, tipping the head backward to stretch the neck, the backbend acrobatic (unless you are a trained gymnast), arm circles with the palms down, and standing toe touches or windmills.

• Avoid stretching muscles that are already over-stretched from poor posture.

• To benefit from static or PNF stretching, you need gravity, force, or a partner to provide sufficient overload. If you use a partner, he or she should be *extremely careful* not to overstretch you. You must tell your partner when the tension is tight enough.

• Your stretch can be more effective if you contract the muscles *opposite* the muscles you are trying to stretch because this makes the stretched muscle relax more and stretch farther.

• Regardless of the type of flexibility exercise you choose for your program, start slowly. Like muscular endurance exercises, even though some flexibility exercises seem easy, it does not take much to make your muscles sore. Begin slowly and gradually increase the time and the number of reps and sets.

guidelines and cautions in mind to help you achieve and maintain flexibility safely.

• It is wise to do mild cardiovascular exercise such as walking or slow jogging to warm up your muscles before you begin stretching.

• Do static or PNF stretching rather than ballistic, if you do not exercise regularly or if you do not need a high performance level of flexibility.

• Do *not* stretch ballistically if you have a recent injury to that muscle or joint, such as a back problem. Do only static or PNF stretches.

• If you do ballistic stretching, do not try to bounce too far. Stretch gently to avoid injury.

• Do *not* stretch joints that are hypermobile, unstable, swollen, or infected.

• Do *not* stretch until you feel pain. The old saying "No pain, no gain" is wrong! Stretch only until the muscle feels tight and a little uncomfortable.

Lesson Review
1. What are the differences among static stretching, PNF stretching, and ballistic stretching?
2. What are the fitness target zones for static and ballistic exercise?
3. List the guidelines for doing flexibility exercises safely.

Activity 10
Flexibility Exercise Program

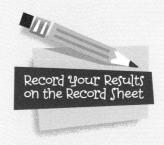

Record your Results on the Record Sheet

This flexibility program will help improve your range of motion. If you did not get a good fitness rating on your evaluation, or if you have been inactive or have joint injuries, choose the static and PNF exercises. If you rated "good" and exercise regularly, then you may add some ballistic exercises to your program. If you add ballistic exercises, be sure to begin with the static and PNF exercises before progressing to the ballistic ones. Review the guidelines on page 142, and then follow these directions. Write your results on your record sheets.

• Refer to the FIT Target Zone chart on page 141 for the appropriate number of reps, sets, and time.

• Perform each of the exercises below and record the date and number of sets or reps on your record sheet. Your instructor will probably specify the number of sets and reps.

• For a PNF exercise, hold a maximum isometric contraction for 3 seconds, relax, then stretch for 10 to 30 seconds.

• A PNF exercise may be done as a static exercise by omitting the contraction phase and doing only the stretch phase for 10 to 30 seconds.

Knee-to-Chest
(PNF or static)

1 Lie on your back with knees bent (hook lying position), arms at sides. (See page 139.)

2 Lift your hips until there is no bend at the hip joint. Squeeze the buttocks muscles hard for 3 seconds. Relax by lowering your hips to the floor.

3 Immediately place your hands under your knees and gently pull your knees to your chest. Hold for 10–30 seconds.

Note: For static exercise, omit step 2.

This exercise stretches the lower back and gluteal muscles.

Backsaver Sit and Reach
(PNF or static)

1 Assume the Backsaver Sit and Reach position (see page 54), with the right knee bent and left leg straight.

2 Bend your left knee slightly and push your heel into the floor as you contract the hamstrings hard for 3 seconds. Relax.

3 Immediately grasp your ankle with both hands and gently pull your chest toward your knee and hold for 10–30 seconds.

4 Repeat on the other leg.

Note: For static stretch, omit step 2.

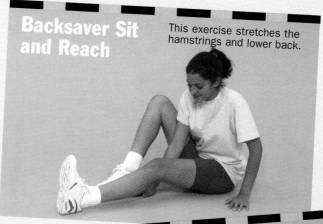

Backsaver Sit and Reach

This exercise stretches the hamstrings and lower back.

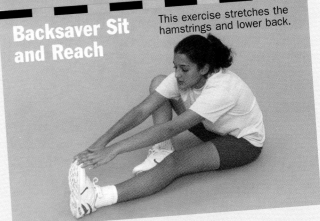

Backsaver Sit and Reach

This exercise stretches the hamstrings and lower back.

Spine Twist (static)

1 Lie on your back with your knees bent (hook lying position), arms extended at shoulder level.

2 Cross your left leg over your right.

3 Keep your shoulders and arms on the floor as you rotate your lower body to the left, touching the right knee to the floor. Stretch and hold 10–30 seconds.

4 At the end of the stretch, reverse the position of your legs (cross your right over your left), and rotate to the right and hold.

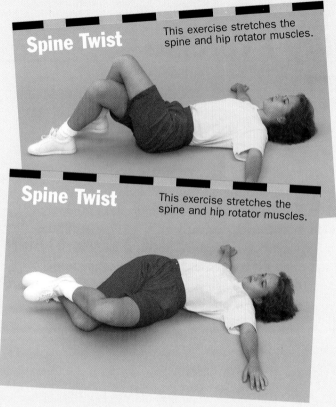

Spine Twist — This exercise stretches the spine and hip rotator muscles.

Spine Twist — This exercise stretches the spine and hip rotator muscles.

Sitting Stretcher (PNF or static)

1 Sit with the soles of your feet together, elbows or hands resting on knees.

2 Contract the muscles on the inside of your thighs, pulling up as you resist with the arms pushing down. Hold 3 seconds. Relax your legs.

3 Immediately lean your trunk forward and push down on your knees with your arms to stretch the thighs. Hold 10–30 seconds.

Note: For static stretch, omit step 2.

Zipper (PNF or static)

1 Stand or sit. Lift your right arm over your right shoulder and reach down the spine. (See page 138.)

2 With your left hand, press down on the right elbow. Resist the pressure by trying to raise that elbow, contracting the opposing muscles. Hold for 3 seconds. Relax.

3 Immediately stretch by reaching down the spine with the right arm, as the left arm assists by pressing on the elbow. Hold 10–30 seconds.

4 Repeat with other arm.

Note: For static stretch, omit step 2.
This exercise stretches the triceps and lattisimus muscles.

Arm Pretzel (static)

1 Stand or sit. Cross your right arm over your left. Turn your right palm toward the back of the left hand and point the thumb down.

2 Grasp your right thumb with the left hand and pull down gently. Stretch and hold 10–30 seconds.

3 Reverse arm positions and stretch the left shoulder.

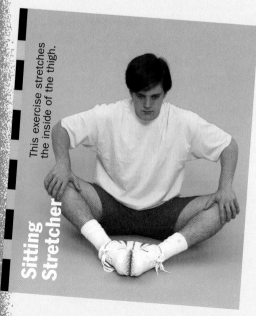

This exercise stretches the inside of the thigh.

Sitting Stretcher

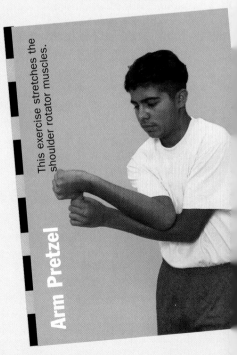

This exercise stretches the shoulder rotator muscles.

Arm Pretzel

Hip Stretcher
(static or ballistic)

1 Take a long step forward on your right foot and kneel on your left knee. The right knee should be directly over your ankle and bent at a right angle.

2 The left knee should be slightly behind your left hip, so that you feel a stretch across the front of the left hip joint.

3 Place your hands on your right knee for balance. Stretch by shifting the weight forward as you tilt your pelvis and trunk backward slightly. Hold 10–30 seconds.

4 Repeat with other leg.

Note: For a ballistic stretch, do a gentle bouncing motion forward as you tilt the pelvis back.

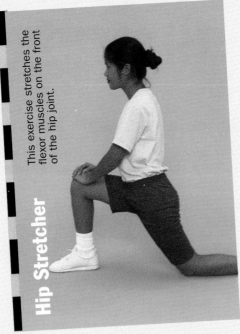

This exercise stretches the flexor muscles on the front of the hip joint.

Hip Stretcher

Chest Stretch
(PNF, static, or ballistic)

1 Stand in a forward stride position in a doorway. Raise arms slightly above shoulder level. Place hands on either side of doorway.

2 Lean body into doorway. Resist by contracting arm and chest muscles. Hold 3 seconds. Relax.

3 Immediately lean farther forward, letting your body weight stretch the muscles. Hold 10–30 seconds.

4 For a ballistic stretch, gently bounce your body forward.

Static stretch: omit steps 2 and 4.

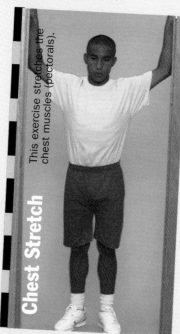

This exercise stretches the chest muscles (pectorals).

Chest Stretch

Arm Stretcher
(static)

1 Sit and cross your right arm over your left with palms facing. Lace your fingers together.

2 Raise your arms overhead to your ears. Straighten your elbows, stretching up and back. Hold 10–30 seconds.

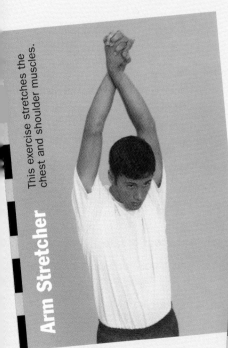

This exercise stretches the chest and shoulder muscles.

Arm Stretcher

Calf Stretcher
(static or ballistic)

1 Step forward with your right leg in a lunge position. Keep both feet pointed straight ahead and the front knee directly over the foot. Place the hands on your right leg for balance.

2 Keep the left leg straight and the heel on the floor. Adjust the length of your lunge until you feel a good stretch in the left calf and Achilles tendon. Hold for 10–30 seconds.

3 Repeat with other leg.

Note: For ballistic stretch, gently bounce heel toward floor.

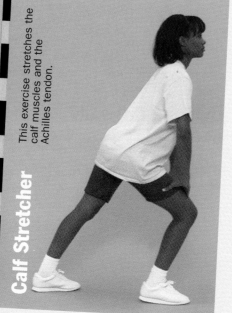

This exercise stretches the calf muscles and the Achilles tendon.

Calf Stretcher

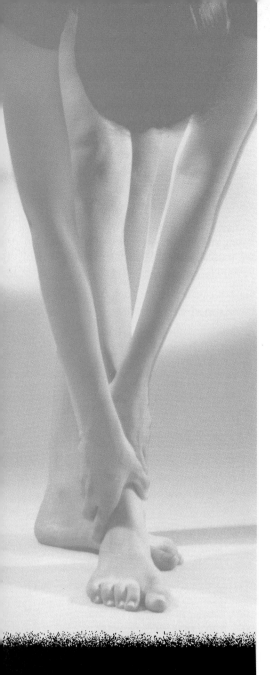

10 Chapter Review

Reviewing Concepts and Vocabulary

Copy the number of each statement on a sheet of paper. Next to each number, write the word or words that correctly completes the sentence.

1. _____ in the body's joints is essential for good health, wellness, and efficient, effective functioning.

2. The amount of movement you can make at a joint is called your _____ .

3. Exercises that involve moving beyond your range of motion are _____ .

4. Doing _____ will help you maintain movement ability in your joints.

5. A _____ involves contracting, then relaxing the muscle before you stretch it.

6. _____ is stretching slowly as far as you can without pain, then holding the stretch for several seconds.

7. Gentle bouncing motions are part of _____.

Number your paper. Next to each number, choose the letter of the best answer.

Column I	Column II
8. hypermobility	a. pain in the front of the shins
9. arthritis	b. place where bones come together
10. joint	c. looseness of the joints
11. laxity	d. the ability to extend the knee, elbow, thumb, or wrist joint past a straight line
12. shin splints	e. disease in which joints are inflamed

On your paper, write a short answer for each statement or question.

13. Why do you have to be especially careful when a partner helps you stretch?

14. Why should you do some mild cardiovascular exercise before stretching?

15. What are the two main kinds of exercises that maintain flexibility?

Thinking Critically

Write a paragraph to answer the following question.

During the first two weeks of volleyball practice, three players suffered shoulder muscle tears and two players are experiencing extreme back pain. The coach thinks the injuries may be due to a lack of flexibility. Why do you think flexibility may be an issue and what advice would you give the coach?

Project

Have students research the kinds of joints in the body (ball-and socket, hinge, gliding, pivot, fixed) and where they are located. Students can make posters or models of the joints, then explain or demonstrate the kind of motion that each joint allows. Help students explain the range of motion possible in each joint when performing flexibility exercises.

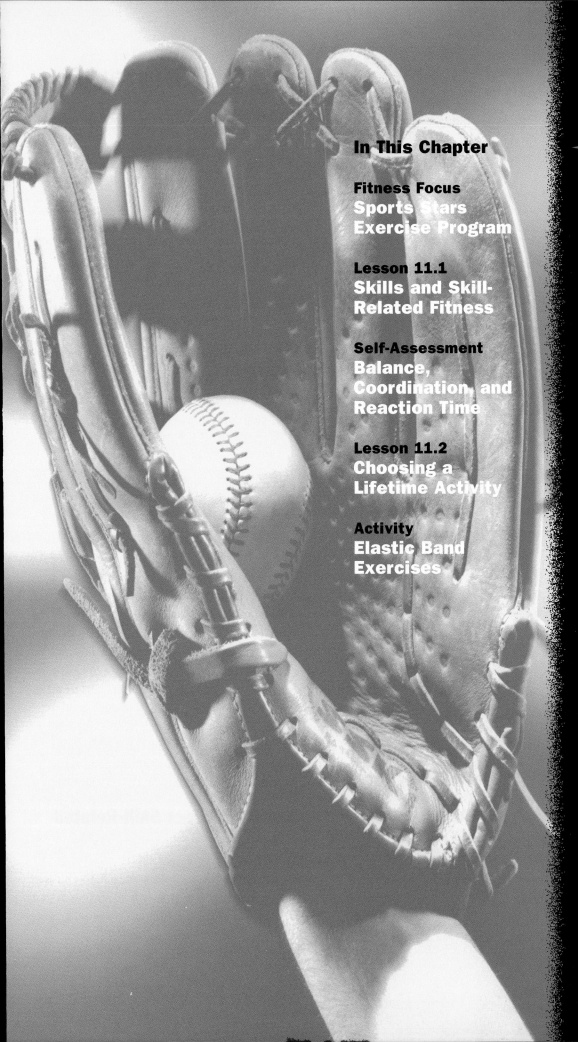

11

Skills and Skill-Related Physical Fitness

Fitness Focus 11
Sports Stars Exercise Program

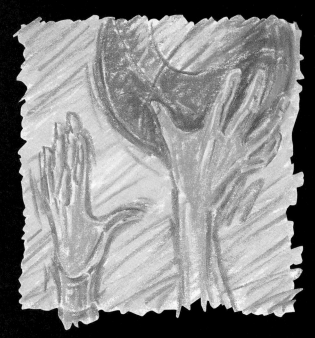

In this chapter you will learn about choosing lifetime physical activities that will provide you with health and wellness benefits. The Sports Stars Exercise Program is designed to help you use sports in your physical activity program. The program is based on earning a certain number of stars, or points, per week as you participate in sports of your choice. Your instruction sheet will show you the number of stars you can earn in a variety of sports.

You should earn 100 stars per week to build good health-related fitness, especially cardiovascular fitness. If you use sports as only part of your exercise, you might earn fewer than 100 stars. If you choose sports that do not build all parts of fitness, you should exercise to build fitness in those parts of fitness not covered by sports.

11.1 Skills and Skill-Related Fitness

Lesson

Lesson Objectives
After reading this lesson, you should be able to:
1. Define *physical skills* and give examples.
2. Explain how skill-related fitness abilities differ from physical skills.
3. Identify and explain factors that affect skill-related fitness and skills.
4. Discuss the importance of assessing personal skill-related fitness.

Lesson Vocabulary
physical skill, practice

You already know that physical fitness is divided into two categories: health-related fitness and skill-related fitness. Health-related fitness is considered the most important because you need it to maintain good health and wellness. Skill-related fitness is less related to good health and more related to your ability to learn sports and other physical skills.

Learning about your own skill-related fitness will help you determine which sports and lifetime activities will be easiest for you to learn and enjoy. Because people differ in their levels of each part of skill-related fitness, different people will find success in different activities. In this lesson you will learn how to assess your own levels of skill-related fitness so that you can choose activities that match your abilities, work to improve your abilities, and find activities you can enjoy for a lifetime.

Factors That Affect Skill-Related Fitness

You learned in Chapter 1 that skill-related physical fitness is a group of basic abilities that help you perform well in sports and activities that require certain physical skills. These abilities include agility, balance, coordination, power, speed, and reaction time.

Notice that skill-related fitness abilities and physical skills are not the same thing. **Physical skills** are specific physical tasks that people perform, such as the sports skills of catching, throwing, swimming, and batting, and other skills such as dancing. Skill-related fitness abilities help you learn particular skills. For example, if you have good skill-related fitness abilities in speed and power, you will be able to learn football running skills easily, or if you have good balance, you will be able to learn gymnastics skills more easily.

Several factors affect your skill-related fitness and your skills. Some of these factors are heredity, practice, and the principle of specificity. The diagram shows how these factors are related.

Heredity Skill-related fitness abilities are influenced by heredity. For example, some people are able to run

fast or react quickly because they inherited these traits from their parents. A person who did not inherit a tendency to excel in these areas may have more difficulty performing skills that require those abilities. Improving your skills is always possible, and often extra practice and desire make up for lack of "natural" ability.

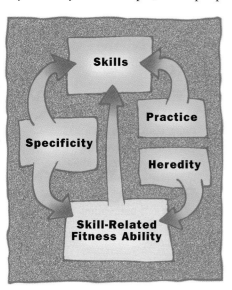

Practice Anyone can learn the skills required for sports, games, and other lifetime activities. **Practice**—repeating a skill over and over—is the key! If you repeat a skill such as a tennis serve and do

it correctly, you will become better at that skill. You probably will learn the skill faster if you have good skill-related fitness in an area such as coordination. While everyone cannot become an Olympic athlete, with practice everyone can learn the basic skills necessary to enjoy some sports and to perform physical tasks efficiently. Learning about your own skill-related abilities can help you choose a sport or activity in which you are more likely to succeed.

Principle of Specificity The principle of specificity applies to all parts of skill-related fitness and to physical skills. Just because you excel in one part of skill-related fitness, you will not necessarily excel in other parts. This is often the case even when abilities seem closely related, such as reaction time and speed. For example, you might have great speed, which helps you run fast, but also lack good reaction time, which prevents you from getting a good start. Apply the principle of specificity to choose a sport or activity that

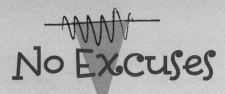

No Excuses

Improving Self-Perception

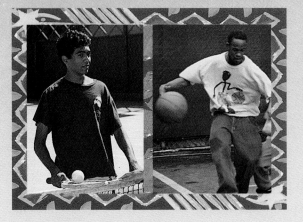

Self-perception is the awareness you have about your own thoughts, actions, or appearance. It is how you think other people view you. Four areas of physical self-perceptions are strength, fitness, skill, and body attractiveness.

Michael wasn't sure that he wanted to go back to school after the summer break. It seemed as if all of his friends had grown several inches taller in the last few months, and he had stayed the same height. Michael felt embarrassed and a little jealous, even though none of his friends seemed to notice. His height certainly didn't alter his ability to play tennis. In fact, friends still called him "King of the Court" because he usually won the match whenever he played.

Raul was one of the shortest in his class, but height didn't stop him from being involved in activities. He realized he'd never be a great basketball player, but

he still liked to play with his friends from school. He discovered that height had nothing to do with his ability to go hiking, and it didn't prevent him from being a good wrestler.

All people have a mental picture of themselves. If you think you do well in a certain activity, you will probably take part in that activity. If you feel embarrassed about your appearance or ability level while doing an activity, you probably will avoid that activity.

For Discussion

Michael's self-perception about his appearance has changed from positive to negative. What can he do to change his negative perception? How does Raul keep a positive self-perception? What else can a person do to develop a positive self-perception? Fill out the questionnaire to find out about your own self-perception.

requires the specific skill-related fitness abilities you perform best.

The principle of specificity also tells you that once you choose an activity or sport that you would like to learn, it is best to practice the specific skills of that activity. With practice you may be able to make some improvement in skill-related fitness, but it is best to use practice time on the skills of the activities in which you want to improve.

Assessing Skill-Related Fitness

A good first step for a person interested in learning a lifetime sport or physical activity is the assessment of skill-related fitness abilities. Assessing each of the abilities can help you identify those you have that will help you succeed in a particular activity. As you perform skill-related fitness assignments, you should be aware

that skill-related fitness has many different subparts. For example, coordination is a skill-related ability that includes hand-eye coordination—the ability to use the hands and eyes together as in hitting a ball—or foot-eye coordination—the ability to use the eyes and feet together as in kicking a ball.

Lesson Review
1. What are some examples of physical skills?
2. How do skill-related fitness abilities differ from physical skills?
3. List and explain three factors that affect skill-related fitness and skills.
4. Why is assessing personal skill-related fitness important?

Balance, Coordination, and Reaction Time

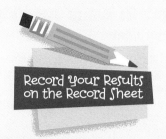

Record Your Results on the Record Sheet

Use these stunts to assess your skill-related fitness abilities in the areas of balance, coordination, and reaction time. You will learn to assess the other parts of skill-related physical fitness in Chapter 12. Keep these points in mind, especially if you score low:

- You can improve all parts of your skill-related fitness.

- Many activities do not require high levels of these abilities.

- You don't need to excel in an activity or sport to enjoy it.

- Many subparts of skill-related fitness are not included in these stunts. You may excel in some of these other subparts. Ask your teacher to help you find stunts to test more specific abilities not measured by these stunts.

Part 1: Stick Balance (Balance)

You may take one practice try before doing each stunt for a score.

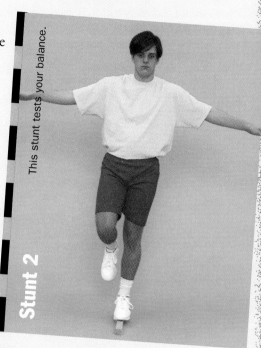

This stunt tests your balance.

Stunt 2

Stunt 1

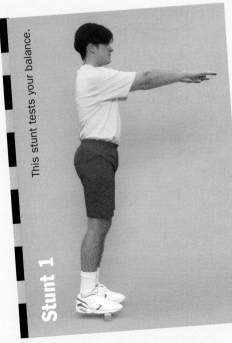

This stunt tests your balance.

Stunt 1

1 Place the balls of both feet across a stick so that your heels are on the floor.

2 Lift your heels off the floor and maintain your balance on the stick for 15 seconds. Hold your arms out in front of you for balance. Do not allow your heels to touch the floor or your feet to move on the stick once you begin. *Hint:* Focus your eyes on a stationary object in front of you.

3 Try the stunt twice. Give yourself 2 points if you are successful on the first try, 1 point if you failed on the first try but succeeded on the second, and 3 points if you were successful on both tries. Try Stunt 2 even if you did not do well on Stunt 1.

Stunt 2

1 Stand on a stick with either foot. Your foot should run the length of the stick.

2 Lift your other foot off the floor. First, balance for 10 seconds with your foot flat. Then rise up on your toes and continue balancing for 10 seconds. *Hint:* Balance on your dominant leg—the one you balance on when you kick a ball.

3 Try the stunt twice. Give yourself 1 point if you balanced for 10 seconds flat-footed, and another point if you balanced on your toes for 10 seconds. Give yourself another point if you successfully balanced both flat-footed and standing on your toes. Your maximum score is 3 points.

Part 2: Wand Juggling
(Coordination)

1 Take three practice tries before doing this stunt for a score. Hold a stick in each hand. Have a partner place a third stick across your sticks.

2 Toss the third stick in the air so that it makes a half turn. Catch it with the sticks you are holding. The tossed stick should not hit your hands.

3 Do this 5 times, tossing the stick to the right, and 5 times tossing it to the left. Score 1 point for each successful catch. *Hint*: Absorb the shock of the catch by "giving" with the held sticks, as you might do when catching an egg or something breakable.

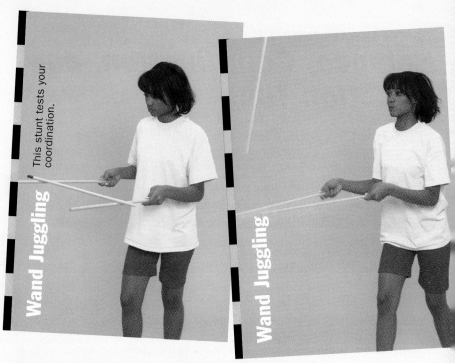

This stunt tests your coordination.

Wand Juggling

Wand Juggling

Part 3: Yardstick Drop
(Reaction Time)

1 You will need a partner for this stunt. Have your partner hold the top of a yardstick with his or her thumb and index finger between the 1-inch mark and the end of the yardstick.

2 Position your thumb and fingers at the 24-inch mark on the yardstick. Your thumb and fingers should *not* touch the yardstick. Your arm should rest on the edge of a table with only your hand over the edge.

3 When your partner drops the stick without warning, catch it as quickly as possible between your thumb and fingers. *Hint:* Focus on the stick, not your partner, and be very alert.

4 Try this stunt 3 times. Your score is the number on the yardstick at the place where you caught it. Record your scores. Your partner should be careful not to drop the yardstick after the same waiting period each time. You should not be able to guess when the yardstick will drop. To get your rating, use the middle score (midpoint between your lowest and highest score).

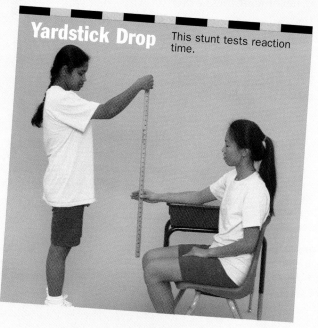

Yardstick Drop — This stunt tests reaction time.

Scoring and Rating

Record your individual scores on your record sheet. Then follow the instructions for each stunt to find your fitness rating.

Rating Chart: Balance, Coordination, and Reaction Time

Performance Rating	Stick Balance	Wand Juggling	Yardstick Drop
High Performance	6	9 to 10	more than 21 inches
Good Fitness	5	7 to 8	19 to 21 inches
Marginal Fitness	3 to 4	4 to 6	14 to 18 inches
Low Fitness	less than 3	less than 4	less than 14 inches

11.2 Choosing a Lifetime Activity

Lesson

Lesson Objectives

After reading this lesson, you should be able to:
1. Develop a personal skill-related fitness profile as a basis for selecting personal lifetime activities.
2. Discuss the guidelines for selecting lifetime activities.
3. List some suggestions for improving sports skills.

Lesson Vocabulary

Once you have assessed your skill-related fitness abilities, you can develop a profile of your results which will help you in selecting lifetime activities and sports. In this lesson you will learn how to use a profile to select lifetime activities and make plans for becoming proficient in those activities.

Developing a Skill-Related Fitness Profile

One student, Sue, did all of the skill-related physical fitness assessments in this chapter and in Chapter 12. You can see the chart she developed to profile her skill-related fitness below. Sue's chart helped her identify her strengths and weaknesses. Sue used her chart to develop her fitness program.

Sue's Skill-Related Fitness Profile

Fitness Part	Skill-Related Performance Rating			
	Low	Marginal	Good	High
Agility				X
Balance		X		
Coordination			X	
Power		X		
Speed		X		
Reaction Time	X			

You can see that Sue has better abilities in some parts of fitness than in others. One way she can use her profile is to see how she can improve her skill-related fitness in areas in which she didn't do so well. She can use the chart on the next page to identify activites that provide the most benefits for each part of skill-related fitness.

The second way Sue can use her profile is to find physical activity that is suited to her abilities. Activities that give the most benefits in a specific part of skill-related finess will also require the greatest amount of fitness in that part. Sue did not do well in power, so she decided to take karate lessons to help her improve. She also didn't do well in speed and reaction time but realized that, because of heredity, she probably would not be a a really fast person with good reaction time. Still, she thought that karate might help these abilities some. She also decided not to worry if she wasn't as able as other people in these parts of fitness.

Sue decided to use her profile to help her choose other activites that would be easier to learn. Since she scored well in coordination, Sue selected bowling because an activity that benefits a certain part of fitness also requires good skill in that part. Since bowling is excellent for building coordination, it is also an activity in which a person with good coordination is likely to succeed.

Sue selected bicycling as another activity she would include in her activity program because it did not require high amounts of skill-related fitness, did not require her to learn new skills, but did have a lot of health benefits.

You can develop your own skill-related fitness profile using a chart similar to the one Sue used. Use your profile to determine which activities might help you improve where you need it and which activities will be the ones you can most easily learn.

Skill-Related Benefits of Sports and Other Activities

Activity	Balance	Coordination	Reaction Time	Agility	Power	Speed
Badminton	Fair	Excellent	Good	Good	Fair	Good
Baseball	Good	Excellent	Excellent	Good	Excellent	Good
Basketball	Good	Excellent	Excellent	Excellent	Excellent	Good
Bicycling	Excellent	Fair	Fair	Fair	Poor	Fair
Bowling	Good	Excellent	Poor	Fair	Poor	Fair
Circuit Training	Fair	Fair	Poor	Fair	Good	Fair
Dance, Aerobic/Social	Fair	Good	Fair	Good	Poor	Poor
Dance, Ballet/Modern	Excellent	Excellent	Fair	Excellent	Good	Poor
Fitness Calisthenics	Fair	Fair	Poor	Good	Fair	Poor
Football	Good	Good	Excellent	Excellent	Good	Excellent
Golf (walking)	Fair	Excellent	Poor	Fair	Good	Poor
Gymnastics	Excellent	Excellent	Good	Excellent	Excellent	Fair
Interval Training	Fair	Fair	Poor	Poor	Poor	Fair
Jogging/Walking	Poor	Poor	Poor	Poor	Poor	Poor
Judo/Karate	Good	Excellent	Excellent	Excellent	Excellent	Excellent
Racquetball/Handball	Fair	Excellent	Good	Excellent	Fair	Good
Rope Jumping	Fair	Good	Fair	Good	Fair	Poor
Skating, Ice/Roller	Excellent	Good	Fair	Good	Fair	Good
Skiing, Cross-Country	Fair	Excellent	Poor	Good	Excellent	Fair
Skiing, Downhill	Excellent	Excellent	Good	Excellent	Good	Poor
Soccer	Fair	Excellent	Good	Excellent	Good	Good
Softball (fast pitch)	Fair	Excellent	Excellent	Good	Good	Good
Swimming (laps)	Poor	Good	Poor	Good	Fair	Poor
Tennis	Fair	Excellent	Good	Good	Good	Good
Volleyball	Fair	Excellent	Good	Good	Fair	Fair
Weight Training	Fair	Fair	Poor	Poor	Good	Poor

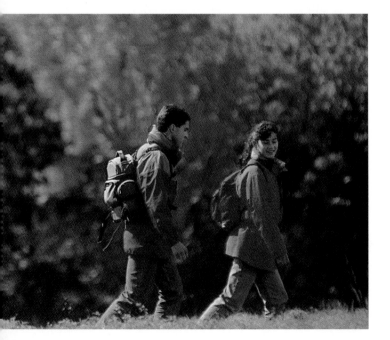

Hiking requires little skill but has many health-related benefits.

Other Guidelines for Activity Selection

Your level of skill-related physical fitness should not be the only basis for making your selection of activities. What other factors should you consider?

• **Your health-related fitness** How well you do in an activity depends on all parts of fitness, health-related as well as skill related. Choose activities that match your abilities in both kinds of fitness.

• **Your interests** If there is an activity that you really enjoy or always wanted to do, don't avoid it just because it doesn't match your fitness profile. However, be aware that it may take you longer than others to learn the activity even with practice. Consider doing the activity with others of your own ability so that you won't be discouraged if you do not learn the activity as quickly as you would like.

• **The benefits of the activity** Sue found that bowling matched her abilities. Bowling is a fun activity in which she could probably do well with practice. But bowling is not a great activity for promoting health and wellness benefits. Sue would probably be wise to select at least one other activity that is good for health-related fitness.

• **Some activities do not require high levels of any part of skill-related fitness.** Of activities in the Physical Activity Pyramid, sports provide the most benefits to skill-related fitness, but they also require relatively high levels of it. In addition to skill-related finess, most sports require considerable skill, so they will require a lot of practice if you are to perform them well. Lifestyle, aerobic, strength/muscular endurance, and flexibility activities generally require fewer skills. Even people with relatively low scores on most or all parts of skill-related fitness can find a life-time activity. Jogging, walking, cycling, and hiking are only a few of these activities. Because they also do not require many skills, extensive practice is not necessary to perform them. You may want to consider one of these activities if you are not willing to take the time necessary to learn more complicated activities. Sue chose to do biking in addition to bowling because it was something that she could easily learn and it met many of her needs.

In the next Chapter you'll learn more about which sports and activities are best for improving the various parts of health-related physical fitness. Sue will wait until she has considered this information before she makes her final decisions about which lifetime activities she will select. In the meantime, she can continue to work on improving her skills in bowling, biking, and other sports and activities she is considering.

Learning Sports Skills

Many sports require practice of more than a few skills if you are to become proficient. For example, the basketball players in the photo must practice shooting, dribbling, passing, catching, and defensive skills. Use these suggestions to improve your sports skills:

• **Get correct instruction.** If you learn a skill incorrectly, it will be hard to improve, even with practice.

• **At first do not worry about details.** When you first learn a skill, concentrate on the skill as a whole. Details can be dealt with after the main skill is learned.

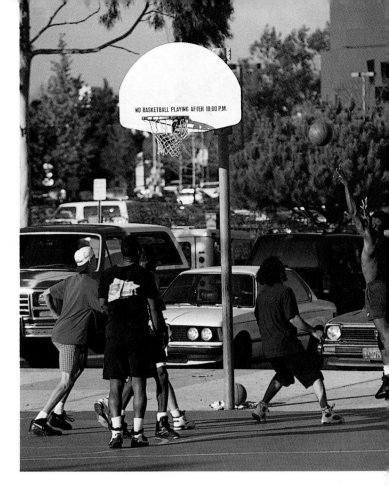

Basketball requires practice of several skills.

• **Keep practicing.** Many people don't like to practice skills; they just want to "play the game." However, just playing the game doesn't provide practice for a particular skill. Also, when you play a game without having the proper skills, you often develop bad habits that hinder your success and enjoyment of the game.

• **Avoid competition when learning a skill.** While competition can be fun, competing when you are learning a skill is stressful and does not promote optimal learning.

• **Choose an activity that matches your skill-related fitness.** Learn an activity that uses the parts of skill-related fitness that you possess.

Lesson Review
1. How can you develop a personal fitness profile?
2. What are four guidelines for selecting lifetime activities?
3. How can you improve sports skills?

Activity 11
Elastic Band Exercises

In previous chapters you learned about various types of resistance training. Another less expensive way of providing resistance for building strength and muscular endurance is by doing elastic band exercise. In this type of exercise, elastic bands are used to provide overload to the muscles. The first people to use elastic band exercises used old bicycle inner tubes or pieces of surgical tubing. You might try using these yourself. The size and thickness of the band you use will depend on your current fitness level.

In this activity you will get the opportunity to try several elastic band exercises and to develop some of your own.

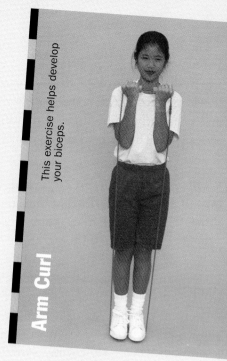
This exercise helps develop your biceps.

Arm Curl

Two-Leg Press

1 Loop the band under the ball of your feet with the ends held with your hands.

2 Begin with your knees near your chest. Press out with your legs against the band to straighten your legs.

3 Return to the starting position. Repeat 7–10 times. Do 1–3 sets.

Arm Curl

1 Loop the band under your feet.

2 With your palms facing up, pull your hands to your chest. Keep your elbows against your sides.

3 Return to the starting position. Complete 7–10 repetitions. Do 1–3 sets.

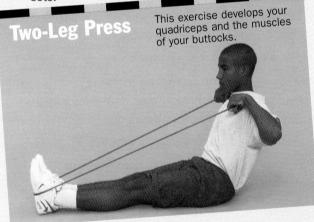
Two-Leg Press
This exercise develops your quadriceps and the muscles of your buttocks.

Upward Row

1 Loop the band under your feet.

2 Hold the band with both hands, your palms facing you. Gradually pull up on the band, keeping your elbows high. Pull until your hands reach your chin or as far as you can pull.

3 Lower your hands to the starting position. Complete 7–10 repetitions. Do 1–3 sets.

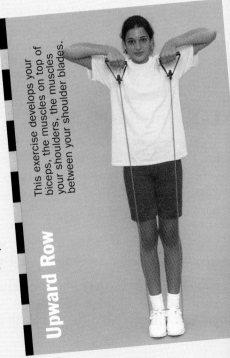
This exercise develops your biceps, the muscles on top of your shoulders, the muscles between your shoulder blades.

Upward Row

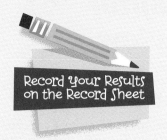

Leg Curl (Prone)

1 Loop the band behind one heel.

2 Have a partner stand on the ends of the bands.

3 Pull backward on the band with your heel until your leg is bent at a 90-degree angle.

4 Repeat with your other leg. Complete 7–10 repetitions with each leg. Do 1–3 sets.

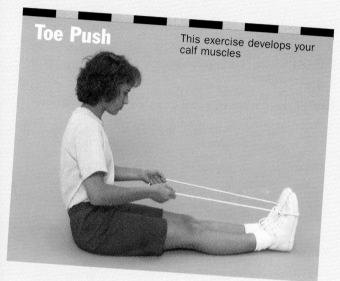

Toe Push

This exercise develops your calf muscles

Toe Push

1 Loop the band under your toes. Hold the ends with your hands.

2 Push with your feet by pointing your toes against the band.

3 Return to the starting position. Repeat 7–10 times. Do 1–3 sets. You might hold the band closer to your feet to make the exercise more difficult.

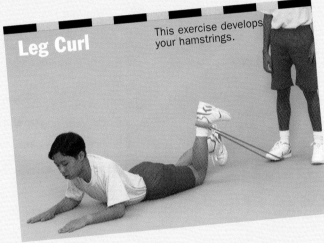

Leg Curl

This exercise develops your hamstrings.

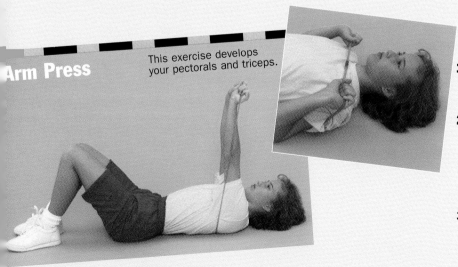

Arm Press

This exercise develops your pectorals and triceps.

Arm Press

1 Loop the band under your back and hold the ends with your hands.

2 With your arms bent, press up against the band. Return to the starting position. You can hold your hand closer to your shoulders to make the activity more difficult.

3 Repeat 7–10 times. Complete 1–3 sets.

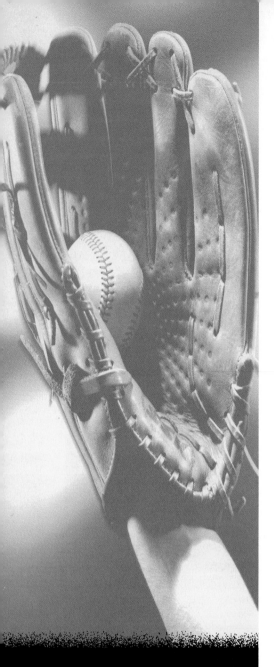

11 Chapter Review

Reviewing Concepts and Vocabulary

Copy the number of each statement on a sheet of paper. Next to each number, write the word or words that correctly complete the sentence.

1. Of the activities in the Physical Activity Pyramid, _____ generally require the most skills.

2. A good first step for a person interested in learning a lifetime physical activity is to _____.

3. Specific physical skills can best be improved by _____.

Number your paper. Next to each number, choose the letter of the best answer.

Column I	Column II
4. skill-related fitness abilities	a. repeating a skill over and over
5. physical skills	b. agility, balance, speed
6. practice	c. catching, batting, dancing

On your paper, write a short answer for each statement or question.

7. What factors affect skill-related fitness and how does each affect it?

8. How do skill-related abilities differ from physical skills?

9. How can developing a skill-related fitness profile help you choose recreational activities?

10. What are some guidelines for improving sports skills?

Thinking Critically

Write a paragraph to answer the following question.

You might be interested in a particular activity that you would like to consider for your lifetime fitness program. What factors should you consider before you make a final decision?

Project

Survey local schools in your area. What lifetime sports and physical activities do they teach? Which sports or activities are the most popular? Which are the least popular? What are some sports or activities that are not taught that students would like to learn? How might you encourage change in the sports curriculum in your school?

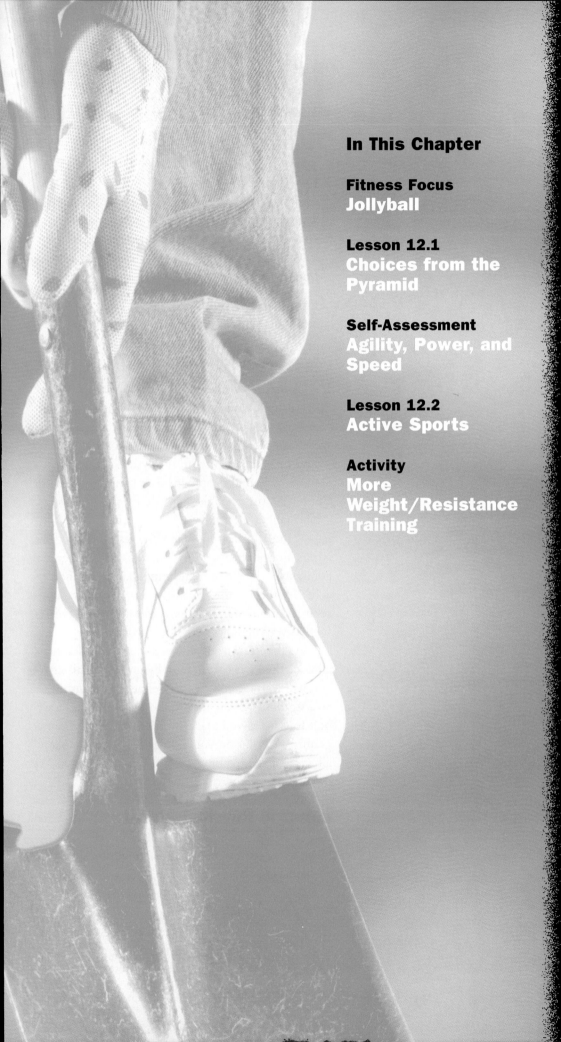

12

Activities for Health-Related Fitness

Jollyball

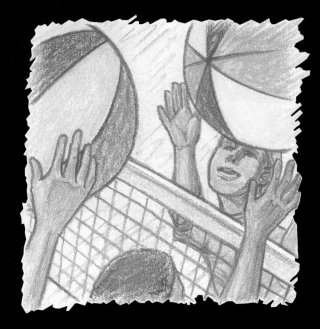

In planning your lifetime physical activity program, you might want to include some sports but feel that you lack the necessary skills. Many people avoid participation in sports for the same reason. However, some sports can be modified to make them more fun for everyone regardless of skill level. For example, jollyball is the name given to several different modifications of volleyball that may make the sport more fun for everyone. Your instruction sheet will show you how to play some jollyball activities.

Keep It Moving
All Touch
No Look Jollyball
Sitting Jollyball
Two Ball Volley

12.1 Lesson — Choices from the Pyramid

Lesson Objectives
After reading this lesson, you should be able to:
1. Describe different types of activities within each area of the Physical Activity Pyramid.
2. Discuss some guidelines for choosing activities from the pyramid.

Lesson Vocabulary
orienteering, parcourse, interval training

If you surveyed students in your school, what percent do you think would indicate they regularly participate in sports and games? Although the figure might vary from school to school, chances are the percent would be high because most physical activity performed by young people involves sports or games. But by the time people graduate from school, sports are no longer their most popular activities. In fact, few of the 10 most popular activities performed by adults are sports. The most popular activities among adults include strength and muscular endurance activities such as home calisthenics, aerobic activities such as home exercise videos, and lifestyle activities such as walking or working in the yard.

In Chapter 2 you learned about the different areas of the Physical Activity Pyramid. In this chapter you will learn about a variety of activities within each area so that you can choose those activities that are best for you as you plan your personal fitness program. In this lesson you will learn about choices in all areas of the pyramid except sports, which will be discussed in the next lesson.

Lifestyle Physical Activity

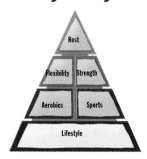

Chances are you already do some physical activities as part of your daily routine. For example, you might walk or ride a bicycle to get to school. In that case, biking and walking can be lifestyle physical activity. When you do activity as part of your daily routine, you are doing lifestyle physical activity.

To gain health and wellness benefits you should do lifestyle activities almost daily. Doing lifestyle activities has a double benefit—you improve fitness while at the same time accomplishing something that has to be done. For example, if you ride your bike to school, you get to school but you also improve your fitness.

Recent evidence suggests that doing lifestyle physical activity is something that you can easily make a habit. Once you form the habit, you are active on a more consistent basis. Some of the most common lifestyle activities are described below.

Bicycling Recreational bicycling is one of the most popular activities for developing and maintaining fitness. To be most effective in building fitness, bicycling should be done at least at moderate intensity.

Walking The American College of Sports Medicine and the United States Centers for Disease Control and Prevention use the example of brisk walking for 30 minutes on most days of the week as an example of how much physical activity is necessary to reduce risk factors. Additional walking—either by walking longer

Have you Heard?

Running speed has little to do with the number of Calories a person burns. Whether you run a mile in eight minutes or in twelve minutes, you will burn approximately the same number of Calories.

or more frequently—has additional health benefits. Even shorter and less vigorous walks can be useful as part of a total physical activity program.

Gardening Gardening is most likely to have an impact on health-related fitness when it involves shoveling, hoeing, and similar more vigorous activities.

Housework Housework such as dusting and light cleaning is probably of little value to health-related fitness. More vigorous activities such as moving furniture no doubt have some benefits and are good if done in combination with other more vigorous types of activity.

Stair Climbing Walking the stairs rather than riding the elevators can contribute to good physical fitness.

Yard Work Shoveling snow or mowing the lawn with a push mower is activity that is beneficial to health. Other less vigorous yard work is better than doing no physical activity at all. The teens in the photo are getting health benefits as they rake leaves.

Aerobic Activity

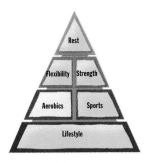

Aerobic activities are among the most popular and the most beneficial of all activities in the Physical Activity Pyramid. Some reasons for the popularity include:
• They often do not require high levels of skill.
• They frequently are not competitive.
• They often can be done at home or near home.
• They often do not require a partner or a group.

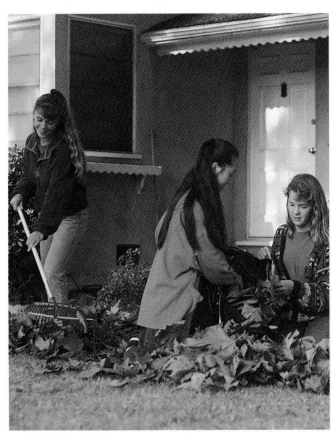

Yard work is a lifestyle physical activity.

Virtually all of the health and wellness benefits described in Chapter 5 can be achieved by performing appropriate amounts of aerobic activity. The benefits of the activity depend on how it is done. In the past some people have felt that for an activity to be aerobic it must be done at a high heart rate. It's true that there are benefits to aerobic activities that follow the FIT formula for increasing heart rate. However, it's also true that an accumulation of Calories expended in activity can result in health and wellness benefits.

Walking, biking, and most other lifestyle activities are aerobic in nature. Aerobic activities not described as lifestyle activities earlier are described below.

Hiking and Backpacking Hiking is a particularly enjoyable activity because it is an outdoor activity that can be done independently or in groups. Most county, state, and national parks have a wide variety of scenic trails for hikers of all levels of experience.

While hiking is usually a one-day trip, backpacking is often a several-day venture. Food, shelter, and other supplies are carried in a pack on your back.

Rope Jumping You did a jump-rope workout in the Fitness Focus in Chapter 6. If people have the fitness to do it continuously—or even in short bouts alternated with rest—jump rope can be a good form of aerobic activity. For some low-fit people, rope jumping can't be done for more than a short period of time, so it may not be effective.

Orienteering Orienteering combines walking, jogging, and map-reading skills. It is usually done in a rural area and might include hiking through rugged terrain. One participant departs from a starting point every few minutes so that he or she cannot follow the person ahead. Each participant has a compass and a map that describes a course from one to ten miles. The compass is used to help locate several checkpoints that are marked by flags or other identification. At each checkpoint the participant marks

a card to indicate that the checkpoint has been located. The goal of each participant is to cover the course in as little time as possible.

Dance Since dance is one of the oldest art forms, it has always been a means of expression by many cultures. Some forms of dance are not only enjoyable but also excellent forms of exercise. Modern dance builds health-related fitness. Ballet develops strength and flexibility. Folk dancing, square dancing, and social dance contribute to cardiovascular fitness as well as skill-related fitness.

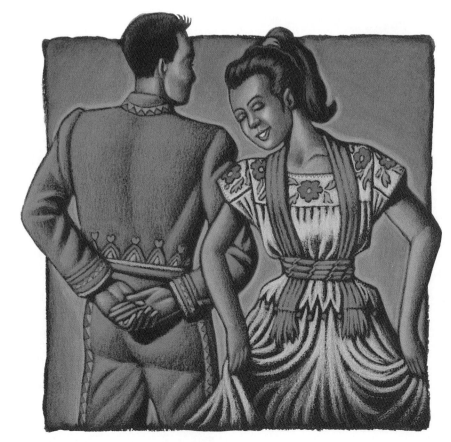

Dance is a form of aerobic activity.

Water Aerobics Water aerobics, also called aqua-dynamics, involves doing calisthenics or dance steps in a swimming pool. This form of aerobic exercise is especially good for people who are overweight, older people, and people with arthritis or other joint problems. The water prevents the exercises from causing stress on the joints. Water also can offer resistance and increase the intensity of exercise for the able-bodied.

Skating Three kinds of skating—ice, roller, and in-line—are aerobic activities. However, skating can also be a competitive sport. Skating is part of the Olympic games, and for Olympic athletes skating is quite competitive. Some people participate in sports such as ice hockey and roller hockey. The teens in the photo are inline skating, one of the fastest growing of all activities.

Other Programs Cooper's aerobics, cycling, swimming, jogging, running, and walking are among other aerobic activities. Information on Cooper's aerobics, aerobic dance, and jogging can be found elsewhere in this book.

Exercise for Strength and Muscular Endurance

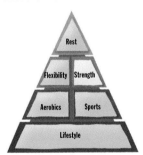

In Chapters 8 and 9 you learned about many of the activities included in the strength/muscular endurance section of the Physical Activity Pyramid. Some sports build strength and muscular endurance as do some lifestyle physical activities. For most people, however, it is necessary to perform special calisthenics or resistance training exercises to build these parts of fitness. Calisthenics and resistance training are discussed in Chapters 8 and 9.

Exercise for Flexibility

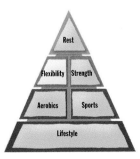

Like strength and muscular endurance, flexibility can be developed in sports such as gymnastics. Unlike other parts of fitness, flexibility is not developed in many other activities. Exercises such as static,

ballistic, and PNF stretching described in Chapter 10 are the best method of developing flexibility. Calisthenics are an appropriate form of flexibility exercise when planned specifically for building flexibility. Exercise circuits often contain activities for developing flexibility.

Other Types of Physical Activity

The Physical Activity Pyramid is one way of classifying various types of physical activity. It helps you understand the differences in types and the advantages and disadvantages of each. But all activities do not fit easily into the pyramid. For example, anaerobic activities are not easily placed in the pyramid.

Some activities are a combination of several different types of activities. The continuous rhythmical exercise program that you did in the Fitness Focus in Chapter 3 is an example of one combination of activities. Other examples are the exercise circuits that you read about in Chapters 4 and 8.

Parcourse and interval training are two other combination activities. A **parcourse** usually has 10 to 20 outdoor exercise stations located at least 100 yards apart. Simple exercise equipment is located at each station along with a sign suggesting the number of repetitions for each exercise. **Interval training** involves alternating several short bursts of high-intensity exercise with a rest period. The exercise and rest periods are of preplanned length and speed.

Inline skating is one of the fastest growing activities.

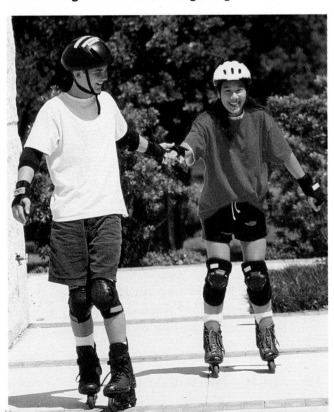

Health-Related Benefits of Exercise Programs

	Develops Cardiovascular Fitness	Develops Strength	Develops Muscular Endurance	Develops Flexibility	Helps Control Body Fatness
Lifestyle Activities					
Bicycling •	excellent	fair	good	poor	excellent
Walking •	good	good	fair	poor	good
Aerobic Activities					
Aerobic Dance •*	excellent	fair	good	good	excellent
Calisthenics •	poor	fair/good	good/excellent	excellent	poor
Circuit Training •	fair	good	excellent	good	fair
Continuous Rhythmical Exercise •	excellent	fair	excellent	good	excellent
Cooper's Aerobics •	excellent	fair	good	poor	excellent
Dance					
Ballet *	fair/good	good	good	excellent	fair/good
Modern *	fair/good	fair	good	excellent	fair/good
Social •	fair/good	poor	fair	fair	fair/good
Hiking/Backpacking •*	good	fair/good	excellent	fair	good
Interval Training •*	excellent	fair	good	poor	excellent
Orienteering	excellent	poor	good	poor	excellent
Parcourse *	good	good	excellent	good	good
Rope Jumping •	good	poor	good	poor	good
Skating					
Ice •*	fair/good	poor	good	poor	fair/good
Inline •*	good/excellent	poor	good/excellent	poor	good/excellent
Roller •*	fair/good	poor	fair	poor	fair/good
Swimiming	excellent	fair	good	fair	excellent
Water Aerobics •	good	fair	good	fair	good
Weight Training•	poor	excellent	good	poor	fair

• Denotes lifetime activity.
* Denotes fitness needed to prevent injury.

Inactivity or Rest

The small area at the top of the Physical Activity Pyramid is inactivity or rest. Whereas activity is something that is encouraged on a regular basis, inactivity is generally discouraged. But if you do regular activity, taking some of your free time to read, listen to music, or just relax is not bad. Inactivity becomes a problem when time spent being inactive keeps you from doing enough activity to become fit and healthy. Consider some inactivity as a normal part of healthy living for those who do enough physical activity for good fitness, health, and wellness. Consider inactivity a problem when it becomes a major part of a person's life.

Choosing a Physical Activity

As you evaluate activities for developing your physical activity program, consider the benefits each activity provides. The above chart summarizes some of the benefits. Also, consider these guidelines.

• **Individualize.** Planned programs are especially likely to contain exercises that are not good for everyone. If another person plans a program that you use, be sure the program meets your personal needs.

• **Avoid risky exercises.** Recall the risky exercises described in Chapter 2. Some exercise programs described in popular magazines and in videos might

No Excuses

Choosing a Good Activity

You can help yourself be active by choosing activities you are likely to do both now and throughout your life. One way to evaluate a physical activity is to find out the number of people who participate and how long they stay involved.

At a recent high school reunion, the alumni enjoyed seeing their former classmates again. Everyone remembered Norma as an active participant in sports. She played soccer, basketball, and softball. What a surprise when her classmates discovered ten years later that Norma did very little physical activity! The closest she got to participating in any sport was to watch her son's T-ball games. According to Norma, "It was too hard to find people who wanted to play the team sports I once enjoyed."

Kim Lee was the opposite of Norma. In high school she'd always go to the games and cheer for the teams, but she never dreamed of taking part in a sport. Kim

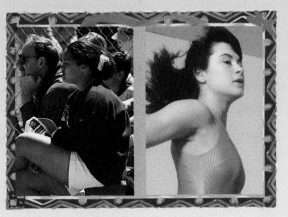

would be the first to admit that she was the original "couch potato." Now Kim goes biking with her two children. She also organizes the neighborhood aerobics class. "Every Tuesday and Thursday morning we all get together and talk while we work out. No one cares how we dress or how good we are at doing the exercises, and we all seem to be energized as we go on to our next activities."

For Discussion

Why was it no longer feasible for Norma to continue participating in the same sports she played in high school? What might help her get involved in a physical activity again? Why do you think Kim Lee started to participate in activities? Fill out the questionnaire to find out what factors determine the popularity of an activity.

contain dangerous exercises. Be sure to avoid doing these risky exercises.

• **Consider more than one activity.** If you typically only do one form of activity, you have nothing to fall back on if you can't do that activity for some reason. Including at least one lifestyle activity would ensure activity even when your free time is limited. Different activities build different parts of fitness; selecting more than one activity will help build all parts of fitness.

• **Alternate muscle groups from one exercise to another.** Avoid performing consecutive exercises that work the same muscles. For example, if you use your arms in one exercise, your next exercise should work a different muscle group, such as your legs.

• **Select activities that complement sports.** Bowling is one of the most popular participation sports, but it

is one of the least beneficial in building health-related fitness. If you bowl or do some other less active sport, consider also doing other more vigorous activities.

• **Have fun.** This book emphasizes the importance of choosing activities that contribute to fitness, health, and wellness. But remember—physical activity can be FUN! It's OK to do an activity just because it's an enjoyable way to spend your time.

Lesson Review

1. Give at least two examples of activities for each area of the Physical Activity Pyramid.
2. What are six guidelines for choosing activities from the Physical Activity Pyramid?

Agility, Power, and Speed

In Chapter 11 you assessed your skill-related fitness in the areas of balance, coordination and reaction time. Use this self-assessment to evaluate your agility, power, and speed.

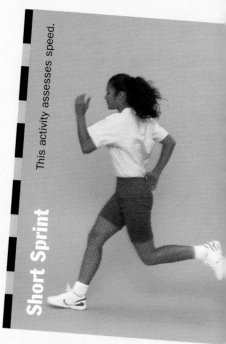

This activity assesses speed.

Short Sprint

Side Shuttle
(Agility)

Use masking tape or other materials to make five parallel lines on the floor, each 3 feet apart. Have a partner count while you do the side shuttle. Then count while your partner does it.

1 Stand with the first line to your right. When your partner says "go," slide to the right until your right foot steps over the last line. Then slide to the left until your left foot steps over the first line. *Note:* Be careful not to cross your feet.

2 Repeat, moving from side to side as many times as possible in 10 seconds. Only one foot must cross the outside lines.

3 When your partner says "stop," freeze in place until your partner counts your score. Score 1 point for each line you crossed in 10 seconds. Subtract 1 point for each time you crossed your feet.

4 Do the side shuttle twice. Record the better of your two scores on your record sheet.

Short Sprint
(Speed)

Use masking tape or other material to make lines two yards apart starting 10 yards from the starting line for a total distance of 26 yards. Work with a partner who will time you and blow a whistle to signal you to stop.

Try this once for practice without being timed; then try it for a score. Record your score on your record sheet.

1 Stand 2 or 3 steps behind the starting line.

2 When your partner says "go," run as far and as fast as you can. Your partner will start a stopwatch when you cross the starting line. Then your partner will blow the whistle 3 seconds later. Do not try to stop immediately, but begin to slow down after the whistle blows.

3 Your partner should mark where you were when the 3-second whistle blew. Measure the distance to the nearest yard line. Your score is the distance you covered in the 3 seconds after crossing the starting line.

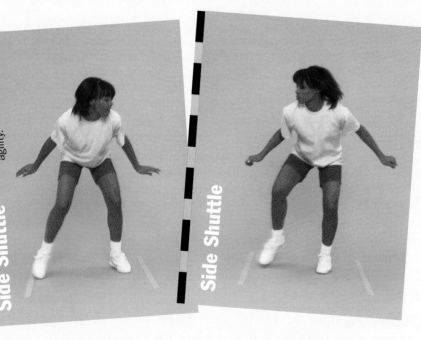

This activity assesses agility.

Side Shuttle

Side Shuttle

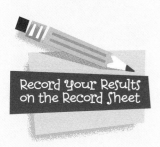

Record your Results on the Record Sheet

Standing Long Jump
(Power)

Use masking tape or other materials to make a line on the floor.

1 Stand with both feet behind the line on the floor. Swing your arms forward, and jump as far as possible. Keep both feet together. Do not run or hop before jumping.

2 Have a partner measure the distance from the line to the nearest point where any part of your body touched the floor when you landed.

3 Do this stunt twice. Record the better of your two scores on your record sheet.

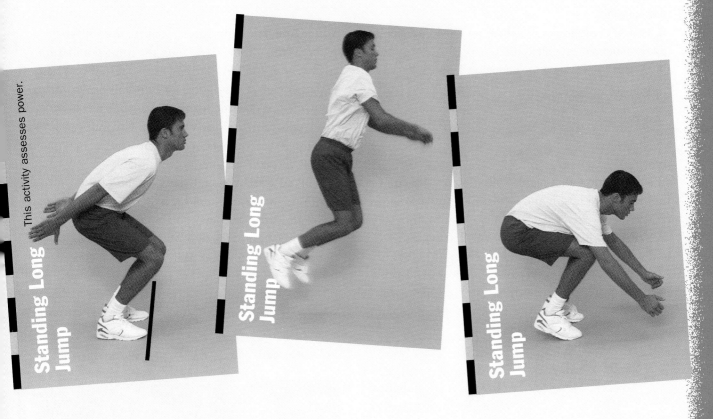

This activity assesses power.

Standing Long Jump

Standing Long Jump

Standing Long Jump

Scoring and Rating

After recording your individual scores on your record sheet, find your scores on the rating chart. Record your ratings.

Rating Chart: Agility, Power and Speed

	Agility (lines crossed)		Power (inches jumped)		Speed (yards run)	
	males	females	males	females	males	females
High Performance	31 or more	28 or more	87 or more	74 or more	24 or more	22 or more
Good Fitness	26–30	24–27	80–86 in.	66–73 in.	21–23 yds	19–21 yds
Marginal Fitness	19–25	15–23	70–79	58–65	16–20	15–18
Low Fitness	less than 19	less than 15	less than 70	less than 58	less than 16	less than 15

12.2 Active Sports

Lesson Objectives

After reading this lesson, you should be able to:
1. Identify four categories of sports.
2. Explain why fitness is important to sports participants.
3. Identify categories of sports for which participants must be especially fit.
4. Discuss guidelines for choosing a sport.

Lesson Vocabulary
sports

You already know that regular physical activity contributes to good health and well-being. You also know that no one activity or set of exercises is best for everyone. An individual's choice of physical activities is based on such factors as age, skill-related fitness abilities, skills, interests, and personal fitness goals. In this lesson you will learn about the many kinds of sports and their benefits. As you read this lesson, think about the sports you think are best for you.

Sports of Many Kinds

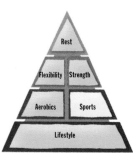

Active sports are activities from the Physical Activity Pyramid that generally are done competitively and have rules that are well established. Typically, winners and losers are determined in sports based on a score or outcome. There are so many different sports that it is impossible to mention them all.

Generally sports are grouped into several categories: team sports, dual sports, individual sports, and outdoor challenge sports. Other sports will not be considered here because they are not among the most popular or because they have little importance to the personal physical activity program of the typical person. Examples include motor sports (car racing), and racing (dogs and horses).

Have you Heard?

Dr. James Naismith invented basketball in 1891 as an indoor exercise for his physical education class. A soccer ball was used for the first basketball game.

Team Sports Team sports, such as the volleyball game in the photo, are among the most popular for high school students and for adult spectators. These activities can be very good for building fitness for participants but do little for the fitness of spectators. Team sports are hard to do after the school years because they require other participants (teammates) as well as special equipment or facilities.

Because relatively few people who play team sports continue to pursue them for a lifetime, you may want to begin learning a new sport or activity that you can enjoy later in life. Some of the health-related fitness benefits that result from different team sports and other sports are identified in the table on the next page.

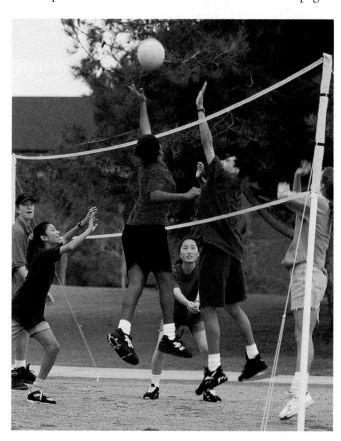

Participation in sports is an enjoyable way to be active.

Health-Related Benefits of Sports

Sport	Develops Cardiovascular Fitness	Develops Strength	Develops Muscular Endurance	Develops Flexibility	Helps Control Body Fatness
Individual Sports					
Badminton •	fair	poor	fair	fair	fair
Bowling •	poor	poor	poor	poor	poor
Golf (walking) •	fair	poor	poor	fair	fair
Gymnastics	fair	excellent	excellent	excellent	fair
Rowing, Crew	excellent	fair	excellent	poor	excellent
Skiing					
Cross-Country •*	excellent	fair	good	poor	excellent
Downhill •*	poor	fair	fair	poor	poor
Dual or Partner Sports					
Handball/Racquetball•*	good/excellent	poor	good	poor	good/excellent
Judo/Karate •*	poor	fair	fair	fair	poor
Table Tennis •	poor	poor	poor	poor	poor
Tennis •*	fair/good	poor	fair	poor	fair/good
Team Sports					
Baseball/Softball*	poor	poor	poor	poor	poor
Basketball					
Half-court •*	fair	poor	fair	poor	poor
Vigorous •*	excellent	poor	good	poor	excellent
Football *	fair	good	fair	poor	fair
Soccer *	excellent	fair	good	fair	excellent
Volleyball •*	fair	fair	poor	poor	fair
Challenge Sports					
Canoeing •	fair	poor	fair	poor	fair
Horseback Riding •	poor	poor	poor	poor	poor
Mountain Climbing •*	good	good	good	poor	good
Sailing •	poor	poor	poor	poor	poor
Surfing •*	fair	poor	good	fair	fair
Waterskiing •*	fair	fair	good	poor	fair

• Denotes lifetime sport.
* Denotes fitness needed to prevent injury.

Dual or Partner Sports Dual sports are those you can do with one other person. Examples include tennis, badminton, fencing, and judo. Because they require fewer people than team sports, dual sports are often referred to as lifetime sports. Dual sports can be practiced individually, so you can get activity in these sports without a partner.

Some dual sports are not activities that large numbers of people do as adults. Wrestling, for example, is a sport which is considered a dual sport but is not often done as a lifetime sport even though it does develop many important parts of health-related fitness. Dual sports that are not done by many adults are not considered lifetime sports.

Individual Sports Individual sports are those that you can do by yourself. Golf, gymnastics, and bowling are truly individual sports because they can be done individually. Many of these types of sports are also lifetime sports because they are more likely to be done

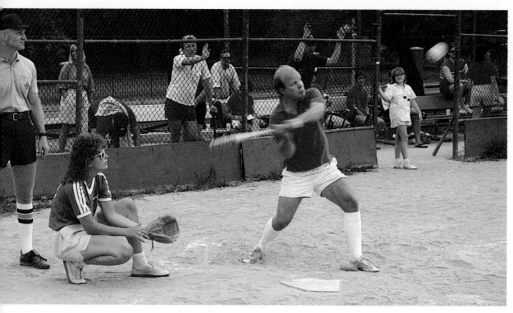
These players must be fit to safely participate in the sport.

- **Physical contact**: football, wrestling, ice hockey
- **Fast sprinting**: baseball, softball, soccer
- **Sudden fast starts and stops**: racquetball, track, basketball
- **Vigorous jumping**: basketball, high jump, soccer
- **Danger of falling**: skiing, skating, judo
- **Danger of overstretching muscles**: tennis, football

Choosing a Sport

If you decide that participation in a sport should be a part of your lifetime physical activity plan, consider these guidelines.

- **Consider your skill-related abilities.** In the previous chapter you learned how to match your abilities to different activities. Consider your abilities as you choose a sport.
- **Consider the health-related benefits of the sport.** Use the information from this lesson to help you choose a sport that will help you build important parts of fitness.
- **Consider a lifetime sport.** Sports that can be done throughout life are good choices because you are likely to stick with them.
- **Learn the skills of the sport.** You learned in Chapter 11 that skill is important if you are going to do an activity on a regular basis. Set aside time to practice your sports skills.
- **Be fit for sports.** Remember you need to be physically fit even for sports that do not build fitness.
- **Choose sports that you enjoy doing.** Sports can be fun. Sometimes it is pleasant and worthwhile to just get away from the pressures of life and do something that you enjoy.

throughout life, although some such as gymnastics are not done by many later in life.

Outdoor Challenge Sports Some activities do not involve competition. An example is mountain climbing. The challenge is to get to the top. The mountain is conquered, not an opponent. These types of sports are usually done outdoors, although some can be done indoors, such as indoor rock climbing.

Fitness for Sports

Just as sports can contribute to good fitness, you also must stay fit to participate actively in sports. A weekend athlete is someone who neither exercises nor plays a sport on a regular basis. For example, some people snow ski only once or twice a year, but otherwise do not exercise regularly. Nevertheless, they believe they are fit enough to ski. Actually, these people should exercise regularly for several weeks before skiing to get ready for it and to avoid injury.

Some individuals mistakenly assume that fitness is not necessary for certain sports, especially if the sports do little to build fitness. For example, softball is not particularly good for developing fitness, but it does require fitness if you are to perform well. A player must sprint between bases, slide into bases, and jump to catch the ball. Each action could result in an injury if the player is not physically fit.

Be fit before actively playing a sport that involves the factors listed below. Each sport could result in injury if you are not physically fit.

Lesson Review
1. What are four categories of sports? Give an example of each.
2. Why is fitness important to sports participants?
3. What are some categories of sports for which participants must be especially fit?
4. List six guidelines for choosing a sport.

More Weight/Resistance Training

You have performed several strength and endurance exercises using resistance training, and you have learned the importance of correct lifting and spotting technique. Also you have learned how to determine the correct amount of weight/resistance for you. In this activity you will learn some different free weight or machine exercises and have an opportunity to find your 1RM and 7RM as you did in Chapter 9. Only two exercises are presented here. Because you are ready to make some decisions about your own program, you will learn these two and then choose from the other exercises described on your record sheet. (You may need to review the lifting and spotting techniques in Chapter 7 and the method for determining your estimated 1RM and 7RM in Chapter 9.)

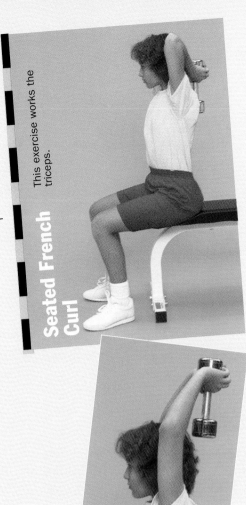

This exercise works the triceps.

Seated French Curl

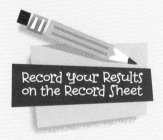

Record your Results on the Record Sheet

Seated French Curl

Weights: Barbell or dumbbells

1 Sit on end of bench, arms extended overhead, palms facing away.

2 Hold one end of a dumbell in both hands above and behind the head; tighten abdominals and back muscles. Slowly lower the weight toward the back of the neck until the elbows are fully flexed. Keep the elbows high.

3 Slowly return to the starting position. Only the elbows move.

Note: A barbell may be substituted for the dumbell. If this is done, spotters should be used: 2 spotters place barbell in the lifter's hands and spot for safety.

The equivalent machine exercise is the Triceps Curl.

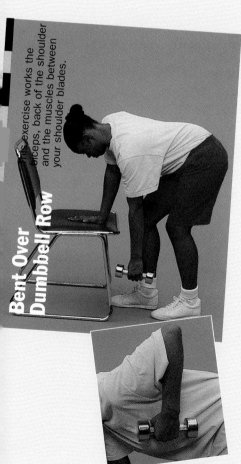

This exercise works the triceps, back of the shoulder and the muscles between your shoulder blades.

Bent Over Dumbbell Row

Bent Over Dumbbell Row

Weights: Dumbbell

Spotters: None needed

1 Hold dumbbell in one hand and rest the free hand on a bench to support the weight of the trunk and protect the back.

2 Pull the dumbbell upward until it touches the side of your chest near the arm pit. and the elbow points toward the ceiling.

3 Slowly lower the weight.

4 Repeat exercise with other arm.

Note: The equivalent machine exercise is Seated Rowing.

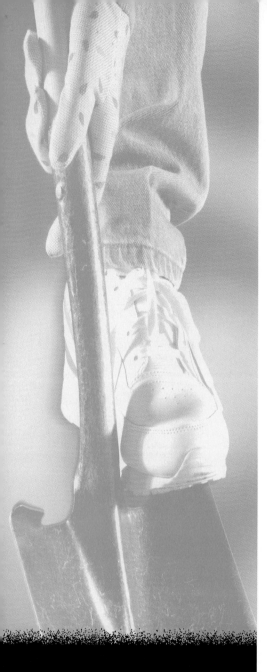

12 Chapter Review

Reviewing Concepts and Vocabulary

Copy the number of each statement on a sheet of paper. Next to each number, write the word or words that correctly complete the sentence.

1. Sports that you can do by yourself are _____.

2. _____ is a problem only when it keeps you from doing enough activity to become or remain fit.

3. The largest age group that plays team sports is _____.

4. Jogging, swimming, and skating are examples of _____ activity.

Number your paper. Next to each number, choose the letter of the best answer.

Column I	Column II
5. static stretching	a. builds strength and muscular endurance
6. orienteering	b. has 10–20 exercise stations
7. parcourse	c. alternates high-intensity exercise with rest
8. interval training	d. uses map-reading skills
9. resistance training	e. builds flexibility

On your paper, write a short answer for each statement or question.

10. What are some guidelines for choosing a physical activity?

11. Why is it important to include in your activity plan choices from the lifestyle physical activities part of the Physical Activity Pyramid?

12. Why is aerobic activity among the most beneficial types of activity?

13. Why might team sports not be good as an only choice for your lifetime activity plan?

14. What are some guidelines for choosing sports?

15. Why is it important to be physically fit when participating in sports?

Thinking Critically

Write a paragraph to answer the following question.

What are some activities you might include in your lifetime activity program? Explain why you made each choice.

Project

Work with a group of students to set up a short orienteering course on the school grounds or in a nearby park. Plan a course in which all members of the class can participate. Decide what equipment you need. Learn how to use a compass and map. Teach others to to use the compass.

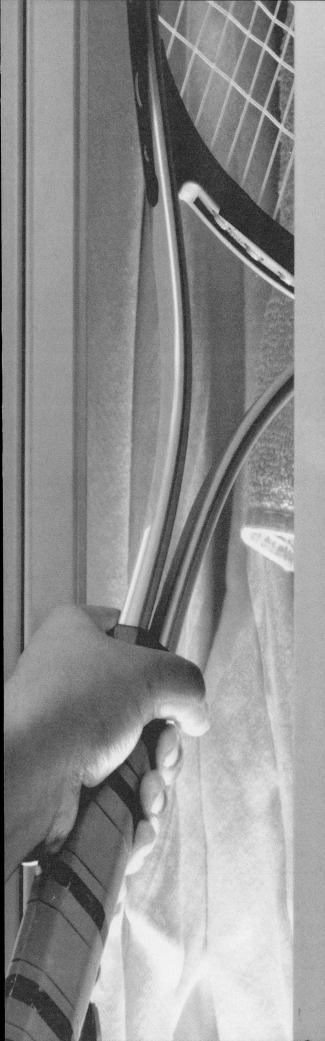

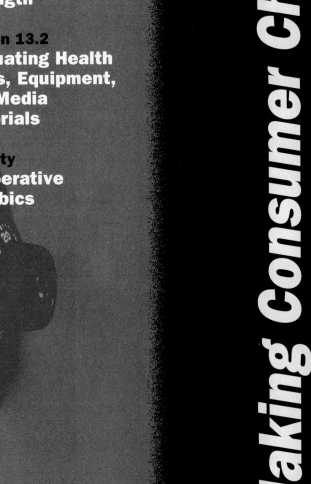

13

Making Consumer Choices

Step Aerobics

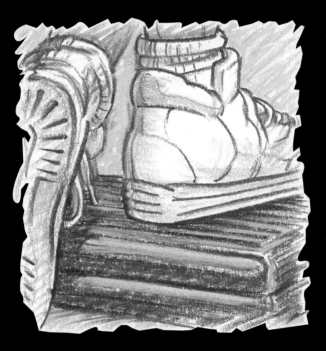

If you performed the aerobic dance routine in Chapter 5, you got an idea of how you can make physical activity fun by using various foot and arm movements. Step aerobics uses similar arm and leg movements to aerobic dance. In step aerobics, you use a step, or an elevated platform, to create interesting additional movements. Stepping up and down on the step during a step aerobics routine can increase the cardiovascular intensity of the exercise without causing stress to the joints. Also, stepping helps increase muscular endurance of the legs. The height of the step can be adjusted to alter exercise intensity. Follow the directions on your instruction sheet to have fun with step aerobics.

Routine 1:	Routine 2:
Basic Right Step	Alternating Basic Step
Basic Left Step	V Step
Turn Step	Step Touch
The Step Over	High Knee Step

13.1

Lesson

Health and Fitness Quackery

Lesson Objectives

After reading this lesson, you should be able to:

1. Explain the importance of being an informed health consumer.

2. Name reliable sources of health-related and fitness-related information.

3. Name and describe examples of health-related and fitness-related misconceptions and quackery.

Lesson Vocabulary

quackery, registered dietitian, food supplement, sports supplement, fad diet, passive exercise

You probably have seen and heard newspaper, magazine, radio, and television advertisements for health and fitness products and services. Is a product or service effective simply because it is advertised? In this lesson, you will learn how to become a wise consumer, or purchaser, of health and fitness products.

What Is Quackery?

Some people are in a hurry to lose body fat or gain muscular strength. Often, people who want quick results are persuaded to purchase useless health and fitness products and services. They may become victims of quackery. **Quackery** is a method of advertising or selling that uses false claims to lure people into buying products that are worthless, or even harmful.

If you have questions about health or fitness, be sure to ask an expert's advice. For medical advice, talk to a physician (M.D. or D.O.) or a registered nurse (R.N.). For questions about general health, ask a certified health education teacher. A physical educator, registered kinesiotherapist (R.K.T.), or registered physical therapist (R.P.T.) is qualified to advise you about exercise and fitness. These experts have college degrees and training in their area of specialization.

A **registered dietitian** (R.D.) is best qualified to advise you about diet, food, and nutrition. Keep in mind that a person who uses the title "nutritionist" is not necessarily an expert. Many states do not require specialized college degrees for that title. Similarly, staff members in health clubs are often not required to have college degrees in physical fitness or health. Neither nutritionists nor health-club employees are considered reliable sources of health or fitness information unless they have the credentials that are described above.

Detecting Quackery

Separating fact from fiction can be difficult. Frequently you can spot health or fitness quackery by identifying sales techniques such as these:

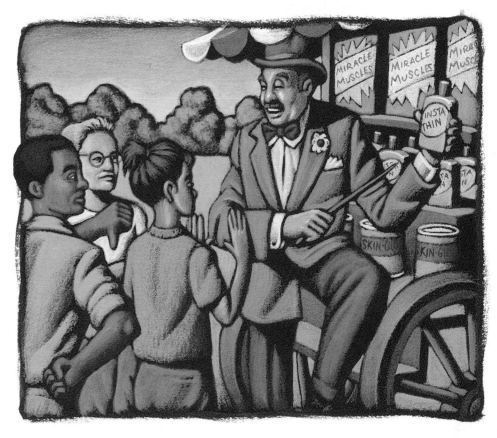

Beware of quacks who promise miracles.

False credentials A quack might claim to be a doctor or to have a college or university degree. However, the degree might be in a subject unrelated to health and physical fitness. It might come from a nonaccredited school, or it might be falsified. You can verify credentials by checking with your local or state health authorities or professional organizations.

Immediate results Be suspicious if a salesperson promises immediate, effortless, or guaranteed results.

Sales pitch Look for words and phrases such as *miracle, secret remedy, breakthrough,* and *clinical studies show.* A quack is likely to use these and similar terms in a sales pitch for an item that is useless. Notice the names of the products shown in the picture above. Would it be wise to buy any of these products?

Mail-order sales Be cautious of mail-order offers and money-back guarantees. You cannot examine mail-order products before buying them. A guarantee is only as good as the company that backs it.

Lack of medical support Some quacks claim that the American Medical Association (or another similar group) is against them only because the organization will not profit from the sale of the product. In reality,

lack of medical support usually indicates that the product is useless or even harmful.

Brand-new (untested) products Quacks do not subject their products to a thorough scientific testing. The product is rushed onto the market in order to make money as quickly as possible. Using such products can pose significant risks for a consumer.

Health Quackery

Many people are willing to try new health products. In fact, the market is flooded with health products, many of which are useless. Although some of these products may not be harmful, false advertising claims give people unrealistic expectations about the benefits these products can provide. Be aware that many advertisers promote myths about health and fitness. You can recognize health quackery when advertisements make unrealistic claims about a product. Examples include claims that a product will increase muscle development, promote hair growth, cure acne, make wrinkles disappear, or remove cellulite (fat tissue).

Food Supplements A **food supplement** is a product intended to add to a person's nutrient consumption.

Such a product usually is unnecessary and sometimes is harmful. For example, health experts consider products such as amino-acid supplements and weight-control supplements a waste of money. Food supplements often are produced as syrups, powders, or tablets. Generally, they are sold in health-food stores or through the mail. In special cases, a physician might prescribe supplements for those who need them. Those persons should use only the prescribed supplement according to the physician's directions.

Sports Supplements A current fad is the use of **sports supplements** or sports vitamins, products sold to enhance athletic performance. These supplements are also called "Ergogenic Aids." Many supplements sold as "Ergogenic Aids" are actually quack products. These quack products include such items as Argentina bull organs, kola nuts, and palmetto berries.

The health and fitness claims made about these products are a myth. There is little, if any, scientific evidence that these substances improve performance. However, there is considerable evidence that they cause serious adverse effects. The chart shows examples of these products and some of their dangerous effects.

Fad Diets "Lose pounds a day on the ice-cream diet!" "Rice diet works wonders!" "Fruit diet dissolves

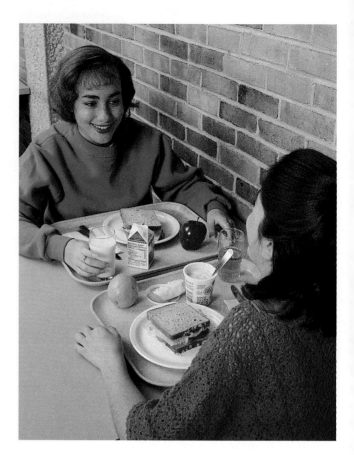

Fad diets are ineffective; healthy eating works.

fat!" How many similar weight-loss claims have you heard? Each claim is false and an example of a **fad diet**. Although fad diets are popular because they usually promise fast results, nearly all fad diets are nutritionally unbalanced. They often restrict eating to only one or two food groups, or even one specific food. As you have learned, a combination of physical activity and eating fewer Calories is the only safe, effective way to reduce body fatness and lose weight. Eating healthful, low-Calorie foods like the teenagers in the picture are doing can help you control your Calorie intake.

Fitness Quackery

Many useless products are being sold to promote fitness. For example, you may have seen advertisements for thigh creams to reduce fat in the thighs. Such claims are a myth. These creams do not reduce body fat. Also be alert for the following worthless fitness devices and methods:

• Exercise programs that use **passive exercises** are ineffective because, instead of using your own muscles, they use machines or other outside forces to move your body. A variety of devices provide passive exercises. For example, rollers are machines that roll along

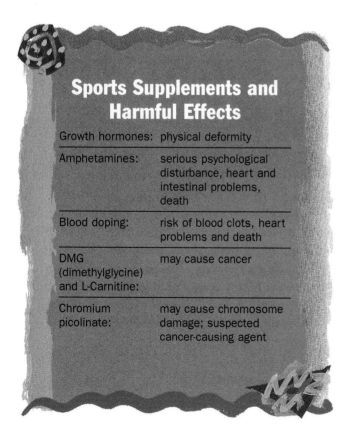

Sports Supplements and Harmful Effects

Growth hormones:	physical deformity
Amphetamines:	serious psychological disturbance, heart and intestinal problems, death
Blood doping:	risk of blood clots, heart problems and death
DMG (dimethylglycine) and L-Carnitine:	may cause cancer
Chromium picolinate:	may cause chromosome damage; suspected cancer-causing agent

No Excuses

Logging Your Activities

An activity log is a written account of the physical activities that you participate in during a period of time. It's a way to keep track of what you do so you can tell if you are meeting your activity goals.

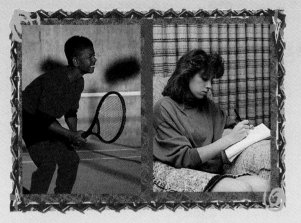

Mark enjoyed playing tennis on the weekends. He'd start out full of energy, but lacked the endurance to play well for a complete match. His instructor suggested that he do some daily activities to improve his endurance. For several weeks Mark reported that he faithfully engaged in the activities. But Mark's instructor was a little skeptical based on his level of improvement. Finally, she suggested that Mark keep a log of all the times he actually did the activities. "Boy, was I surprised. I rarely spent as much time as I thought on each activity. I really thought I was doing well until I actually saw the results written down."

Erica's situation was different. She had knee surgery and was ordered to limit the kinds and amount of activity she engaged in and follow a schedule of rehabilitation exercises. She was also supposed to elevate her leg whenever possible. Erica's leg was often swollen and sore at the end of the day. Her therapist suggested that she keep a daily log. Erica discovered that she spent much more time on her feet than she realized. She knew that she had to curtail more activities in order for her knee to heal, yet still continue to do her rehabilitation exercises.

For Discussion

How did the logs help both Mark and Erica? What are some other ways in which a log could help people? What are some good suggestions that can help people keep up with their activity log? Set a one-week physical activity goal for yourself. Use the weekly log to keep track of how well you meet your goal.

---

your hips or legs. Vibrating machines shake body areas and are said to "break up" fat cells. Motorized belts, cycles, tables, and rowing machines are advertised for fat reduction and weight loss. These claims are false.

• Figure wrapping, wearing nonporous garments, and soaking in baths are often advertised for weight loss. These practices can cause overheating and dehydration and can be extremely dangerous to your health.

• An unqualified fitness instructor might recommend spot exercises. You can do spot exercises to strengthen muscles in a certain part of the body, but these exercises do not remove fat at that location. Remember that physical activity helps reduce fat all over the body.

Reaching Goals Safely Remember that you need to use more Calories than you consume in order to decrease body fat and lose weight. Physical activity, such as doing exercises for cardiovascular fitness, can help you use Calories.

Attaining health and fitness goals takes planning and time. No diet, product, or exercise program can work magic. Recognizing myths and misconceptions, such as those described here, can help you save your money and your health. Education is the best safeguard against quackery.

Lesson Review

1. Why is learning to recognize quackery important?
2. To whom should you direct questions about health and fitness?
3. Name and describe two examples of health-related or fitness-related quackery.

Self-Assessment 13
Reassessing Body Composition, Flexibility, and Strength

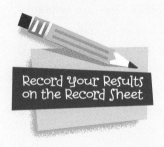

Record Your Results on the Record Sheet

You can determine your present state of fitness by reassessing the five health-related components. Reassessing your fitness is important for several reasons. First, practicing self-assessments will help you know how to do self-assessments properly throughout your life. Second, you can select the self-assessments that you think you will most likely use when you are doing them independently. Finally, these reassessments will allow you to see if your fitness in any category has changed since the assessments you did earlier in the class. If you do not see changes, keep in mind that it normally takes about six weeks for any significant improvement to occur in physical fitness. You can do periodic reassessments of fitness throughout your life to determine your personal fitness progress.

In this Self-Assessment, you will reassess your body composition, flexibility, and strength. Choose assessment items that you think are best for you personally. Refer to the page references following each self-assessment for instructions on doing the assessment and for determining your ratings. If time allows, perform more than the designated number of self-assessments from the list below. When you are finished with your reassessment items, record your results and ratings on your record sheet. Also, indicate the reasons for performing the assessment items that you chose.

Part I: Body Composition

Choose either Skinfolds, Body Mass Index, or the Height-Weight Chart to reassess your body composition:

Skinfolds (pages 93-94)

• Triceps

• Calf

Body Mass Index (page 53)

• Height

• Weight

Height-Weight Chart (page 95)

Part II: Flexibility

Choose at least one assessment from each category to reassess your flexibility.

Upper Body

• Arm Lift (page 138)

• Zipper (page 138)

• Wrap Around (page 139)

Lower Body

• Knee to Chest (page 139)

• Back Saver Sit and Reach (page 54)

Trunk

• Trunk Rotation (page 139)

Ankle

• Ankle Flexion (page 139)

Part III: Strength

Choose either free weights or machine measures to reassess your strength. If time allows, you may want to choose one or more of the assessments listed in the optional categories below.

1RM Strength Assessment (free weights)

• Biceps Curl (page 101)

• Bench Press (page 101)

• Half Squat (page 100)

1RM Strength Assessment (machine)

• Biceps Curl (page 125)

• Bench Press (page 125)

• Leg Press (page 124)

Optional 1RM Strength Assessments (free weights)

• Hamstring Curl (page 100)

• Seated Overhead Press (page 100)

• Heel Raise (page 101)

Optional 1RM Strength Assessments (machine)

• Hamstring Curl (page 124)

• Seated Overhead Press (page 124)

• Heel Raise (page 125)

If no weights are available, use grip strength to reassess strength.

Isometric Grip Strength (page 126)

13.2

Evaluating Health Clubs, Equipment, and Media Materials

Lesson Objectives

After reading this lesson, you should be able to:

1. Evaluate health-related and fitness-related facilities.

2. Describe the proper clothing and equipment that you need for physical activity.

3. Evaluate printed and video material that is related to health and fitness.

Lesson Vocabulary

Growing emphasis on health and fitness has led to an increase in related facilities, literature, and other products. In this lesson, you will learn about health and fit-ness clubs as well as exercise clothing and equipment. You also will learn how to evaluate literature and other materials. Finally, you will read about reliable consumer organizations.

Health Clubs

You do not need to join a health club, spa, or gym to attain or maintain fitness. In fact, you can design your own fitness program so that no special facility or equipment is required. School classes and after-school programs offer good opportunities to achieve and maintain fitness.

Some people find that joining a group helps motivate them to exercise and remain physically active. Many low-cost programs are offered through community centers, schools, universities, churches, and other groups. If you do prefer to join a commercial club, spa, or gym, keep in mind the following guidelines:

• Join on a pay-as-you-go basis, if possible. If you do sign a contract, make it a short-term one. Read the fine print carefully. Do not sign a contract right away.

• Choose a well-established club. Such a club is less likely to go out of business. Make sure the facility has qualified fitness experts, such as those described earlier in the chapter. Be alert for signs of fitness quackery. If you notice signs of quackery, quit the club.

You do not have to join a health club to be fit. You can exercise at home.

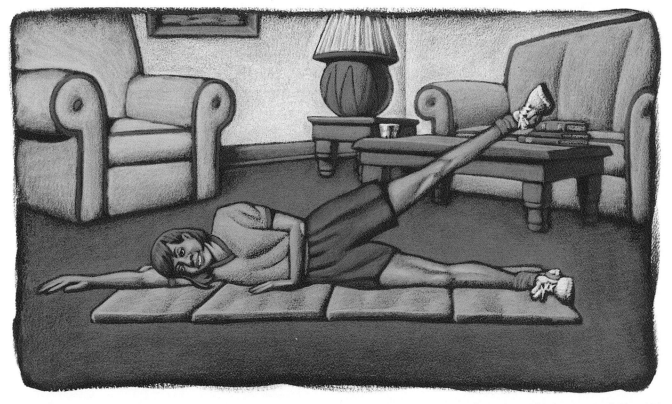

• Make a trial visit to the club at a time when you would normally use it. Make sure you feel comfortable with the employees and other patrons. Also make sure the equipment and facilities are available for your use.

• If weight loss is your primary goal, consider joining a program recommended by your physician or sponsored by a hospital, rather than joining a health club.

Special Clothing and Equipment

A good fitness program requires a minimum of clothing and equipment. Review what you learned in Chapter 4 about proper clothing and footwear for safe physical activity. Fashionable exercise clothing and footwear are popular, but not necessary. You need only wear what is comfortable and safe.

In some cases, such as those listed below, special facilities or equipment is desirable for certain kinds of physical activity.

• A person who has joint pain may prefer to avoid activities such as jogging, choosing instead to swim for cardiovascular fitness. In such a case, a facility that includes a swimming pool would be necessary.

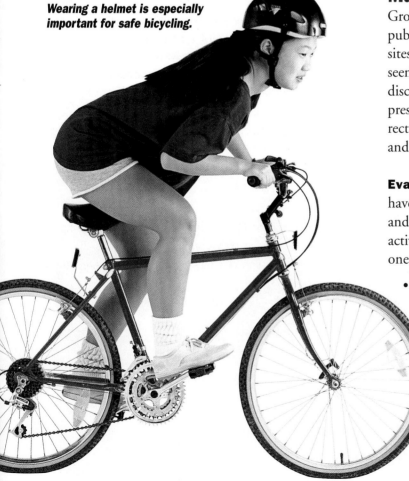

Wearing a helmet is especially important for safe bicycling.

• A person who does bicycling needs a bicycle that is in good condition. In addition, a helmet is necessary for safety and often required by law. Serious cyclists, such as the one shown, often wear tight spandex clothing to control chafing and reduce air resistance.

• For strength and endurance, homemade weights, inner tubes, or latex bands can be used for resistance. Serious weight trainers or body builders may choose to purchase free weights or pulleys.

Purchasing Exercise Equipment Avoid investing money in exercise equipment until you are sure you will use it. Many people buy equipment but do not use it after the first few months. Evidence of this can be seen in the many ads for slightly-used equipment found in the classified sections of newspapers.

Consult with a fitness expert before buying equipment. Do not rely on sales clerks and do not purchase equipment through the mail. Buy from a well-established company that will honor the warranty, service the product, and have replacement parts available.

Evaluating Printed and Other Media Materials

Growing emphasis on health and fitness has led to the publication of many books, articles, videos, and web sites on weight control and exercise. You may also have seen or heard television and radio shows presenting discussions on these topics. Much of the information presented through the media is misleading or incorrect. How can you evaluate information about health and fitness that you read, see, and hear?

Evaluating Books and Articles Chances are, you have seen, read, or heard about a wide variety of books and articles about weight control, fitness, and physical activity. These guidelines can help you decide which ones are worthwhile:

• The author(s) or consultant(s) should be a registered dietitian, an individual who has completed advanced study in nutrition, a physical or health educator, physical therapist, or exercise scientist.

• The book or article should contain information about a balanced diet and recommend physical activity as well as a diet plan.

• Information should be included on how to reduce Calories and fats by choosing healthful, low-fat foods.

• The diet plan should include servings from the food groups shown in the Food Guide Pyramid. You will learn about the Food Guide Pyramid in Chapter 17. Methods for correcting unhealthful nutritional habits also should be provided.

• A weight-loss plan should call for at least 1,000 to 1,200 Calories per day and no more than two pounds of weight loss per week.

Evaluating Books and Articles About Fitness

Books and articles about physical fitness fill the shelves of bookstores and newsstands. The following guidelines can help you evaluate them:

• The author(s) or consultant(s) should be a physical educator, physical therapist, or an individual who has completed advanced degrees in exercise physiology.

• Exercise discussions should include the principles of overload, progression, and specificity, in addition to the FIT Formula.

• The recommended exercises should be safe and effective. The exercises should require the use of your own muscles and should not recommend *effortless* devices.

Evaluating Exercise Videos

You probably have noticed many exercise videos for sale. The following guidelines can help you evaluate an exercise video:

• The video should include appropriate warm-up and cool-down exercises (cardiovascular and flexibility).

• Make sure the video does not contain exercises identified in Chapter 2 as questionable.

• The video should rotate the use of muscle groups. For example, use arms, then legs, then back, then abdominal muscles, and so on.

• If the video claims to be a total fitness program, it should include activities for all parts of fitness. Exercises for the different parts of fitness should be rotated.

• The activities on the video should be appropriate for beginners, intermediate, or advanced, as labeled.

• The exercises should start gradually and then progress in intensity.

• The routine should be fun and interesting.

• If the video does not meet all of the guidelines, modify it. For example, change the order of the routine to make it better.

Reliable Consumer Organizations

Many organizations work to protect consumers from misleading advertising and quackery. These organizations include the Federal Trade Commission, the Food and Drug Administration, the Consumer Product Safety Commission, the United States Postal Service, the Better Business Bureau, Consumers Union, the National Council Against Health Fraud, the American Medical Association, the American Dental Association, and the American College of Sports Medicine. These agencies receive and investigate consumer complaints and provide information to consumers.

As a consumer, you need to be informed about the products and services you use. Do not assume that every advertised product is safe and effective. While agencies such as the ones named above can provide information, you make the final decision about buying a product or service.

Lesson Review

1. What are some guidelines to consider regarding the joining of an exercise group?
2. What should you consider before buying exercise equipment?
3. Describe three guidelines for evaluating exercise videos.

Activity 13
Cooperative Aerobics

In the Fitness Focus in Chapter 5, you learned an aerobic dance. Maybe you had previously participated in aerobic dance classes or exercised with an aerobic dance video. Perhaps you found this activity a new experience. In either case, you probably learned that aerobic dance is a fun way to get a cardiovascular workout. The only skill required is keeping rhythm with the music.

During this activity, you will be divided into squads. Each person in the squad will make up an arm and leg pattern to teach to the squad and then to the class. Listen to the music your instructor plays as you invent your combinations.

Look at the arm movements and leg movements that are listed below. You can use these movements in any combination to create a dance step. On the other hand, you may prefer to use your imagination and make up your own movements.

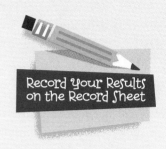

Record Your Results on the Record Sheet

Leg Movements

Note that *R* stands for right, and *L* stands for left.

1 Step-Heel
- Step R, touch L heel to floor.
- Repeat with L step and R heel.

2 Step, Close-step, Heel
- Step R, slide L foot to R.
- Step R, point L heel forward.

3 Step, Close-step, Kick
- Follow directions for step, close-step, heel (above), except kick instead of pointing heel forward.

4 Step-Close
- Step R, slide L foot to R.
- Repeat with step L, close R.

5 Stair-Step
- Walk forward—R, L.
- Walk back—R, L.

6 Step-Kick
- Step R, kick L.
- Step L, kick R.

7 Step Knee-Lift
- Step R, lift L knee.
- Step L, lift R knee.

8 Grapevine
- Step R.
- Cross L behind R, and step.
- Step R.
- Cross L in front of R, and step.

9 Box Step
- Step forward R.
- Cross L over R, and step.
- Step back R.
- Step back L.

10 "Pony"
- Step R, slow.
- Step L, quick.
- Step R, slow.
- Repeat, starting L. (similar to dance called Cha-Cha)

11 Rocker
- Step R, point L heel forward, lean back.
- Step L, point R heel backward, lean forward.

12 Hustle Forward and Back
- Step forward, R, L, R.
- Hop R, lift L knee.
- Step backward, L, R, L.
- Hop L, lift R knee.

13 Elbow to Knee
- Step R, lift L knee to R elbow.
- Step L, lift R knee to L elbow.

14 Charleston
- Point L toe forward, step back L, toe then heel.
- Point R toe back, step forward R, toe then heel.
- Repeat.

15 Mambo
- Step forward R, back L.
- Step R, L, R,. in place.

Arm Movements

1 Arm Press

- Push arms down and up from chest to waist.

2 Biceps Curl

- Move as though weight-lifting.

3 Triceps (French) Curl

- Move arms overhead as in weight-lifting.

4 Front Scissors

- Swing arms across each other in front of chest then out to sides.

5 Back Scissors

- Scissor arms behind back.

6 Double Arm Swing

- Swing arms together across front of chest.

7 Arm Circles

- Alternate circling R arm clockwise and L arm counter-clockwise.

8 Chicken Wings

- Bend elbows and flap them up and down at your sides.

9 Windshield Wipers

- Bend elbows and move hands in front of face like windshield wipers.

10 Rowing

- Move arms as though rowing a boat.

11 Cheerleader

- Pump arms up and down alternately overhead.

12 Hustle Arms

- Swing both arms backward, then forward, with a clap on the hop.

13 Elbow to Knee Arms

- Twist and touch R elbow to L knee.
- Twist and touch L elbow to R knee.

14 Drive a Big Truck

- Move both arms as if turning a very large steering wheel.

15 Picking Cherries

- Reach up with both arms to "get a cherry and put it in your pocket."

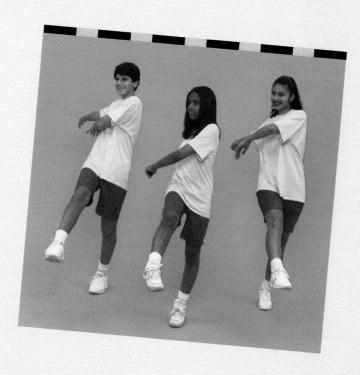

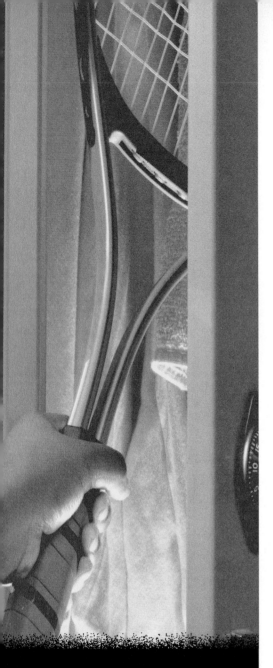

13 Chapter Review

Reviewing Concepts and Vocabulary

Copy the number of each statement on a sheet of paper. Next to each number, write the word or words that correctly completes the sentence.

1. Many products sold as _____, or Ergogenic Aids, are quack products.

2. A _____ exercise uses machines or outside forces to move your muscles.

3. A method of advertising or selling that uses false claims is _____.

4. A food _____ is a product intended to add to a person's nutritional intake.

5. A _____ diet often promises quick results but is usually nutritionally unbalanced.

Number your paper. Next to each number, choose the letter of the best answer.

Column I	Column II
6. medical doctor	a. may not be an expert
7. certified health education teacher	b. provides medical advice
8. registered physical therapist	c. offers advice about diet and nutrition
9. dietitian	d. has information about fitness
10. nutritionist	e. answers concerns about general health

On your paper, write a short answer for each statement or question.

11. Describe three ways you can recognize quackery.

12. Explain the effect of spot exercises on levels of body fat.

13. What factors should you consider if you are thinking about joining a health club?

14. What kinds of clothing and equipment do you need for a good fitness program?

15. List three guidelines you should follow when evaluating a book or article about weight control.

Thinking Critically

Write a paragraph to answer the following question.

Your friend Lee is interested in joining a health club that provides figure wraps and steam baths. The club also encourages use of motorized rowing machines and other such devices. What advice would you give your friend? Explain your reasons.

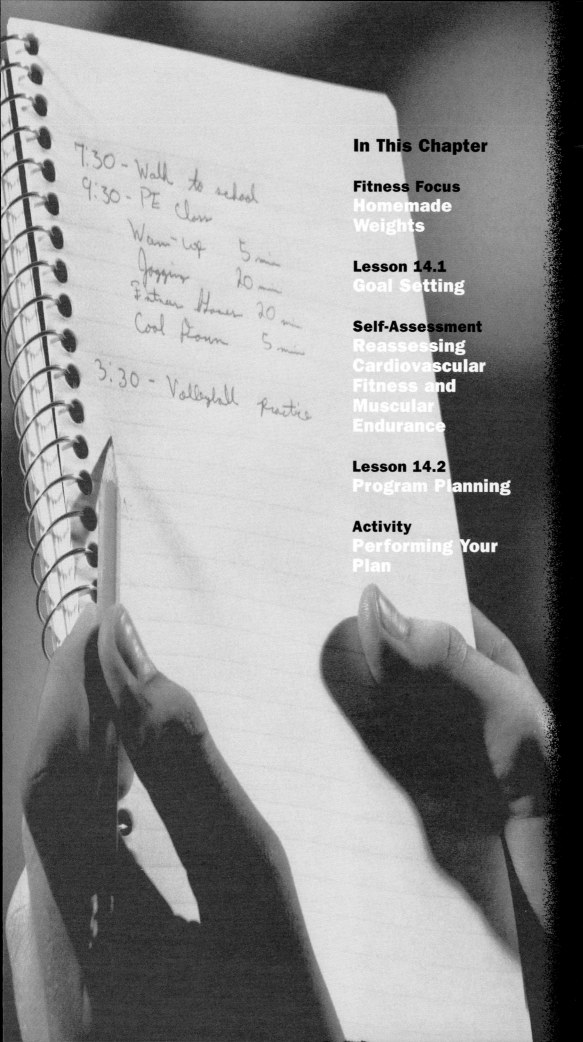

7:30 - Walk to school
9:30 - PE Class
      Warm-up   5 min
      Jogging   20 min
      Fitness Stations 20 min
      Cool Down   5 min

3:30 - Volleyball Practice

14

Personal Program Planning

Fitness Focus 14
Homemade Weights

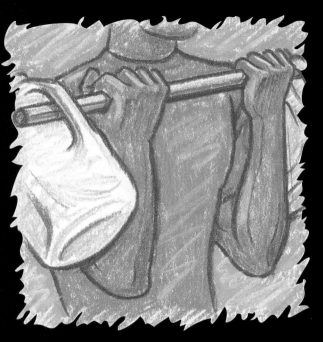

In previous chapters you learned how to properly perform free-weight exercises to build muscular endurance and strength. If your school has weights and keeps the weight room open for recreational use, you can perform weight training at school. Of course, you can buy weights or join a health club so that you have the equipment to do free-weight training, but either can be expensive. An alternative is to use homemade weights made of bottles filled with water and a broomstick or piece of plastic pipe. If done properly, this alternative can be a safe and inexpensive way to do free-weight training.

Biceps Curl	Jogging in Place
Heel Raise	Sitting Stretcher
Lateral Raise	Jump Rope
Half Squat	Calf Stretcher
Shoulder Shrug	Stride Jump
Lunge	Zipper

14.1 Lesson · Goal Setting

Lesson Objectives
After reading this lesson, you should be able to:
1. Explain how goal setting can help you plan your fitness program.
2. Identify some guidelines you should follow when setting goals.

Lesson Vocabulary
goal setting

Suppose you wanted money for a specific purpose. It might be to buy a CD player, a bicycle, or a car. Or you might want to go on a trip or need money for college. Most likely you would develop a plan to get money. You might decide to babysit after school or work on weekends. You identify your goal—to make money—and then develop a plan to reach your goal.

Successful people use **goal setting** as part of their overall planning to achieve success; they decide ahead of time what they plan to accomplish and then establish how they will go about doing it. You can use goal setting to plan your personal fitness program. In this lesson you will learn how to use long-term goals and short-term goals to plan your personal program.

Long-Term Goals
Some goals might take a long time to reach, perhaps even years. For example, if your goal is to save money for college, you might have to work on weekends and summers all through high school. When you plan your fitness program, include some long-term goals, especially after you have had some success in achieving some short-term goals.

Long-Term Physical Activity Goals When setting physical fitness goals, a long-term goal is usually considered to be more than one month and up to several months or even a year. An example of a long-term physical activity goal would be to expend 1500 Calories in activities from the Physical Activity Pyramid each week for the next six months. You should examine your long-term goals periodically to see if you need to adjust them in any way.

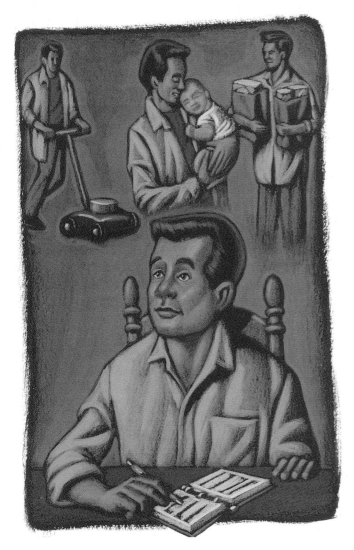

Successful people set goals to help them accomplish many tasks.

Obviously, long-term goals are sometimes hard to accomplish because they may require a lot of effort and dedication. For this reason, you are more likely to succeed if you perform activities that you enjoy. Fun activities not only build fitness, but they also enrich life.

Long-Term Physical Fitness Goals Setting long-term fitness goals is a good idea, especially if the goals are consistent with your long-term physical activity goals. If you do the right kind of physical activity, your fitness will improve automatically. For example, a person who meets a long-term activity goal of doing flexibility exercises 15 minutes a day for three months would no doubt meet a long-term fitness goal to improve flexibility by the end of three months.

Long-term fitness goals are important because they increase the probability that fitness improvement will occur. Of course, doing the right kind of activity and

doing it regularly (meeting long-term activity goals) is critical to meeting long-term physical fitness goals.

Short-Term Goals
Short-term goals can be reached in a short period of time, such as a few days or a few weeks. You might set a series of short-term goals to help accomplish a long-term goal. For example, to meet your long-term goal of making money, you may set a short-term goal of finding a job. After completing this short-term goal, you can re-examine your long-term goal, decide on the next step, and establish your next short-term goal.

Short-Term Physical Activity Goals Most physical activity goals make good short-term goals. Walking 30 minutes a day for the next two weeks is a short-term activity goal. It can be accomplished in a short time— two weeks—and with effort virtually anyone can accomplish it. Your participation, rather than your performance, determines whether you meet the goal.

Short-Term Physical Fitness Goals Although physical activity goals are good short-term goals, achieving fitness takes time. A realistic short-term fitness goal is one that can be accomplished in four to six weeks because it takes at least this many weeks of regular exercise to produce fitness improvement. An example of a short-term physical fitness goal would be to be able to do ten push-ups.

Every year millions of Americans set unrealistic short-term fitness goals. They choose to waste their money on products that promise to give them "quick" fat loss or "fast" muscle gain. These products do not work because fitness does not come quickly.

The best way to meet short-term fitness goals is to do regular exercise and to allow yourself enough time to accomplish each goal. A person who does regular strength and muscular endurance exercises can expect to increase the number of push-ups that he or she can perform. But several weeks should be allowed for improvement. The goal of doing ten push-ups may be reasonable for one person but not for another. For this reason individual goals are important.

Beginners are advised to set the short-term goal of increasing activity in one area of the pyramid. Beginners are not asked to set short-term physical fitness goals until they have learned more about fitness and how to set goals. You will see later in this chapter that you are now ready to set some short-term goals for both physical fitness and physical activity because you are well beyond the beginning stage.

Guidelines for Goal Setting

You may be a little confused about how to go about setting goals. The guidelines below can help you as you identify and develop your goals.

General Guidelines Whether you are a beginner in physical fitness or have been active for some time, these guidelines can help you:

• **Be realistic**. Realistic goals are ones that can be accomplished easily by those willing to give effort but difficult enough to be challenging. Set goals you know you can attain. People who set goals that are too hard doom themselves to failure before they begin.

• **Be specific.** Vague or very general goals are hard to accomplish. Specific goals help you determine if you have accomplished what you set out to do.

• **Personalize.** What is a realistic goal for one person can be unrealistic for another. Base your goals on your own individual needs and abilities. Meeting health standards or setting your own performance standards makes more sense than trying to be like others.

• **Know your reasons for setting your goals.** Those who set goals for reasons other than their own personal improvement often fail. Ask yourself "why" when setting goals. Make sure you are setting goals for yourself based on your own needs and interests.

• **Consider activities for all parts of fitness.** If you want to reap the health and wellness benefits described in this book, do activity for all parts of health-related fitness and reach the good fitness zone in all parts.

• **Self-assess periodically or keep logs.** Keeping logs will help you determine if you have met physical activity

goals. Doing self-assessments will help you determine if you met your physical fitness goals.

• **Set new goals periodically.** Achieving a personal goal is rewarding. You feel good. Don't be afraid to congratulate yourself for your accomplishment. Now you can set a new goal.

• **Revise if necessary.** Set smaller, more realistic goals rather than goals that are too hard. If you do find that your goal is too hard to accomplish, don't be afraid to revise the goal. When you try hard and fail, the chances that you will give up increase.

Guidelines for Beginners In addition to the above guidelines, beginners should follow these additional guidelines:

• **Focus on short-term activity goals.** Beginners often don't know enough about their own fitness to set meaningful fitness goals. Building fitness takes time. Persistence in doing regular activity should be the goal of beginners. You now are advanced enough to set fitness goals, but if later you want to start doing activity after a long layoff, use short-term goals at first.

• **Reward yourself.** If you decide to walk every day for two weeks and you accomplish your goal, tell someone! Your effort deserves credit. Keeping an activity log is a good way to reward yourself.

• **Participate in activities with others who have similar abilities.** This may help you meet your short-term activity goals. Friends can keep friends going and can give each other a pat on the back whenever a goal is achieved.

Guidelines for Intermediates These guidelines will be helpful if you are an intermediate exerciser:

• **Focus on short- and long-term physical activity goals.** Expand to longer-term goals. You may want to keep track of the total minutes of activity, or the total Calories burned. Keep an exercise log.

• **Use your self-assessments to set realistic short-term fitness goals.** After you have made assessments of each part of fitness, use your results to set short-term fitness goals. Set goals in the areas in which you need the most improvement because you are most likely to see faster gains in these areas.

• **Focus on improvement.** Set goals at one level higher than your current fitness level. For example, if you

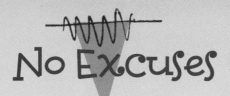

No Excuses

Setting Goals

Chances are good that you've heard someone say something like this: "I know I should exercise, but I'm tired of setting goals and never reaching them. Sometimes I feel like a failure." The key to reaching goals is to set the right goals for you.

As the physical education teacher passed the weight room, he couldn't help noticing Kevin, who was struggling to do one more bicep curl. Anyone could see that he was discouraged. "What's up, Kevin?" Mr. Booker asked.

Kevin put down the weights and pushed up the sleeves on his T-shirt. "Look at my arm. I've been doing bicep curls and bench presses for two weeks. I wanted my arms to be at least an inch bigger by the

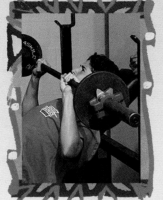

end of the month." He shook his head. "It doesn't look like I'm going to reach my goal. I might as well give up."

Mr. Booker just smiled. "It takes a while to build muscle, and you need to find out about goal setting. Why don't you stop by my office after school and maybe I can help you?"

Kevin decided to go talk to Mr. Booker the next day.

For Discussion
Was the goal Kevin set a realistic one? What kinds of advice do you think Mr. Booker gave Kevin about goal-setting? What kind of goal did Kevin set? What other kinds of goals do you think Kevin should set for himself? What else could Kevin do to make sure that he set realistic goals for himself? You can use the goal-setting worksheet to plan some realistic goals for yourself.

are in the low fitness zone, aim for the marginal zone. If you are very far from moving to the next zone, set smaller short-term goals.

Guidelines for the Advanced Exercisers Even advanced exercisers can benefit from these goal-setting guidelines:

• **Consider using all four types of goals.** Fit and active people generally are able to set long-term fitness goals based on fitness profiles. If set properly, all four types of goals can motivate advanced exercisers.

• **Set comprehensive goals.** Make sure that all parts of fitness are developed through activities from all parts of the pyramid. Advanced exercisers sometimes focus only on the parts of fitness in which they excel.

• **Consider maintenance goals.** An active, fit person cannot continue to improve in fitness forever. At some point "enough is enough!" Following a regular workout

schedule and maintaining fitness in the good fitness zone are reasonable goals for fit and active people.

Write It Down

Since you have assessed all of the parts of fitness and have been doing some activity in this class, you are considered at least an intermediate exerciser and can use either the intermediate or advanced category when setting personal goals. Now consider what you learned in this lesson and write your physical activity and fitness goals on a sheet of paper. Save your goals to use in planning your fitness program in the next lesson.

Lesson Review
1. How can you use long-term and short-term goals to plan your fitness program?
2. List some guidelines you should follow when setting goals. Be sure they are appropriate for your level.

Reassessing Cardiovascular Fitness and Muscular Endurance

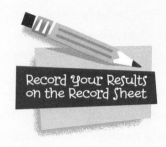

Record Your Results on the Record Sheet

In Chapter 13 you had the chance to reassess your body composition, flexibility, and strength. Remember—reassessments can be good because they give you a chance to practice self-assessment procedures, they allow you to choose those fitness assessments you think meet your personal needs best, and they allow you to see if your fitness changes over time.

In this Self-Assessment you will reassess your cardiovascular fitness and muscular endurance. All of the assessments are good, but you will have a choice. Choose those assessments you think are best for you. Refer to the page references following each self-assessment for instructions on doing the assessment and for determining your ratings. If time allows, perform more than the designated number of self-assessments from the lists below. When you are finished doing the reassessments, write your results and ratings on your record sheet. Also indicate the reasons for performing the assessments you chose.

Part I: Cardiovascular Fitness

Choose one of the following to reassess your cardiovascular fitness.

- PACER (page 40)
- Step Test (page 79)
- One-Mile Run (page 80)

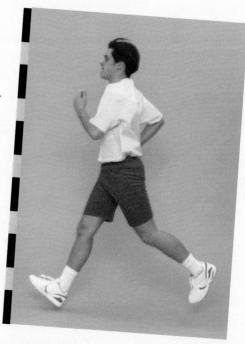

Part II: Muscular Endurance

Choose at least one item from each area below to reassess your muscular endurance.

Upper body

- Push-Up (90-degree) (page 26)
- Bent-Arm Hang (page 110)

Lower Body

- Leg Change (page 110)
- Side Stand (also measures upper body) (page 108)

Abdominals

- Curl-Up (page 25)
- Sitting Tuck (page 109)

Back

- Trunk (Upper Back) Lift (page 108)

Note: These items also assess strength, but since they are typically done for more than a few repetitions, they are included in the muscular endurance section of this reassessment.

14.2 Program Planning

Lesson Objectives

After reading this lesson, you should be able to:

1. Explain how to use a fitness profile to plan a personal fitness program.

2. Describe six steps in planning a personal fitness program.

Lesson Vocabulary

fitness profile

In the preceding chapters you learned about the many activities that can be used as part of a personal activity program and about which of these types of activities is most appropriate for building each part of health-related physical fitness. In the first part of this chapter you learned some basic information about goal setting. Now you have the opportunity to use this information as you go through the six steps in planning your personal physical activity program. Your teacher will provide you with worksheets to help you plan.

Step 1: Construct a Fitness Profile

A **fitness profile** is a brief summary of your fitness. A health-related fitness profile is useful in program planning because it helps you determine the areas in which you need improvement.

You can build a health-related physical fitness profile by summarizing all of your self-assessment results. On Application Worksheet 14B, record the ratings from all the self-assessments you have done in this course. Then use the guidelines below to determine one rating for each part of health-related fitness and record that rating on the worksheet.

• If the ratings for all self-assessments for any fitness part are similar, use that rating.

• For flexibility, strength, and muscular endurance you could determine a rating for each different part of the body. For this profile, determine an upper-body and lower-body rating for each of the fitness parts.

• If the ratings are different for different assessments of any fitness part, choose the rating you think is most

representative of your fitness. Consider any reasons why one result might be better than another.

• Be sure to consider your reassessment results as well as all other self-assessment results.

• For strength (1RM) you can use Application Worksheet 14A to help determine a rating.

Step 2: List Activities You Will Do

In the first lesson you had the opportunity to establish your physical activity and fitness goals. Use the goals you established in that lesson to help you with the remaining steps of your program planning.

Your physical activity goals should indicate most of the activities you will do in your program. On Application Worksheet 14C, check off all of the activities you plan to do in your program based on your goals. You might enjoy some activities that you have not included in your activity and fitness goals. For example, you might consider activities that you selected based on your skill-related fitness profile in Chapter 11. Check these also. Check any other activities you plan to do (or write them in if not listed), including those that you currently do on a regular basis. It is also important to consider your fitness profile at this point. Make sure you have selected activities in the areas for which you have less than good fitness ratings.

Step 3: Rate Your Activity Benefits

List the activities you plan to do (from Step 2) on Application Worksheet 14D. Rate each activity for its ability to produce each of the parts of health-related physical fitness. The charts on pages 164 and 169 of Chapter 12 will help you. Be sure that all of your activity and fitness goals are likely to be met with the activities you have selected. If all goals are not likely to be met, add activities to the list as necessary.

Step 4: Structure Your Program Plan

Using the list of activities you will include in your exercise program, decide when and where you will exercise. You already know that you should exercise several days a week to achieve and maintain all parts of fitness. Decide which days you will exercise. Pick at least three days of the week during which it would be easiest and most convenient for you to exercise. Remember that exercise for some parts of fitness, such as strength, should not be done every day. Some people rotate the parts of fitness they work on each day.

Review the FIT formula charts in this book before you decide on which days to exercise.

The best time of day for you to exercise is when you most enjoy exercising—a time when you are not likely to be interrupted. Keep in mind that you might complete different activities at different times.

Step 5: Write It Down

Now you are ready to write your program. On Application Worksheet 14E, list your warm-up exercises. Chapter 1 includes information about a warm-up and

Chapter 10 includes stretching exercises that you might consider. Include exercises that stretch the muscles you will use while exercising. You might plan more than one warm-up to vary your program.

Now list the activities you will do in each workout session. If you plan special exercises, include them in your workout. If you play sports, include practice as part of your program. Next, list your cool-down exercises. Remember to include stretching exercises for muscle cool-down and a cardiovascular cool-down.

Look at the program written by one student, Neal. He especially wanted to lose body fat and improve cardiovascular fitness, but he does not have high skill-related fitness scores, so he chose jogging. Neal enjoys tennis and, through practice, built enough skill to enjoy playing the game. However, he was not especially skilled in other sports, so he chose jogging which he knows is good for both cardiovascular fitness and reducing body fat. Special exercises were included to maintain strength, muscular endurance, and flexibility.

Step 6: Evaluate Your Program

After you have tried your program for a period of time (depending on your goals), evaluate your program. Go through the first five steps to revise your program.

Lesson Review
1. How can you use your fitness profile to plan your fitness program?
2. What are the six steps in planning a personal fitness program?

Weekly Exercise Plan for *Oct* 20 **to** *Oct* 27
Month Day   Month Day

Day	Activity	Time of Day	How Long?	
M O N	Warm up	7:30 a.m.	5	min.
	Jogging	7:35 a.m.	20	min.
	Special exercises for	8:00 a.m.	10	min.
	flexibility			min.
	Cool down	8:15 a.m.	5	min.
T U E	Warm up	4:00 p.m.	5	min.
	Special exercises for	4:05 p.m.	20	min.
	strength			min.
	Cool down	4:30 p.m.	5	min.
				min.
W E D	Warm up	7:30 a.m.	5	min.
	Jogging	7:35 a.m.	20	min.
	Special exercises for	8:00 a.m.	10	min.
	flexibility			min.
	Cool down	8:15 a.m.	5	min.
T H U	Warm up	4:00 p.m.	5	min.
	Special exercises for	4:05 p.m.	20	min.
	strength			min.
	Cool down	4:30 p.m.	5	min.
				min.
F R I	Warm up	7:30 a.m.	5	min.
	Jogging	7:35 a.m.	20	min.
	Special exercises for	8:00 a.m.	10	min.
	flexibility			min.
	Cool down	8:15 a.m.	5	min.
S A T	Warm up	10:00 a.m.	5	min.
	Tennis	10:05 a.m.	60	min.
	Cool down	11:00 a.m.	5	min.
				min.
				min.
S U N	Bicycle ride	2:00 p.m.	60	min.
				min.
				min.
				min.
				min.

Neal's exercise program.

Activity 14
Performing Your Plan

In this chapter you completed a personal program plan. In this Activity you will perform one day of your plan.

Choose a day from your program that includes enough activities to fill a full class period. Perform the activities in class. If no single day's activities last as long as one class period, supplement your program with activities from another day. If equipment is not available for the activity of your choice, select an activity that is similar in its benefits and one that you are likely to enjoy. Remember to warm up, then do your personal workout, and finish with a cool-down. On the appropriate record sheet write down those activities you performed in class.

In Chapter 13 you learned about keeping an activity log. Keeping a log will help you keep track of how you are doing with your personal physical activity program.

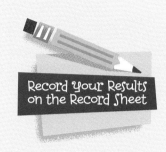

Record Your Results on the Record Sheet

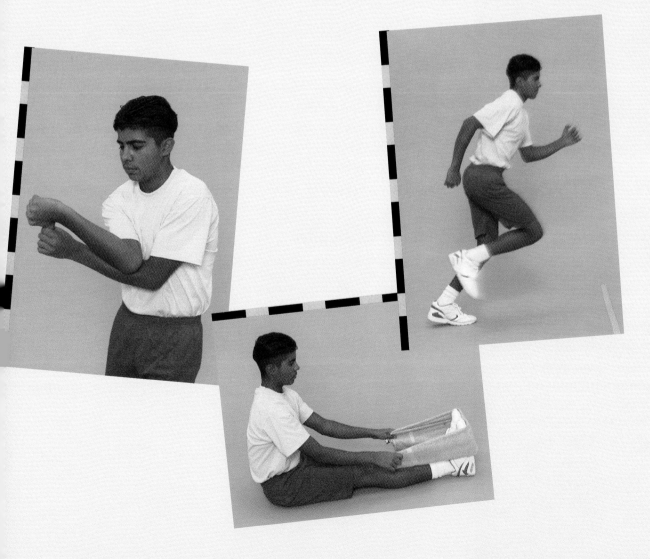

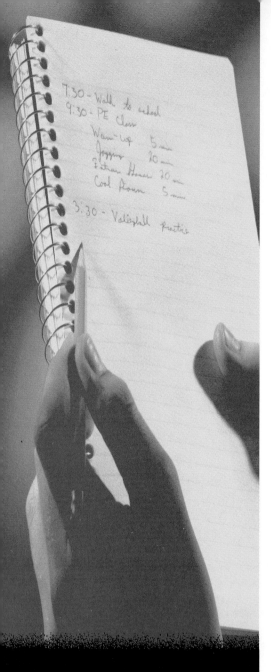

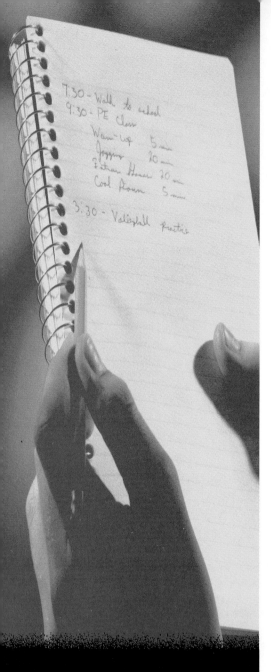

14 *Chapter Review*

Reviewing Concepts and Vocabulary

Copy the number of each statement on a sheet of paper. Next to each number, write the word or words that correctly complete the sentence.

1. A _____ is a brief summary of your fitness.

2. Successful people use _____ to decide what they want to accomplish and how to do it.

3. The best time of day to exercise is _____.

Number your paper. Next to each number, choose the letter of the best answer.

Column I

4. short-term physical activity goal

5. long-term physical activity goal

6. short-term fitness goal

7. long-term fitness goal

Column II

a. be able to do 10 push-ups

b. improve your bench press 10 pounds in 10 weeks

c. walk 30 minutes a day for 2 weeks

d. expend 1500 Calories in activity each week for 6 months

On your paper, write a short answer for each statement or question.

8. Explain why constructing a fitness profile is an important first step in program planning.

9. Why is it wise to keep a fitness log?

10. Why is it necessary to periodically reevaluate your fitness program?

Thinking Critically

Write a paragraph to answer the following question.

Why is it important to develop your own fitness program and not just use one developed for someone else?

Project

Research where in your community activities that require special equipment or grounds could be carried out. Compile a directory that provides phone numbers, addresses, facilities, and equipment. Distribute the directory to your class.

15

Fitness and Your Future

Fitness Focus 15
Exercise at Home

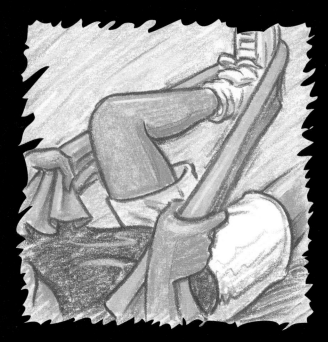

In previous lessons you learned about many different ways to exercise to build various parts of health-related physical fitness. Many of these activities require special equipment. Some equipment can be found at school, the YMCA or YWCA, at fitness clubs, or you can buy the equipment for use at home. But everyone can't afford to join a fitness club or to buy all the equipment they want. Common household items can be substituted for more expensive exercise equipment at home. Your instruction sheet will show you how to use these household items in a variety of exercises.

Stairstep Exercises
Towel Exercises
Broomstick Exercises
Food Can and/or Book Exercises
Rope Exercises

Lesson 15.1 Staying Fit and Active

Lesson Objectives
After reading this lesson, you should be able to:
1. Identify characteristics that help people become active and stay active.
2. Explain action strategies that you can use to develop the characteristics of an active person.
3. Describe five types of people in terms of their activity level.

Lesson Vocabulary
self-management skills

Think about the people you know, both young and old. Some of them are probably very active, some less active, and others not active at all. As you think about each group, can you identify any common characteristics the people in each group might share? Researchers have discovered that certain personal characteristics help people get active and stay active. In this lesson you will learn about some of those characteristics and what you can do to develop them.

What Makes People Active?
You probably possess many of the characteristics that help people become active and stay active. To strengthen those characteristics or build new ones, use the action strategies below.

Self-Confidence You most likely are familiar with the children's story "The Little Engine That Could." The story's message—*If you think you can, you often can*—applies to becoming fit and active, especially if you do not set standards that are too high for success. Self-confidence is the most important characteristic in becoming and staying active. People who think they are able to do activities usually are active. People who think they can't, aren't.

Recognizing factors that reduce your self-confidence is important. Some of these factors are comparing yourself to others, setting unrealistic goals or standards, thinking that your behavior is inappropriate, and fearing that people will make fun of you.

Action Strategies: Avoid negative thoughts and self-talk—thinking or saying to yourself "I can't do that." Instead concentrate on positive self-talk—saying "I can do that no matter what any one else thinks." Learn about stereotypes and avoid them. For example, some women feel that certain activities, such as weight training, are not appropriate for women, so they lack the confidence to try them. These women need to learn that, like the woman in the picture, they can and should do these activities. Both men and women sometimes feel that they are not able to get involved in certain activities because they didn't do them when they were young. Don't let these feelings keep you from activity.

Also, don't let your appearance reduce your confidence in your abilities. Wear a jogging suit or a type of clothing that helps you look your best while you are improving. To avoid feelings that exercise "does not work," be sure your goals are realistic. When it comes to weight and fat control, many adults have unrealistic goals. Remember—it takes time to change fitness and body fatness.

Knowledge Knowing that an activity is good for you is important in making a decision to do it. For this reason much space in this book has been used to help you learn the facts about physical fitness and physical activity. Knowledge has other advantages too. If you choose to be active, knowledge helps you do your activity properly and avoid injury, which, in turn, helps maintain your activity. Also, as more people learn the benefits of activity, they give social support to encourage activity among others.

Action Strategies: Keep up with the most recent facts about activity. Be sure that the activity you do is helpful rather than harmful. Be prepared to do fitness self-assessments and to plan your own program.

Beliefs Many people believe that activity makes them so hungry that they have to eat more Calories than they burn in activity. This is not a fact (what is true); it's a belief (what some people *think* is true). But for those people who believe that activity makes them hungry, the belief is a reason to avoid activity. When it comes to making decisions about what you will do in life, scientists have shown that what you think is true often is as powerful as what actually is true.

Action Strategies: Make sure your beliefs are backed up by facts. Check out the claims of others about fitness before you make them your personal beliefs.

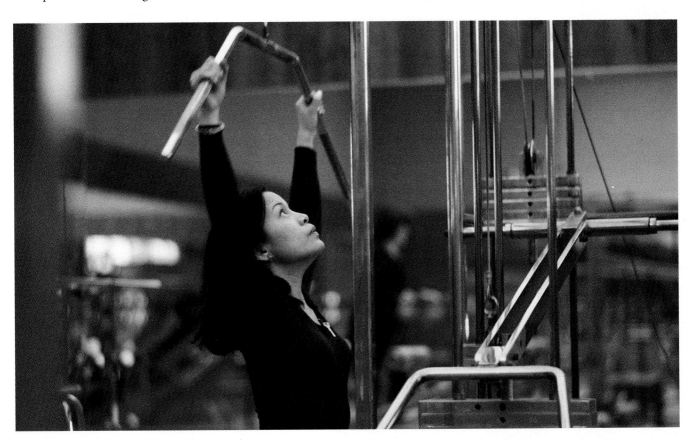

Self-confidence helps you be active.

reasonable goals and standards of success also helps. Doing activity with other people of similar ability can make some activities more enjoyable.

Skill The more skill you have in an activity, the more likely you are to do it. People who participated in sports when young are more likely to do them as adults. But don't believe the theory that "You can't teach an old dog new tricks!" You can learn new skills if you practice. The guidelines in Chapter 11 can help you when learning new skills.

Action Strategies: If you don't have a lot of physical skill in an activity, find one that matches your skill-related fitness abilities and practice the skills of that activity. Another alternative is to find an activity that does not require a lot of skill.

Physical Fitness Fit people, or those who need exercise the least, are the most likely to exercise. Unfit people, or those who need it most, are less likely to do it. Part of the reason is that unfit people lack confidence and often lack skill. Because they are unfit, they also may fatigue quickly.

Action Strategies: Begin slowly. Set activity goals rather than fitness goals using the guidelines you learned in Chapter 14. Choose lifestyle activities from the pyramid and gradually work up to more difficult activities (principle of progression). Use the information in this text to plan a personal program.

Enjoyment Most likely if your doctor told you to exercise, you would do it—at least for a while. In fact, the number one reason why inactive people start exercising is because of a doctor's advice. Knowing or believing that exercise is good for you might get you started. But starting an activity and staying with it are two different things. If you don't enjoy the activity, you probably won't stay with it. Over a lifetime it is important to find activity that you enjoy.

Action Strategies: Give yourself time to "learn to enjoy" an activity. Sometimes it takes a while. Setting

Self-Motivation How many of the active people you know are self-starters? People who are self-starters are more likely to be active than those who need others to get them started. The reason why some people are more self-motivated is not known. But a common belief for some who are not self-starters is that they should "be given something for what they do." This belief leads them to do things only when they are paid or rewarded. Scientists tell us that pay or external rewards such as trophies can get people to be active, but in the long run they may reduce self-motivation.

Action Strategies: Set your goals based on your own reasons rather than rewards from others. Avoid competition when you are first learning skills or first starting exercise; you might do (or not do) activity because of the competition rather than the activity itself. Promise yourself to meet your goals and make sure your goals are realistic.

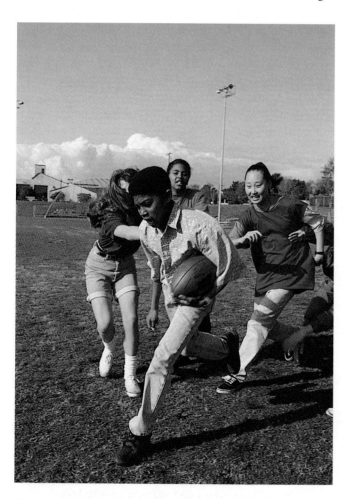

You are likely to stay with activities that are fun.

Support When you were young, you had a lot of support for being active—it was the "in thing to do." But as you entered your high-school years, some of your friends might have considered exercising less acceptable. One study revealed that among high-school teens "hanging out" was far more popular than any kind of exercise. If your friends are active, you are more likely to be active. If your parents do activity, you are more likely to do it.

Action Strategies: Find friends who are active, and encourage your friends to be active. Discuss activities with friends to see which ones you could all do together. Start an exercise club or join one that already exists. Encourage your friends to do lifestyle activity such as walking to school. Be supportive of people who you see doing exercise. Don't make fun of unfit people who are trying to become active.

Convenience You are probably pretty busy in this stage of your life, and as you get older you might get even busier. If this is true, convenience is likely to be an important factor in determining how physically active you are.

Action Strategies: Consider choosing some activities you can do by yourself that do not need special equipment and that can be done at home or near home. Save your money, if necessary, to buy the equipment needed to do the activities you enjoy. Scout the area to find safe and convenient areas to exercise. Find friends who live near you and who have similar interests and abilities. Adults can try to find a workplace that has a fitness or wellness program and workout facilities. You and your friends may be able to create such a program at school.

Success How many things do you enjoy doing that you don't do well? Probably not many because we all like doing things in which we succeed. If you repeatedly fail in a activity, you will probably drop out. On the other hand, if you find ways to feel successful, you will be more likely to be active for a lifetime.

Action Strategies: Set realistic goals—this is the most important factor! Review Chapter 14 if you need help in goal setting. Set your own standards of success. Avoid competition when you're

learning new activities or skills. If you lack confidence, avoid competition.

Self-Management Skills You know that those who have good physical skills are likely to be active. But physical skills are just one type of skill. Another type—**self-management skills**—also can help you be active. *Self-management* means "managing yourself or taking control of yourself." You can use self-management skills to improve those areas that help you be active. If you learn to use the action strategies described in this lesson and in the No Excuses feature in each chapter, you are learning self-management skills. You are learning how to help yourself be active both for now and the future.

Inactive to Active: How Do We Change?

Fitness experts tell us that there are five types of people. The first type is totally inactive and the fifth is regularly active. The rest are somewhere in between. Understanding the different types of people and how you can change from one to another will help you be active in the future. Generally, a person does not move from one type to another quickly. A worthwhile goal is to move to Type 5 and stay there, but any movement upward is better than being at Type 1.

Type 1: I don't do it and I don't plan to. You know people of this type—those who don't currently possess many of the characteristics necessary to be an active person. They are inactive and do not intend to

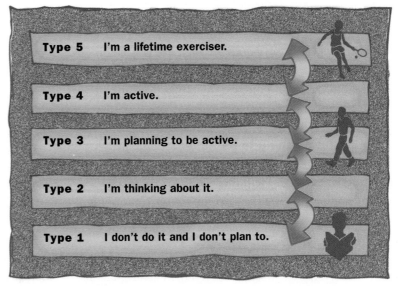

Which of these five types best describes you and your activity level?

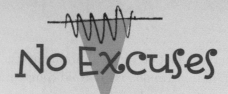

No Excuses

Managing Time

Why can some people always find time for an added activity while others barely have time to do their regularly scheduled activities? For a lot of people the answer is time management. People who are good time managers know how to make the best use of their time. They efficiently control their daily schedule in order to complete their activities without wasting time. These people are more likely to find time for regular physical activity.

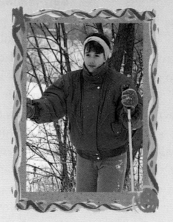

Jennifer lives near some good cross-country ski trails . Her friends spend a few hours skiing every Monday and Wednesday after school in the winter. They often go skiing on weekends as well. Although they always ask her to join their fun, Jennifer usually refuses. Her common excuse is, "I just don't have the time. I really love skiing, but with three honors classes, homework, and my job at the mall, I barely have time to eat, let alone ski. I wish I could go with you, but I can't. It's impossible! I'll ski next year when my schedule is easier. Then I'll have more spare time."

Jennifer's friends are used to her excuses. In fact, she used many of the same excuses last year. Her friends have the same classes and work hours that Jennifer has, but they complete their homework assignments and handle their jobs with time to spare. They cannot understand why Jennifer can't manage to find the time to go skiing with them.

For Discussion
What is different about how Jennifer and her friends manage their time? Consider the time management strategies presented in Lesson 15.2. What strategies might Jennifer follow to better manage her time? How will these strategies help her free some time for physical activities? Complete the questionnaire to find out how well you manage your time so that you have enough left for regular physical activity.

become active. It takes a long time to become a Type 1 person, and it often is hard to change those who are.

Type 2: I'm thinking about it. Inactive people do not become active over night. If you can get them to move from having no interest in activity to thinking about it, you've made progress!

Type 3: I'm planning to be active. Some people make a commitment to be active but do only small amounts of exercise. Help those who are Type 3 to recognize that this is a big step forward because some physical activity is better than none at all.

Type 4: I'm active. A Type 4 person is active, but the activity may be sporadic. This type person may be active for a while and then drop back to a Type 3.

Type 5: I'm a lifetime exerciser. A lifetime exerciser does regular activity most days of the week, most weeks of the year, and all of the years for a lifetime. If you are a Type 5, you are most likely to experience all of the benefits that come with being physically active.

Lesson Review
1. List at least six characteristics that help people become active and stay active.
2. Explain at least six action strategies that you can use to develop the characteristics of an active person.
3. Describe five types of people in terms of their activity level.

Body Measurements

In earlier chapters you learned how to assess all of the parts of health-related physical fitness because good levels of health-related fitness are related to good health and wellness. The two assessments that you will do in this chapter do not measure physical fitness, but the factors that you will assess are very much related to health and wellness.

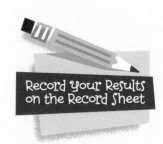

Record Your Results on the Record Sheet

You will use a tape measure to do both assessments. Keep the following in mind as you do the assessments:

• Use a non-elastic tape to make the measures.

• Pull the tape snugly against the skin but not so tight as to cause an indentation in the skin.

• Be sure that the tape is horizontal when measures are made. If the tape sags, measurements will be larger than they should be.

Part 1: Estimating Body Fat

You already know that having too much body fat can cause health problems. You can use body measurements to estimate your percentage of body fat. Males use weight and waist measurements. Females use height and hip measurements. Work with a partner to take the measurements.

Males: Waist and Weight

1 Measure your waist even with your navel.

2 Weigh yourself while fully clothed, but without shoes. Find your weight to the nearest pound.

3 Use the Body Measurement table to estimate your percentage of body fat. To do so, place a ruler so that it cuts across the left vertical line at the mark for your weight and across the right vertical line at the mark for your waist measurement. Your estimated percentage of body fat is the number where the ruler intersects the center vertical line. Write this information on your record sheet.

4 Find your rating in the body fatness rating chart on page 94. Record your rating.

Body Measurement: Males

BODY WEIGHT (pounds)	% FAT	WAIST (inches)
120		45
140	40	40
160	30	
	25	
180	20	35
200	15	
220	10	
240	5	30
260		25

Females: Hip and Height

1 With clothes on, measure your hips at the widest point. Measure to the nearest half inch.

2 Remove your shoes and measure your height to the nearest half inch.

3 Use the Body Measurement table to estimate your percentage of body fat. To do so, place a ruler so that it cuts across the left vertical line at the mark for your hip measurement and across the right vertical line at the mark for your height. Your estimated percentage of body fat is the number where the ruler intersects the center line. Record this information.

4 Find your body fatness rating in the rating chart on page 94. Record your rating.

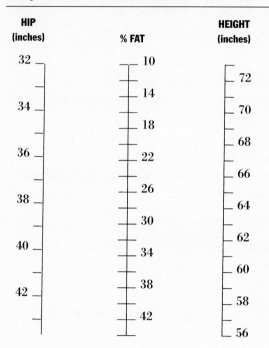

Body Measurement: Females

Part 2: Waist-to-Hip Ratio

Scientists now know that people who have more weight in the middle of their bodies have a higher risk of disease than people who have more weight in their lower body (legs and hips). Those who have too much weight in their mid-section are said to have an "apple" body type, while those who have more weight in their hips are said to have a "pear" body type. Overfat people who have a pear body type have less risk than overfat people with apple body types. In general, women are more likely to be a pear type, and men are more likely to be an apple type. This may in part explain why women have less risk of heart disease than men. The hip-to-waist ratio is a simple method of assessing the risk associated with your body type.

1 Measure your hips at the largest point (largest circumference of the buttocks). Make sure that measurements are made while standing with your feet together. Record your measurement.

2 Measure your waist at the smallest circumference (called the natural waist). If there is no natural waist, measure at the level of the umbilicus. Measure at the end of a normal inspiration (just after a normal breath). Do not suck in to make your waist smaller. Record your measurement.

3 Calculate your waist-to-hip ratio using the formula on your record sheet.

4 Find your ratio in the rating chart. Record your rating.

Rating Chart: Waist to Hip Ratio

	males	females
Good Health Zone	less than .90	less than .80
Borderline Risk	.91 to 1.0	.80 to .85
Higher Risk	more than 1.0	more than .85

15.2 Lesson Time Management

Lesson Objectives

After reading this lesson, you should be able to:
1. Explain the difference between free time and committed time.
2. List and explain four guidelines for time management.

Lesson Vocabulary

committed time, free time

How many times do you hear yourself and others say, "I don't have time?" It seems to be a common complaint. If you are one of those who seems to have too little time, how can you remedy the problem? Many experts believe that learning to manage time is one way to become more active. Because time management is so important, in this lesson you will learn how to manage your time so that you will be more active.

Free Time and Committed Time

In the year 1900, the average person worked more than 60 hours a week. Now the average work week is approximately 40 hours. Likewise, in 1900 many young people were not enrolled in school and were already working long hours in factories and on farms. Now most teens are in school, and even those who work in addition to going to school are usually involved for less than 60 hours a week.

It would seem that free time is much more abundant now than it was years ago. But this isn't always true—most of us make other commitments for our time when we aren't working or going to school. For example, you may have to care for brothers and sisters, or you might have made commitments to school or community activities such as clubs, band, chorus, or sports. You might have a job after school or on weekends. Time is also spent on things such as eating, sleeping, dressing, and getting to and from school or work. The time spent in all of these activities is called **committed time.**

Free time is the time left over when work, school, and committed time have been accounted for. Some people have very little free time because they have so many commitments or have many responsibilities.

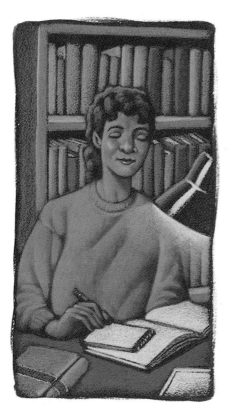
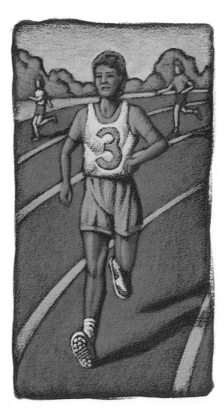
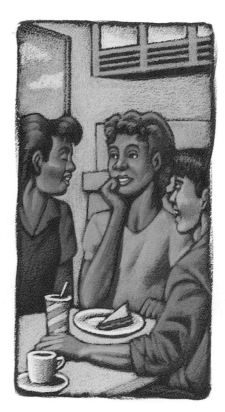

Managing your time can help you accomplish more, including being more active.

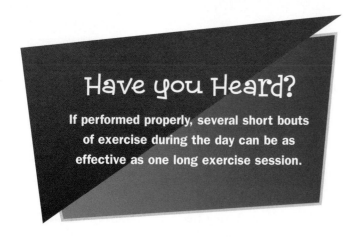

- What activities did you spend more time on than you wanted to?

- How much less time could you spend on each?

- Are the activities you would like to change under your control?

- What activities do you want to spend more time on?

- How much more time would you spend on these activities?

Time for Physical Activity

The people who say they don't have time for activity are often people who have not planned the use of their time carefully. Active people manage their time effectively so that they can commit time on a regular basis to being active. If you are in the group of people who often say "I don't have time," the guidelines below can help you.

Keep Track of Your Time. The best way to start to manage your time more efficiently is to check to see what you do with it. Keeping records will help you do this. Write down what you do during the course of each day. Record when you sleep, when you eat, when you are in school, when you are at work, and when you do all of the other things you do. You might use three categories: school/work, committed time, and free time. Most people who keep records of their time are surprised with the results. For example, some people who say they don't have time to exercise spend several hours a day watching television. Others find that they spend relatively large periods of time doing nothing.

Analyze Your Time Use. Once you have kept records of your time for several days, you can review your records to see how many hours you spend in each of the three categories. You can also determine exactly how you spend your committed time and your free time. This determination will help you decide if you are using your time the way you would like to use it.

Decide What to Do With Your Time. After you determine how much time you spend in various activities, decide whether you are managing your time efficiently. Efficient time management occurs when you get to do all the things you think are important. Here are some questions you can use to decide what is important:

Schedule Your Time. After you decide how you would like to spend your time, you can make a schedule to help you be sure that you have time for the things you think are important. If you feel that regular physical activity is important, you will commit time to doing it. Plan a schedule for one day, making sure you have time to do the things you think are important.

You can sometimes "kill two birds with one stone" with good scheduling. For example, you have to get to school somehow, so you might be able to spend committed time to getting to school on a bicycle or walking. You commit the time to two different purposes. Or you might commit yourself to a sports team or an activity club. This time is committed, but it is committed to a form of physical activity.

Lesson Review
1. Explain the difference between free time and committed time.
2. List and explain four guidelines for time management.

Activity 15
Your Exercise Circuit

In Chapter 4 you did a total fitness circuit which included exercises for all of the health-related parts of fitness. In Chapter 8 you had the opportunity to do a circuit designed primarily for building strength and muscular endurance. Now that you've had some experience with circuits, you can plan your own total fitness exercise circuit.

To plan the circuit, follow the guidelines you used to evaluate a video in Chapter 13. These guidelines help you make sure that you don't have two stations in a row that work the same muscles and that you provide safe exercises.

Your exercise circuit should have eight stations so that you have two stations for flexibility, two stations for cardiovascular fitness/body composition, and four stations for strength and muscular endurance. Choose from the exercises below. Use your record sheet to plan your circuit. Then try out your circuit.

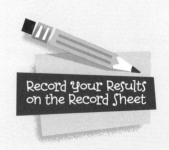

Record Your Results on the Record Sheet

Station 1: Cardiovascular #1

(Limit choices to these to avoid duplication with Station #5.)

- Self-Assessment (Chapter 3)
- Fitness Focus: Bench Stepping (this chapter)
- Fitness Focus (Chapter 5)
- Student-created activities

Station 2: Flexibility

(Choose only upper body stretches.)

- Activity (Chapter 5)
- Fitness Focus (Chapter 9)
- Activity (Chapter 10)

Station 3: Strength/Muscular Endurance

(Choose only upper body isotonic exercises to avoid overlap.)

- Fitness Focus (Chapter 8)
- Activity (Chapter 8)
- Activity (Chapter 9)
- Activity (Chapter 12)
- Fitness Focus (Chapter 14)

Station 4: Strength/Muscular Endurance

(Same as Station 3 except use only lower body isotonic exercises.)

Station 5: Cardiovascular #2

- Fitness Focus: Jump Rope (Chapter 6)
- Self-Assessment (Chapter 16)
- Fitness Focus (Chapter 13)
- Student-created activities

Station 6: Flexibility

(Same as Station 2 but limit to lower body stretches.)

Station 7: Strength/Muscular Endurance

(Limit to upper body isometric exercises.)

- Chapter 17

Station 8: Strength/Muscular Endurance

(Limit to lower body isometric exercises.)

- Chapter 17

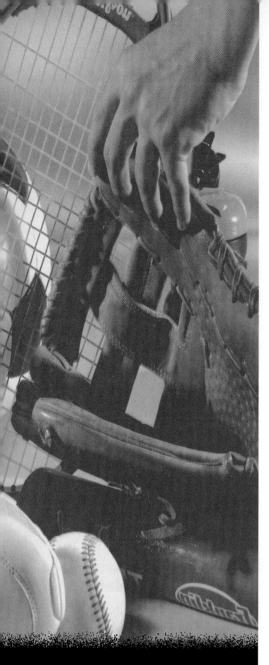

15 Chapter Review

Reviewing Concepts and Vocabulary

Copy the number of each statement on a sheet of paper. Next to each number, write the word or words that correctly complete the sentence.

1. Factors that reduce self confidence include _____.

2. _____ is one of the most important characteristics in becoming and staying active.

3. Skills that help you take control of yourself are _____.

Number your paper. Next to each number, choose the letter of the best answer.

Column I	Column II
4. beliefs	a. what is true
5. facts	b. what people think is true
6. free time	c. eating, dressing, sleeping
7. committed time	d. left-over time

On your paper, write a short answer for each statement or question.

8. How can you use committed time to stay active?

9. Explain how time records can help you manage your time.

10. What are some action strategies that you can use to help inactive people become active?

Thinking Critically

Write a paragraph to answer the following question.

List several characteristics of an active person that you possess. How can these characteristics help you be active? What are four characteristics that you should try to improve? What action strategies can you use?

Project

Interview active people. Include those from all age groups. Ask what strategies they use to stay active. Which do they think are most important? Report your findings to the class.

16

A Wellness Perspective

Walking for Wellness

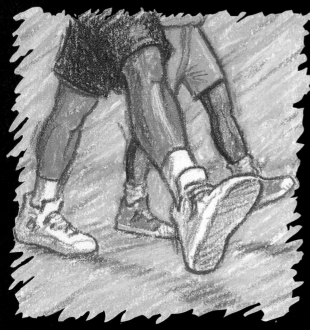

Two major organizations, the Centers for Disease Control and Prevention and the American College of Sports Medicine, recently issued a statement indicating that for good health and wellness all adults should perform regular physical activity equal to 30 minutes of brisk walking on most, if not all, days of the week. In this Fitness Focus you will get the opportunity to perform a 30-minute walk. You may want to determine how many Calories you expend when you do this activity. The chart on your instruction sheet will help you determine how many Calories are expended for the 30-minute walk.

16.1 All About Health and Wellness

Lesson

Lesson Objectives
After reading this lesson, you should be able to:
1. Explain how wellness relates to good health.
2. Identify the components of good health and describe the positive and negative aspects of each.
3. Explain how the positive aspect of each component can contribute to good health.

Lesson Vocabulary
none

What would you wish for if you could only have one wish? Some people would say $1,000,000. Some would wish for other material things, such as a new car or a new house. But after thinking about it, many people indicate that they would wish for good health for themselves and their family. If you possess health and wellness, you can enjoy life to its fullest. Without health, no amount of money will allow you to do all the things you would like to do. In this lesson you will learn about the components of good health and the relationship of wellness to good health.

Good Health Includes Wellness
Did you know that a person born in 1900 had a life expectancy of only 47 years? But a person born today could expect to have a lifespan of 75 years. What is the reason for such an increase in life expectancy? One major reason is the advances in medical science. Prior to 1900, "killer diseases" such as pneumonia, small pox, and polio killed thousands, resulting in a relatively short life for the average person. During that same time, treatment of illness was a major concern because cures such as the antibiotics and vaccines we have today were not available. But as medical science conquered many diseases, research began to focus more on how lifestyles affected disease. The focus shifted from treatment to the prevention of illness and the promotion of wellness.

Recognizing the shift in focus from treatment to prevention, the World Health Organization issued a statement in 1947 indicating that health was more than disease or illness treatment. This recognition led to the development of a more comprehensive definition of health, which now includes a wellness, or positive, element. The illustration to the right shows a model of health that incorporates all three elements—treatment, prevention, and promotion of wellness.

With this expanded definition of health in mind, national health goals were first published in 1980 by the U.S. Department of Health and Human Services. Every ten years national health goals are revised. In 2000 a new agenda, *Healthy People 2010*, was published. The focus of these goals is to prevent unnecessary disease and disability and to promote wellness, the positive component of health, as evidenced by a better quality of life for all Americans.

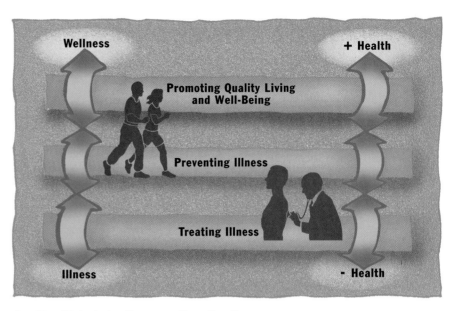

Good health includes the promotion of wellness.

Components of Good Health

In Chapter 5 you learned about many of the health and wellness benefits of physical activity. Most of these benefits were physical, which might lead you to conclude that good health and wellness is only a "physical thing." It's true that good physical fitness is important to overall health and wellness, but you now know that health and wellness have many different components. The health and wellness chain that you first saw in Chapter 1 is shown below. Recall that the links in the chain represent different components of health and wellness, and for a strong chain each link must be strong. Because health and wellness have many different components, it is important not to focus on just one. The physical component is one that has been

emphasized in this book because physical activity is so important to health and wellness. But other components are equally important.

The goal for good health and wellness is to promote the positive in each component and to avoid the negative. Look at the positive and negative aspect of each component shown in the chart below.

Components of Health and Wellness

Negative Aspect (avoid)	Component	Positive Aspect (goal)
Depressed	Emotional	Happy
Ignorant	Intellectual	Informed
Lonely	Social	Involved
Unfit	Physical	Fit
Unfulfilled	Spiritual	Fulfilled
Negative	Attitude	Positive
Illness	Health	Wellness

Adapted from *Concepts of Fitness and Wellness*, Corbin, Lindsey.

If you achieve the positives of each component, you will be well on your way to the quality of life and sense of well-being that the *Healthy People 2010* goals suggest are important. If you are happy, informed, involved, fit, and fulfilled, you have incorporated the positive aspects of the health components into your life. You will possess wellness, and your risk of illness will be decreased.

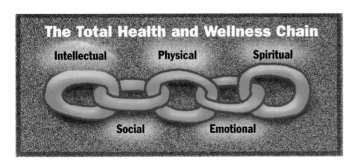

The Total Health and Wellness Chain

Intellectual   Physical   Spiritual

Social   Emotional

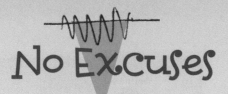

No Excuses

Preventing Relapse

Anyone can begin a program to increase physical fitness. However, just beginning a program is not enough. Some people are active for awhile and then drop out for awhile. This is called a relapse. Those who stay active all of their lives learn how to avoid relapses that can lead to becoming a "couch potato."

Luis missed his old school, especially his old friends. Now he usually came straight home after school instead of heading for the neighborhood basketball court to play a little one-on-one with his buddies. For the first month after he moved, Luis ate dinner, did his homework, and then clicked on the television to fill the time.

Early one evening, Luis's mom said, "Luis, why are you lying around? You like to be active. So get up and get moving!"

Luis yawned. "Where am I going to go? Who am I going to go with? I don't have any friends here."

"What about that boy who lives down the hall? I saw him leave with a gym bag the other day. He must have

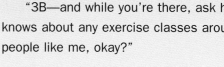

been going somewhere you'd like to go."

"Well, maybe," Luis said. "But maybe he was going to play handball or something like that—something I don't know how to do."

"And maybe he was going to play basketball, huh? And maybe it wouldn't kill you to learn how to play handball or another new sport, right?"

Luis smiled up at his mom. "Maybe. What's his apartment number?"

"3B—and while you're there, ask his mom if she knows about any exercise classes around here for old people like me, okay?"

For Discussion

What caused Luis to have an "activity relapse"? What could he do if it turns out that the boy down the hall likes to swim and hates basketball? What are some other things that cause relapses? What can be done to avoid them? Fill out the questionnaire to find out how you might respond if something begins to interfere with your level of physical activity.

Wellness for All

Because wellness often is considered the opposite of illness, people sometimes think wellness is impossible for a person with a disease or medical problem. Most experts now agree that anyone can have wellness, even if he or she has a disease that is being treated. For example, a person who has had diabetes since birth does have a disease. However, with treatment, the person can live a relatively normal life. By practicing healthy lifestyles and developing the positive aspect of each health component, a diabetic can develop good health and wellness. This, in turn, will enable the person to reach his or her fullest potential.

Most of us have health problems at some point in our lives. These problems may be short- or long-term. However, even with problems, you can develop and practice healthy lifestyles to enhance your sense of

well-being and your quality of life. Maintaining a positive attitude, for example, can help you overcome physical problems that are beyond your control.

One way to gain the information and support you need is to join a health club. Throughout this chapter your class will work together to create a health club. Your teacher will provide you with the information you need to begin.

Lesson Review

1. How does wellness relate to good health?
2. Identify five components of health and wellness. Describe the positive and negative aspects of each.
3. How can the positive aspect of each component contribute to good health?

The Walking Test

Many of the self-assessments you did earlier in this course required very intense physical activity. The cardiovascular fitness self-assessments, such as the Mile Run, can be good assessments but they are not for everyone. Beginners and people who do not enjoy running may prefer doing another type of assessment. The Walking Test gives you an alternative to the Mile Run, the PACER, and the Step Test.

If you are a very active person and are quite fit, the Mile Run or PACER may be best for estimating your cardiovascular fitness, but the Walking Test is also a good test. The test is especially good for people who are beginners, who haven't been doing a lot of recent activity, and who are regular walkers. It is also good for older people and for those who cannot do running tests because of joint or muscle problems. Try all of the assessments because by using results of several different assessments you will have a better overall view of your fitness.

Because you are walking, a warm-up is not necessary. The walk itself is a warm-up. Some people prefer to do some preliminary walking and a warm-up stretch before this test.

Record your Results on the Record Sheet

1 Walk a mile at a fast pace (as fast as you can while keeping approximately the same pace for the entire walk).

2 Immediately after the walk, count your heart rate for 15 seconds. Calculate your one-minute heart rate by multiplying by 4. Record your rate on your record sheet.

3 Locate your walking rating using the appropriate chart. Record your rating.

Rating Chart: Walking Test (females)

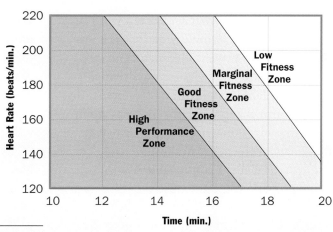

Adapted from the *One Mile Walk Test*, with permission of the author, James M. Rippe, M.D.

Rating Chart: Walking Test (males)

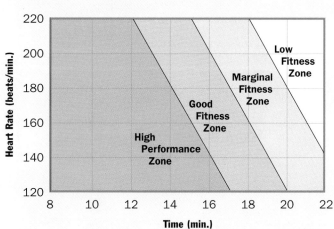

Adapted from the *One Mile Walk Test*, with permission of the author, James M. Rippe, M.D.

16.2 Lesson Healthy Lifestyles

Lesson Objectives

After reading this lesson, you should be able to:

1. Explain the difference between controllable risk factors and noncontrollable risk factors.

2. Identify and explain some healthy lifestyles.

Lesson Vocabulary

controllable risk factor, noncontrollable risk factor

If you asked every person you know, you would probably find that all of them would like to have good health and wellness. But how many of them are aware of all the things they can do to achieve it? In this lesson you will learn about healthy lifestyles and how they can help you achieve good health and wellness.

Healthy Lifestyles and Controllable Risk Factors

You probably know by now that *lifestyle* is a word that refers to the way you live. A healthy lifestyle is a way of living that helps you prevent illness and enhance wellness. In fact, healthy lifestyles are ways that you can reduce **controllable risk factors**—risk factors that you can act upon to change. Healthy lifestyles are in your control and, if you practice them, they reduce your risk of many of the major health problems. For example, a high-fat diet is a controllable risk factor, but by eating properly you can reduce the risk associated with high-fat diets.

As you can see in the diagram at the top of the page, four major factors contribute to early death. The largest number of early deaths results from unhealthy lifestyles. This means that these problems could be prevented if people would change the way they live. It is important to know that practicing healthy lifestyles not only reduces the risk of disease and death from disease but also enhances wellness. For example, not smoking greatly reduces the risk of heart disease and cancer and also increases your quality of your life. You can breathe better, have a keener sense of smell, and spend less money on tobacco and medical care.

Some risk factors are not in your control, such as age and gender. These factors are called **noncontrollable risk factors**. Since there is nothing you can do about these risk factors, focus on those than you can control. For this reason, this chapter focuses on healthy lifestyles over which you have some control.

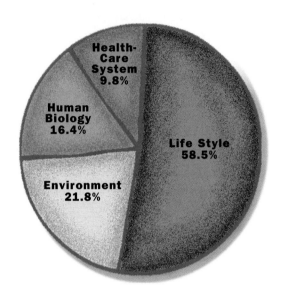

Four main factors contribute to early death.

Identifying Healthy Lifestyles

Doing regular physical activity is a healthy lifestyle that health experts feel is among the most important. Not only does it help you prevent many of the major illnesses and enhance your physical fitness and health, but it can contribute to good health in other areas as well. Though doing physical activity is the healthy lifestyle that is emphasized in this book, other healthy lifestyles also are important. The chart below lists some things you can do for a healthy lifestyle.

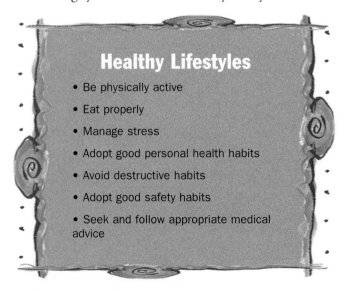

Healthy Lifestyles

- Be physically active
- Eat properly
- Manage stress
- Adopt good personal health habits
- Avoid destructive habits
- Adopt good safety habits
- Seek and follow appropriate medical advice

Be physically active. You have been learning throughout this book why physical activity is important to good health. The benefits to good health and wellness were outlined in detail in Chapter 5. Among the health goals set forth in *Healthy People 2010*, being physically active is one of the most important. It is one of the primary goals because changing inactive people to active people (changing lifestyles) would do more for the health and wellness of people than any other change. For example, being physically active can help you manage stress, which in turn can contribute to more healthy lifestyles.

Eat properly. What kinds of food do you typically eat? Are your meals generally high in fat? Do you eat plenty of fruits and vegetables, as well as grains and meats? Many children, teens, and adults eat more fat than they should and, in general, do not eat a balanced diet. Another major health goal is to improve the nutrition of all citizens. The goals set forth in *Healthy People 2010* outline ways to improve health and wellness by changing eating habits. You will study the healthy lifestyle of eating properly in greater detail in Chapter 17.

Manage stress. You probably have had periods of stress and know how it can affect you for the short term. But did you know that stress can cause health problems and detract from personal well-being and quality of life? While most people are well aware of the stress experienced by business people, elected officials, and other people in "high stress" jobs, many sometimes forget that stress effects everyone—including teens. Learning to manage stress is a healthy lifestyle that is important to good health and wellness. You will study stress in greater detail in Chapter 18.

Adopt good personal health habits. In kindergarten or first grade you most likely learned about personal health habits, such as regularly brushing and flossing your teeth, washing your hands before meals and after using the bathroom, and getting enough sleep. But how many of these habits have you adopted? Using good health habits is one way you can prevent illness and promote optimal quality of living. For example, if you have an illness which could have been prevented through proper health habits, you will feel ill and you will have at least a temporary reduction in the quality of living.

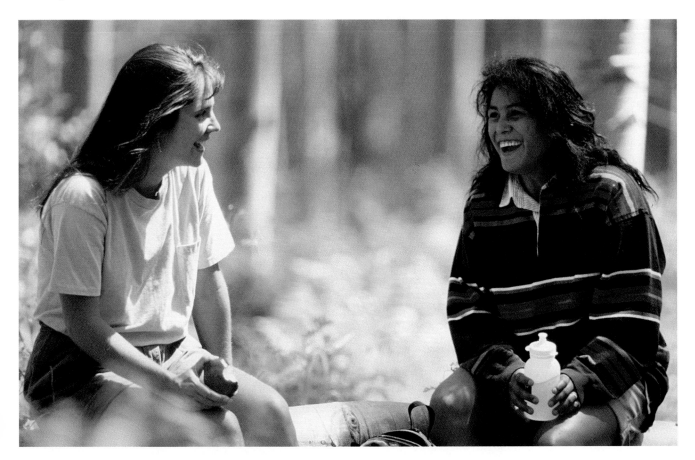

Healthy lifestyles reduce your risk of many health problems.

Avoid destructive habits. Just as adopting healthy habits contributes to good health, possessing destructive habits detracts from health and wellness. Smoking, other tobacco use, abuse of illegal or legal drugs, and the abuse of alcohol are just a few of the destructive habits that detract from total health. These destructive habits can inhibit your fitness, detract from your performance of physical activities, and result in various diseases, lowered feelings of well being, and reduced quality of life.

Adopt good safety practices. News accounts of injuries or deaths due to motor vehicle accidents fill the newspapers each day. Other common causes of death or injury include falls, poisonings, drowning, fires, bicycle accidents, and accidents in and around home. Many of these injuries or deaths could have been prevented if simple safety rules had been followed. A national health goal is to reduce the number of deaths and injuries from accidents. Things you can do to adopt healthy lifestyles include wearing seat belts, wearing helmets while riding bikes or inline skating, locking up poisons, installing and maintaining smoke detectors, practicing water safety, and keeping your home in good repair to reduce the

risks of accidents. And don't forget—being physically fit can help prevent accidents too!

Seek and follow appropriate medical advice. Even if you follow healthy lifestyles, you may become ill occasionally. In those cases, seeking and following appropriate medical advice is important. In fact, for best results, regular medical and dental checkups are recommended to help prevent problems before they start. Consult with your own physician and dentist to determine how often you should have a checkup. Some people avoid seeking medical help because they fear they may be ill. Since early detection of health problems is important to an ultimate cure, this practice can be dangerous.

Practice other healthy lifestyles. Other lifestyles that will help improve health and wellness include protecting the environment (recycling, not polluting the air, land, or water), being an informed consumer (not buying quack products), and learning first aid (learning CPR).

Lesson Review

1. What is the difference between controllable risk factors and noncontrollable risk factors? Give examples.
2. Identify and explain some healthy lifestyles.

Wearing proper safety equipment reduces the risk of injury.

Activity 16
Your Health and Fitness Club

Some people who want information about fitness, health, and wellness join a health and fitness club. These clubs can offer opportunities to engage in healthy lifestyles, such as being active. Many of these clubs are now offering advice and opportunities about other healthy lifestyles such as eating properly, managing stress, and avoiding destructive habits. As you learned in Chapter 13, some of these clubs may have people who are qualified to give sound information and others do not. You can use many of the guidelines you learned in this course to evaluate these clubs and their employees.

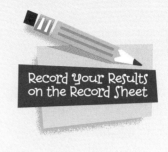

Record your Results on the Record Sheet

If you haven't already joined a health and fitness club, you may later decide to do so to help you adopt healthy lifestyles. One way to learn more about healthy lifestyles and about health and fitness clubs is to establish one of your own.

In this chapter, your class will create a health and fitness club. The class will name the club, select appropriate physical activities to be offered, and prepare materials about wellness and healthy lifestyles that will be available to club members. After these general decisions are made, groups will plan club activities for the club. During your activity class, you will have an opportunity to share your group's information with other class-mates. You will also learn about the other groups' topics. Follow the instructions on your record sheet as you plan your health and fitness club.

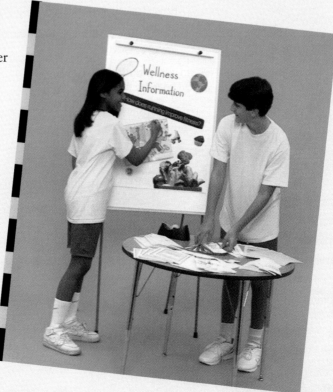

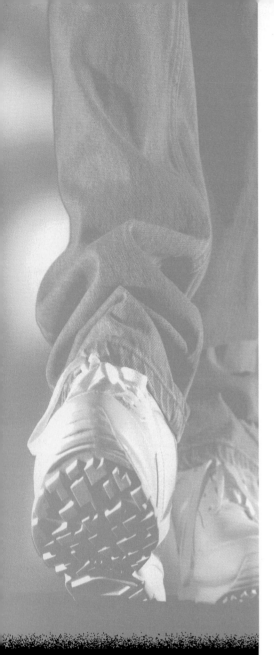

16 Chapter Review

Reviewing Concepts and Vocabulary

Copy the number of each statement on a sheet of paper. Next to each number, write the word or words that correctly complete the sentence.

1. A _____ is a way of living that helps you prevent illness and enhance wellness.

2. _____ are the largest contributors to early death.

3. _____ would do more to improve the health and wellness of American people than any other change.

Number your paper. Next to each number, choose the letter of the best answer.

Column I	Column II
4. fulfilled	a. positive aspect of social component of health
5. informed	b. positive aspect of intellectual component of health
6. involved	c. positive aspect of spiritual component of health

On your paper, write a short answer for each statement or question.

7. How has the definition of *health* changed during this century?

8. Explain the difference between controllable and noncontrollable risk factors. Give examples.

9. What is the focus of the national health goals as set forth in *Healthy People 2000*?

10. What is wellness?

Thinking Critically

Write a paragraph to answer the following question.

What are some healthy lifestyles you now practice? How do they contribute to good health?

Project

Develop a "Health and Wellness Contract" that encourages a commitment to a lifetime of health and wellness. You might want to develop this contract as part of a health and wellness support group. Distribute your contract to the class.

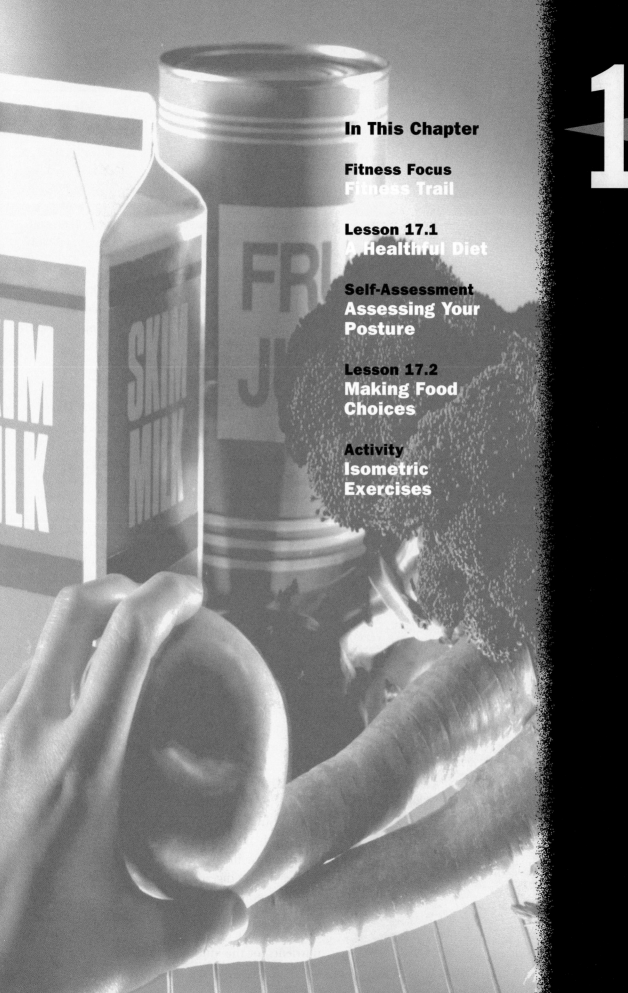

17

Choosing Nutritious Food

Fitness Trail

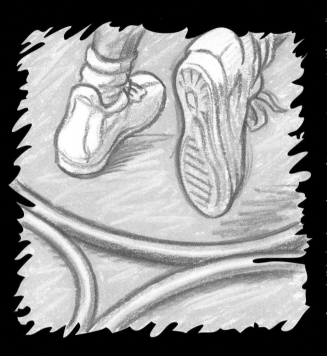

A fitness trail is a form of a physical fitness workout in which you follow a circular path and stop at exercise stations along the way. You jog from station to station and perform the exercise described on the posted sign, using the number of repetitions recommended for your fitness status. These stations are designed for a complete workout— a warm-up and cool-down, with flexibility, strength, and endurance exercises in between. Jogging between stations takes care of the cardiovascular component. Follow the directions on your instruction sheet.

Stride Jump	**Vault**
Backsaver Sit and Reach	**Side Stretch**
Trunk Twister	**Curl-Up**
Knee Lift	**Push-Up**
Hop Scotch	**Reverse Curl**
Chain Swing	**Hand Walk**
Chin-Up/Bent-Arm Hang	**Calf Stretcher**

17.1 A Healthful Diet
Lesson

Lesson Objectives
After reading this lesson, you should be able to:
1. Name functions of each kind of nutrient.
2. Explain how to use the dietary guidelines and the Food Guide Pyramid to plan a balanced diet.

Vocabulary:
nutrient, carbohydrate, simple carbohydrate, complex carbohydrate, nutritionally dense, fiber, protein, amino acid, complete protein, incomplete protein

What kinds of foods are important for your health? How much food do you need to eat? In this lesson, you will learn about healthful foods. You also will learn how to select foods for a balanced diet.

Nutrients Your Body Needs
Scientists have identified 45 to 50 different **nutrients**—food substances required for the growth and maintenance of your cells. These nutrients have been divided into six groups—carbohydrates, proteins, fats, vitamins, minerals, and water.

Food scientists have developed guidelines, called the United States Recommended Daily Allowances (U.S. RDA). These guidelines list the recommended daily nutritional requirements of vitamins, minerals, proteins, and Calories for people according to sex, age, height, and weight. By following these guidelines and eating the right amounts of foods containing all the nutrients, you should get a healthful diet.

Carbohydrates
Carbohydrates are nutrients that provide you with energy. **Simple carbohydrates** are sugars found in foods such as fruits, milk, molasses, and honey. Your body can use them for energy with little or no change during digestion. **Complex carbohydrates** are sugars found in foods such as breads, vegetables, and grain. Complex carbohydrates are called **nutritionally dense** because they contain large amounts of nutrients for the number of Calories they provide.

Fiber is a type of carbohydrate that your body cannot digest. Fiber supplies no energy. Fiber sources include the leaves, stems, roots, and seed coverings of fruits, vegetables, and grains. Examples of foods high in fiber are whole-grain breads and cereals, the skin of fresh fruits, raw vegetables, nuts, and seeds. Fiber helps you avoid intestinal problems and might reduce your chances of developing some forms of cancer.

Protein

Proteins are the group of nutrients that builds, repairs, and maintains body cells. They are called the building blocks of your body. Animal products, such as milk, eggs, meat, and fish, contain proteins. Some plants, such as beans and grains, also contain proteins.

During digestion, your body breaks down proteins into simpler substances called **amino acids,** which your small intestine can absorb. Your body can manufacture 11 of the 20 amino acids. You need to get the other nine amino acids—known as the *essential amino acids*—from food.

Foods with all nine essential amino acids are said to contain **complete proteins.** They come from animal sources, such as meat, milk products, and fish. Foods that contain some, but not all, essential amino acids are said to contain **incomplete proteins.** Beans, nuts, rice, and certain other plants contain incomplete proteins. A daily diet that includes foods with both complete and incomplete proteins usually provides ample essential amino acids. People who do not eat

meat need to eat a variety of incomplete proteins that provide all the essential amino acids.

Fats

Fats provide twice as much energy per ounce as carbohydrates do. Fats are in animal products and in some plant products, such as nuts and vegetable oils.

Fats are necessary for the growth and repair of cells. Fats dissolve certain vitamins and carry them to body cells. In addition, fats enhance the flavor and texture of foods.

Fats are classified as *saturated* or *unsaturated*. In general, saturated fats are solid at room temperature; unsaturated fats are liquid at room temperature. Saturated fats come mostly from animal products, such as lard, butter, milk, and meat fats. Unsaturated fats come mostly from plants, such as sunflowers, corn, soybeans, olives, almonds, and peanuts. Also, fish produce unsaturated fats in their cells.

Foods from the six nutrient groups

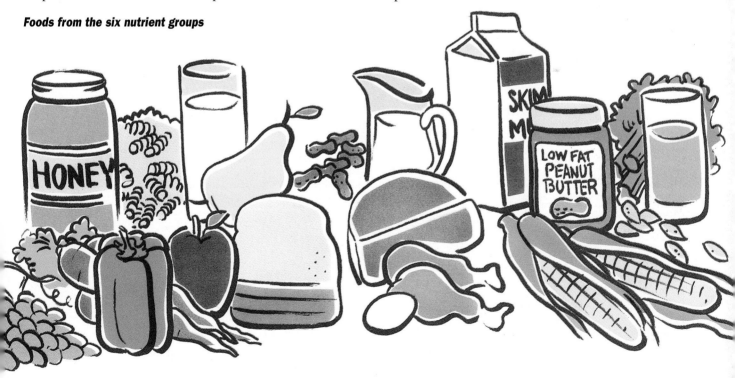

Cholesterol is a waxy, fat-like substance found in the saturated fats of animal cells, including those of humans. You not only produce your own cholesterol, you consume cholesterol in certain foods. High levels of cholesterol can contribute to atherosclerosis and other heart diseases. Medical experts recommend eating foods low in cholesterol and low in saturated fat.

Minerals

Minerals are essential nutrients that help regulate the activities of cells. Minerals have no Calories and provide no energy.

Minerals come from elements in the earth's crust. They are present in all plants and animals. You need 25 different minerals in varying amounts. The table below shows some major functions of the most important minerals as well as some food sources for them.

If you eat a balanced diet, you will most likely be getting the proper amounts of minerals. However if you take a vitamin-mineral supplement, you need to be careful not to exceed the recommended daily allowance (RDA) for any mineral. An excessive amount could lead to health problems. For example, too much calcium could interfere with other medications you may take. Too much magnesium can deplete the body of calcium and phosphorus. Too much zinc can deplete the body of copper.

Calcium Eating calcium-rich foods is important for health. An important function of calcium is building and maintaining bones. At about age 20, your bones become less efficient in getting calcium out of the food you eat and your bones begin to lose calcium. Because of a change in hormones when women reach about age 55, they have much more bone loss than men. A large percentage of older women develop *osteoporosis,* a condition in which the bones become porous and break easily. Men can have this disease, but they get it less often and much later in life. Getting enough calcium and doing weight-bearing exercises all of your life help reduce the risk of osteoporosis.

Iron Iron is a mineral needed for proper formation and functioning of your red blood cells. The red blood cells carry oxygen to your muscles and other body tissues. Iron deficiencies are especially common among girls and women. When you have insufficient iron in your body, you have *iron deficiency anemia.* This condition causes a person to feel tired all the time.

The best sources of iron are meat (especially red meat), poultry, and fish. Iron from these foods is more easily absorbed than iron from other foods. An adequate amount of Vitamin C also helps your body absorb iron. Eating a variety of foods that contain iron is the best way to get an adequate amount.

Functions and Sources of Minerals

Minerals	Function in the body	Food sources
Calcium	Builds and maintains teeth and bones; helps blood clot; helps nerves and muscles function	Cheese; milk; dark green vegetables; sardines; legumes
Phosphorus	Builds and maintains teeth and bones; helps release energy from nutrients	Meat; poultry; fish; eggs; legumes; milk products
Magnesium	Aids breaking down of glucose and proteins; regulates body fluids	Green vegetables; grains; nuts; beans; yeast
Sodium	Regulates internal water balance; helps nerves function	Most foods; table salt
Potassium	Regulates fluid balance in cells; helps nerves function	Oranges; bananas; meats; bran; potatoes; dried beans
Iron	Helps transfer oxygen in red blood cells and in other cells	Liver; red meats; dark green vegetables; shellfish; whole-grain cereals
Zinc	Aids in transport of carbon dioxide; aids in healing wounds	Meats; shellfish; whole grains; milk; legumes

Functions and Sources of Vitamins

Vitamins	Function in the body	Food sources
B1 (Thiamin)	Helps release energy from carbohydrates	Pork; organ meats; legumes; greens
B2 (Riboflavin)	Helps break down carbohydrates and proteins	Meat; milk products; eggs; green and yellow vegetables
B6 (Pyridoxine)	Helps break down protein and glucose	Yeast; nuts; beans; liver; fish; rice
B12 (Cobalamin)	Aids nucleic acid and amino acid formation	Meat; milk products; eggs; fish
Folacin	Helps build DNA and proteins	Yeast; wheat germ, liver; greens
Pantothenic acid	Involved in reactions with carbohydrates and proteins	Most unprocessed foods
Niacin	Helps release energy from carbohydrates and proteins	Milk; meats; whole-grain or enriched cereals; legumes
Biotin	Aids formation of amino, nucleic, and fatty acids and glycogen	Eggs; liver; yeast
C (Ascorbic acid)	Aids formation of hormones, bone tissue, and collagen	Fruits; tomatoes; potatoes; green, leafy vegetables
A (Retinol)	Helps produce normal mucus, part of chemical necessary for vision	Butter; margarine; liver; eggs; green or yellow vegetables
D	Aids absorption of calcium and phosphorous	Liver; fortified milk; fatty fish
E (Tocopherol)	Prevents damage to cell membranes and vitamin A	Vegetable oils
K	Aids blood clotting	Leafy vegetables

Sodium Sodium is a mineral that helps your body cells function properly. Sodium is present in many foods. It is especially high in certain foods, such as snack foods, processed foods, fast foods, and cured meats such as ham. For many people, sodium in the diet comes primarily from table salt (sodium chloride).

Most people eat more sodium than they need. It is wise to limit the amount of sodium in your diet. People with high blood pressure, or hypertension, need to be especially careful to limit sodium. It can cause their bodies to retain water, helping keep their blood pressure high.

Vitamins

Vitamins are needed for growth and repair of body cells. Like minerals, vitamins contain no Calories and provide no energy. If you eat a balanced diet, you most likely will get the proper amounts of vitamins.

Vitamin C and the B vitamins are water-soluble.

They dissolve in blood and are carried to cells throughout your body. Your body cannot store excess B and C vitamins. You need to eat foods containing these vitamins every day. Vitamins A, D, E, and K dissolve in fat. Excess amounts of these vitamins are stored in fat cells in your liver and other body parts. The table above gives you more information about specific vitamins.

Water

Dietitians usually say that water is the single most important nutrient. It carries the other nutrients to your cells, carries away wastes, and regulates body temperature. Most foods contain water. In fact, your own body weight is 50 to 60 percent water.

Your body loses two to three quarts of water a day through breathing, perspiring, and eliminating wastes from the bowels and bladder. In very hot weather, or when you exercise vigorously, you lose even more water than usual. Then you need to drink plenty of extra fluids. The best beverages for this purpose are water, fruit juice, and milk. Avoid soft drinks that contain caffeine because caffeine is a diuretic which increases fluid loss. Also, "sports drinks" sold commercially usually contain sodium and other ingredients that you do not need unless you exercise for several hours in high temperatures.

Planning a Balanced Diet

As you have learned, you need to eat foods containing all six nutrients in order to get a healthful, balanced diet. In addition, other guidelines have been developed to help you choose healthful foods.

Health Goals in America America has national goals, called *Healthy People 2010* goals to promote health and prevent disease. These are the goals related to nutrition:
• Reduce dietary fat, especially saturated fat.
• Increase the servings of food from levels 1 and 2 of the pyramid.
• Increase the amount of calcium in the diet.
• Decrease the amount of salt and sodium in the diet.

• Reduce the incidence of iron deficiency.
• Increase dietary quality of snacks and meals away from home.

Dietary Guidelines for America The Human Nutrition Information Service of the U.S. Department of Agriculture has established important dietary guidelines for Americans:

• Eat a variety of foods.
• Balance the food you eat with physical activity — maintain or improve your weight.
• Choose a diet with plenty of grain products, vegetables, and fruits.
• Choose a diet low in fat, saturated fat, and cholesterol.
• Choose a diet moderate in sugars.
• Choose a diet moderate in salt and sodium.

The Food Guide Pyramid The Food Guide Pyramid, shown here, provides an outline of what you need to eat each day. The Pyramid is based on the dietary guidelines, and it can help you choose foods for a healthful diet. The Pyramid calls for eating a

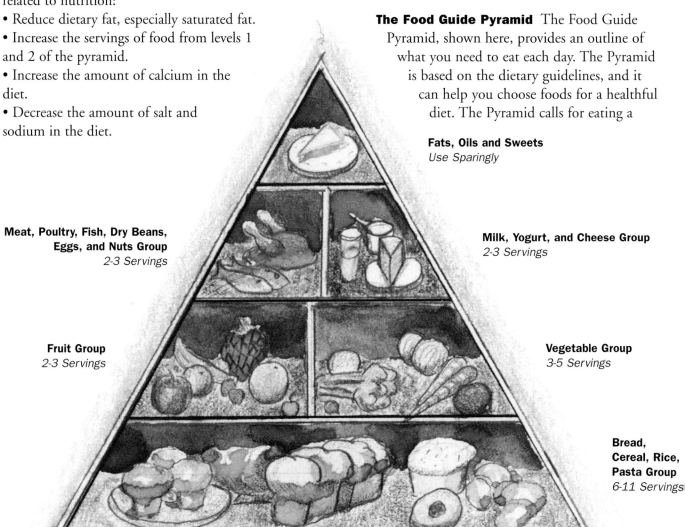

Fats, Oils and Sweets
Use Sparingly

Meat, Poultry, Fish, Dry Beans, Eggs, and Nuts Group
2-3 Servings

Milk, Yogurt, and Cheese Group
2-3 Servings

Fruit Group
2-3 Servings

Vegetable Group
3-5 Servings

Bread, Cereal, Rice, Pasta Group
6-11 Servings

The Food Guide Pyramid

variety of foods that provide the nutrients you need and contain the proper amount of Calories to help you maintain a healthy weight.

The Food Guide Pyramid emphasizes eating foods from the five major food groups that are shown in the lower sections of the Pyramid. Each food group provides some, but not all, of the nutrients you need. For good health, you need to eat the recommended number of servings of foods from each group.

It is especially important to eat more servings from the lowest level of the Pyramid. These foods are from the bread, cereal, rice, and pasta group. These foods contain many essential nutrients and are low in fat. The next greatest number of servings should come from the vegetable group and the fruit group. The foods in these groups are especially rich in vital nutrients. Some evidence indicates that eating fruits and vegetables, particularly those that are dark green, dark yellow, and orange, can significantly reduce the risk of cancer. Choose fewer servings from the meat, poultry, fish, dry beans, eggs, and nuts group, as well as the milk, yogurt, and cheese group. Eating the recom-

mended number of servings from these groups is important to good health and fitness because these foods are high in protein. These foods also tend to be high in fat, so be careful to choose lean meats and low-fat dairy products.

The foods at the top of the Pyramid contain large amounts of fats and sugars and a large number of Calories. They usually contain few, if any, other nutrients such as vitamins and minerals. For this reason, limiting these foods in your diet is wise. Among these foods are cookies, cakes, soft drinks, jellies, butter, margarine, mayonnaise, and salad dressings.

Recommended Servings How much do you need to eat? It depends on your caloric needs. The chart below lists the recommended servings from each food group for each of the following Calorie groups:
• 1,600 Calories: primarily sedentary women
• 2,200 Calories: most children, teenage girls, active women, and sedentary men
• 2,800 Calories: usually teenage boys, active men, and very active women.

Recommended Number and Size of Servings

Calorie Range	1600	2200	2800	Serving Size
Bread/Cereal/ Rice/Pasta	6 servings	9 servings	11 servings	1 slice bread, 1/2 cup cooked cereal, rice, or pasta 1 cup cold cereal 1/4 cup wheat germ 1 6-inch tortilla
Vegetables	3 servings	4 servings	5 servings	1 medium potato 1/2 cup cooked vegetable
Fruit	2 servings	3 servings	4 servings	1 orange 3/4 cup fruit juice 1/2 cup cooked fruit
Milk/Yogurt Cheese	2-3 servings	2-3 servings	2-3 servings	1 cup milk/yogurt 1/2 cup cottage cheese 1 1/2 ounces cheese
Meat/Poultry/Fish Dry Beans/Eggs/Nuts	2 servings	2-3 servings	3 servings	1 serving=2-3 ounces of any cooked meat, poultry, or fish Equivalent=either 1/2 cup of cooked dried beans, 2 tablespoons peanut butter or whole egg=1 ounce of meat/poultry/fish. Quantity and type of fat will vary in each protein source.

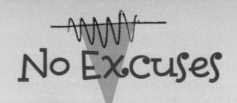

No Excuses

Saying "No"

Sometimes the single act of saying "no" is the best way to avoid a situation that is potentially harmful. While it may seem easy to say this simple word, the action may actually be very difficult to carry out successfully.

Manny was invited to spend the holiday with his girlfriend's family. Plans were made to spend the afternoon water-skiing at a nearby lake followed by a big party. His girlfriend, Rita, warned Manny that her mother always prepared huge amounts of food for the party. It was her family's tradition to "stuff themselves until they couldn't move." She told him to make sure he came with a big appetite. Unfortunately, Manny's doctor had just instructed him to restrict the amount of fats and Calories he consumed.

Manny arrived at the party just as Rita's mother was setting out the food. The table was loaded with tortilla chips, guacamole, beef and bean burritos, chiles rellenos, and fresh corn, as well as cakes, pies, and cookies. Manny knew that he faced a difficult

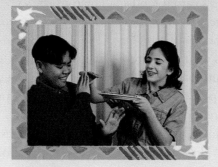

situation as Rita came forward with a plate piled with cookies. "Manny, you're just in time. The food is great!."

Manny replied, "Everything looks good, but I have to watch my diet."

Rita offered him a cookie, knowing they were Manny's favorite. "But you've got to try my mother's cookies. Everyone says they're the best. You'll hurt my mother's feelings if you don't eat one."

For Discussion

In what way does the party put Manny in a "difficult situation?" How can Manny say "no" to Rita without embarrassing her or hurting her feelings? What can he do so that his refusal won't hurt Rita's mother? What could he have done before actually going to the party to prepare for this situation? In what other situations would saying "no" be the best response? Fill out the questionnaire to find out if you are more likely to say "no" and mean it or give in under pressure.

Hidden Fats and Sugars Using fats, oils, and sweets sparingly is not always easy to do. Fats, oils, and sweets are often hidden in foods. For example, a potato is a nutritious, low-fat food. However, french fried potatoes are cooked in oil, so they are high in fat content. Think about other kinds of foods sold in fast-food restaurants. In fact, most of these fast foods are high in fat.

Also, many sauces and toppings that people add to food are high in fats, oils, and sugar. Such sauces include ketchup and mayonnaise. Many salads made of healthful vegetables are topped with dressings that are high in fats, oils, and sugars. You need to keep in mind the ingredients in a food as well as the method used to cook the food in order to limit the fats, oils, and sugars in your diet.

You learned in Chapter 7 that many factors,

including metabolism, heredity, maturation, and physical activity, influence body fatness. These factors also influence the amount of Calories you need to eat. You need to balance the number of Calories you consume with the number of Calories you expend in order to maintain a healthy weight. Your body burns Calories for energy. The more vigorous activity you do, the more energy your body uses and the more Calories you need.

Lesson Review

1. Explain how each of the six kinds of nutrients is important for good health.
2. What are the five major food groups and how many servings are needed daily from each group?

Assessing Your Posture

You need to practice good posture at all times. You can use this Self-Assessment to determine whether your posture is as good as it should be. Wear a gym suit, swimsuit, or shorts and a T-shirt when taking this self-evaluation. Work with a partner to determine each other's scores. Write your results on your record sheet.

Record Your Results on the Record Sheet

1 Stand sideways next to a string hung from at least one foot above your head. The string should be weighted at the bottom so that it hangs straight. Position yourself so that the string aligns with your ankle bone.

2 Have your partner answer *yes* or *no* to each question below.

• Head: Is the ear in front of the line?

• Shoulders: Are the shoulders rounded? Are the tips of the shoulders in front of the chest?

• Upper back: Does the upper back stick out in a hump?

• Lower back: Does the lower back have excessive arch?

• Abdomen: Does your abdomen protrude beyond the pelvic bone?

• Knees: Do the knees appear to be locked or bent backwards?

3 Now stand with your back to the string so that the string is aligned with the middle of your back.

• Head: Is more than one-half of the head on one side of the string?

• Shoulders: Is either shoulder higher than the other shoulder?

• Hips: Is either hip higher than the other hip?

4 Total the number of yes answers. Check the score against the rating chart. Do you think your posture is as good as it should be? How might you improve your posture all of the time, not just when standing?

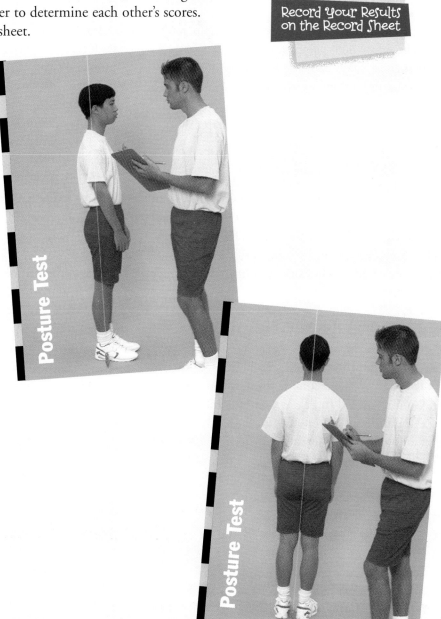

Posture Test

Posture Test

Rating Chart: Good Posture Test

Score (yes answers)	Rating
0 – 1	Good posture
2 – 4	Posture can use some improvement
5 or more	Posture definitely needs improvement

17.2 Lesson Making Food Choices

Objectives

After reading this lesson, you should be able to:

1. Explain how to use the FIT formula to meet your nutritional needs.
2. Explain how reading food labels can help you make healthful food choices.
3. Recognize some common myths about nutrition and explain why they are not factual.

Vocabulary

You have learned how to use the Food Guide Pyramid to choose foods for a nutritious diet. You also learned how following the Dietary Guidelines can help you attain and maintain good health. In this lesson, you will learn more about choosing healthful foods for a balanced diet.

The FIT Formula and Nutrition

The table below shows how you can use the FIT Formula as a guideline for nutritional fitness. Note that the FIT Formula recommends that you use the Food Guide Pyramid to help you choose foods.

Keep in mind that you need to eat foods with the proper amounts of all the nutrients in order to have a healthful diet. Remember that a steady diet of "junk food," fad diets, fast foods, and incorrect use of vitamin and mineral supplements can all be harmful to your health. Also remember that eating properly and doing regular physical activity are important for maintaining a proper amount of body fatness. Be aware of the signs of eating disorders that you learned in Chapter 7.

When selecting foods, you need to determine your own nutritional requirements. As you learned, a person's nutrient needs vary according to age, sex, height, and weight.

Young people who are going through puberty and those who are still growing have special nutritional needs. They need to eat foods high in potassium, calcium, and iron. These minerals aid in the development of bones and blood. By eating the correct number of servings from each of the food groups, you probably are consuming a diet that will meet your nutritional needs.

Food Choices

Many teenagers do not plan meals, shop for groceries, or cook for a family. However, maybe you do help with these activities. Most likely, you do sometimes purchase snacks for yourself. How do you know if the food you are purchasing is nutritious? Reading food labels can help you determine how nutritious a food is. In fact, according to law, manufacturers must now use a standard format for food labels.

Food Labels

You probably have noticed that most foods have a nutrition label and an ingredient list. Look at the food label shown on the next page. First notice the serving size. Keep in mind that if you double the serving size listed, you need to double the nutrient and caloric values. On the other hand, if you eat only one-half the serving size, you need to cut the nutrient and caloric values in half. Find the number of Calories per serving. This information can help you keep track of how many Calories you consume.

You can see that information about a variety of nutrients is provided on the label. Find the information about carbohydrates. You learned in the last lesson, that carbohydrates are important sources of energy. However, remember that you should eat sugars

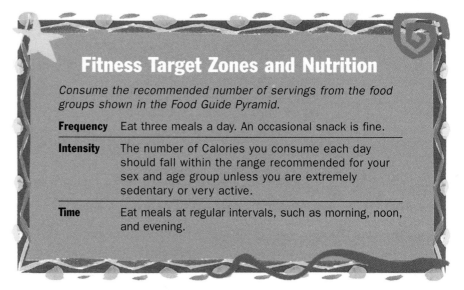

Fitness Target Zones and Nutrition

Consume the recommended number of servings from the food groups shown in the Food Guide Pyramid.

Frequency	Eat three meals a day. An occasional snack is fine.
Intensity	The number of Calories you consume each day should fall within the range recommended for your sex and age group unless you are extremely sedentary or very active.
Time	Eat meals at regular intervals, such as morning, noon, and evening.

Nutrition Facts

Serving Size 1/2 cup (114g)
Servings Per Container 4

Amount Per Serving

Calories 90	Calories from Fat 30

	% Daily Value*
Total Fat 3g	**5%**
Saturated Fat 0g	**0%**
Cholesterol 0mg	**0%**
Sodium 300mg	**13%**
Total Carbohydrate 13g	**4%**
Dietary Fiber 3g	**12%**
Sugars 3g	
Protein 3g	

Vitamin A	80%	•	Vitamin C	60%
Calcium	4%	•	Iron	4%

* Percent daily Values are based on a 2,000 calorie diet. Your daily values may be higher or lower depending on your calorie needs:

		Calories	2,000	2,500
Total Fat	Less than		65g	80g
Sat Fat	Less than		20g	25g
Cholesterol	Less than		300mg	300mg
Sodium	Less than		2,400 mg	2,400mg
Total Carbohydrate			300g	375g
Fiber			25g	30g

Calories per gram:

Fat 9	•	Carbohydrate 4	•	Protein 4

More nutrients may be listed on some labels.

Food Label

you what percent of your daily requirements for a nutrient are met by this food. For fat, saturated fat, cholesterol, and sodium, choose foods with a low percent daily value. For total carbohydrate, dietary fiber, vitamins, and minerals, your goal is to reach 100 percent of your daily value.

Claims on Food Labels You might have noticed terms such as those shown in the chart below on many food containers. These terms can be displayed on food containers only if the food meets legal standards set by the government.

You also might see health claims such as "good for heart health" on some food labels. Manufacturers must comply with government regulations regarding such labeling. For example, if a product advertises that its fat content is good for the heart, the product must be low in fat, saturated fat, and cholesterol. Fruits, vegetables, and grain products that make such claims must not only be low in fat, saturated fat, and cholesterol, but also contain at least the minimum amount of fiber per serving. Foods that display health claims related to blood pressure must be low in sodium.

Common Food Myths

You may have heard a number of incorrect or misleading statements about nutrition. Some common nutrition myths are listed here.

Myth Honey is more nutritious than sugar.
Fact Chemically, honey is quite like refined sugar. Honey contains a few other nutrients, but they are in

sparingly. Fruits, vegetables, whole-grain foods, beans, and peas are all good sources of fiber.

Notice that this label gives information about vitamins and minerals. Other food labels may even list additional information about nutrients.

Now find information on the label about fat, saturated fat, cholesterol, and sodium. What suggestions about these substances are made in the dietary guidelines on page 222?

Look at the column that lists Percent Daily Values. This tells

Key Words	What They Mean
Fat Free	Less than 0.5 gram of fat
Low Fat	3 grams of fat (or less) per serving
Lean	Less than 10 grams of fat, 4 grams of saturated fat, and 95 milligrams of cholesterol
Light (Lite)	1/3 less calories or no more than 1/2 the fat of the higher-calorie, higher-fat version; or no more than 1/2 the sodium of the higher-sodium version
Cholesterol Free	Less than 2 milligrams of cholesterol and 2 grams (or less) of saturated fat per serving

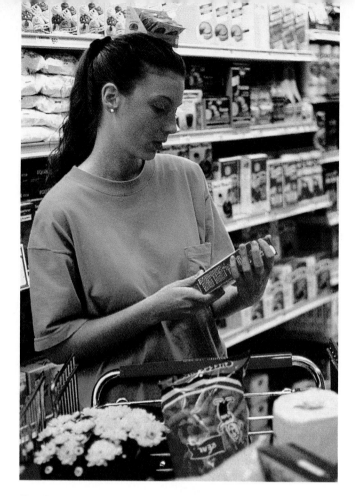

Read food labels to select healthy foods.

(AMA), the American Heart Association, and the American Cancer Society.

Eating Before Physical Activity

Most people can do moderate activity after a meal if they wait about 30 minutes to an hour. Persons who have problems doing activity after eating may have to wait longer or modify what they eat.

If you plan to do vigorous physical activity or participate in a highly-competitive athletic event, you may have to modify your eating patterns. Some guidelines are presented below.

• **Special diets are typically not necessary before athletic competitions.** Some athletes think they need a steak or a food supplement before they compete. Steak is high in protein and fat, both of which are digested slowly. Steak eaten within two hours of the event might interfere with a person's performance. In general, you can eat what you like as long as it does not disagree with you.

• **Allow extra time between eating and activity before vigorous competitive events.** Eat one to three hours before competing. Allow more time if the foods you have eaten are difficult to digest.

• **Before competition, reduce the size of your meal.** Small meals are easier to digest than large ones. If you get very nervous or often have an upset stomach before competition, try a liquid meal of about 900 Calories in 16 ounces of liquid. In general, liquid meals are not recommended.

• **Drink fluids before, during, and after activity.** Whether you are competing or not, it is important to drink water. Added salt or sugar are not typically needed. Using drinks with too much sugar can actually detract from performance.

such small amounts that they are of no benefit. You should limit your use of sugars, including honey.

Myth Foods labeled "natural" or "organic" are more nutritious than other foods.
Fact Often, such foods are not nutritious. For example, some of the "natural" granola-type cereals contain as much sugar and fat as other cereals.

Myth A poor diet causes acne and other skin problems.
Fact Most skin problems are caused by rapid changes in hormones that occur during adolescence. Hormones control oil glands, which can be very active during teenage years. Anxiety and emotional stress can aggravate this problem.

Because health and nutrition quackery is so commonplace, many other myths also exist. When making choices about nutrition, be sure to follow the Dietary Guidelines and the guidelines presented in the Food Guide Pyramid. Use information that comes from reliable sources. Some of these sources include: the Food and Drug Administration (FDA), the United States Department of Agriculture, the American Dietetic Association, the American Medical Association

Lesson Review
1. How can the FIT Formula help you determine how often to eat?
2. List three examples of information you can find on a food label.
3. Explain how two common food myths are incorrect or misleading.

Activity 17
Isometric Exercises

You already know that isometric exercises help develop muscle strength. You can use your own body, a wall, or a towel as immovable resistance when performing isometric exercises. This activity includes examples of isometric exercises good for strengthening muscles. Write your results on your record sheet.

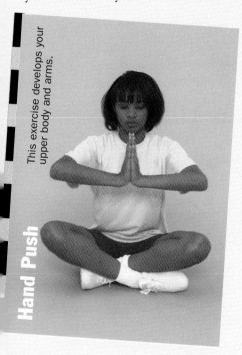

This exercise develops your upper body and arms.

Hand Push

Hand Push

1 Sit on the floor with your back straight. You may cross your legs if you prefer. Place the palms of your hands together.

2 Raise your hands and elbows to shoulder height. Push your hands against each other as hard as your can. Hold for 7 seconds; rest 30 seconds.

3 Repeat 2–3 times as time allows.

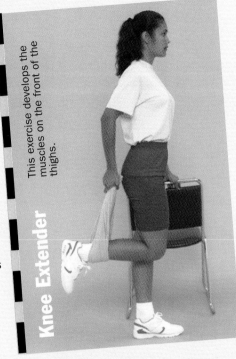

This exercise develops the muscles on the front of the thighs.

Knee Extender

Knee Extender

1 Hold something for support and stand on your left foot. Lift the right foot behind you, bending the knee to a 90-degree angle.

2 Loop a towel under your right ankle; hold the ends of the towel in your right hand.

3 Push downward with your foot, trying to straighten your leg against the resistance of the towel.

4 Repeat 2–3 times with each leg as time allows.

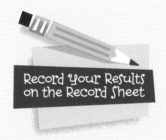

Record your Results on the Record Sheet

Back Flattener

1 Lie on your back with your knees bent.

2 Pull in your abdomen by contracting your abdominal muscles as tightly as possible. Flatten your lower back against the floor. Hold for 7 seconds; rest 30 seconds.

3 Repeat 2–3 times as time allows.

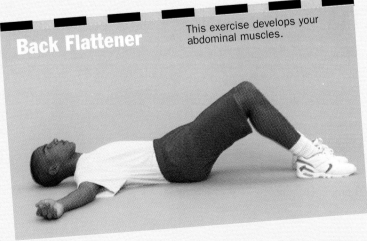

Back Flattener

This exercise develops your abdominal muscles.

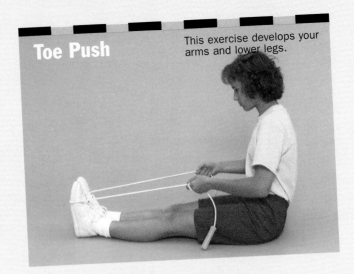

Toe Push

This exercise develops your arms and lower legs.

Toe Push

1 Sit on the floor with good posture.

2 Hold the end of a jumprope or towel in each hand. Loop it over the balls of your feet so it is tight against the soles.

3 Push with the balls of your feet as you pull on the rope or towel. Keep your back straight. Hold for 7 seconds; rest 30 seconds.

4 Repeat 2–3 times as time allows.

Biceps Curl with Towel

1 Stand with your back straight and knees slightly bent.

2 Loop a towel under the back of your thighs.

3 Grasp the towel ends with your palms up. Keep your elbows against your sides.

4 Pull up on the towel as hard as possible. Hold for 7 seconds; rest 30 seconds.

5 Repeat 2–3 times as time allows.

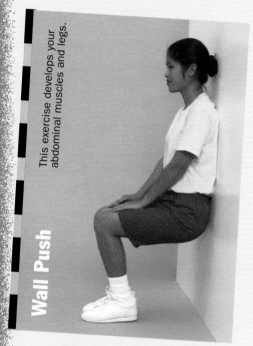

This exercise develops your abdominal muscles and legs.

Wall Push

Wall Push

1 Stand with your back against a wall.

2 Move your feet out as you lower yourself into a half squat. Keep your thighs parallel to the floor.

3 Push your back against the wall by pushing with your legs as hard as you can. Hold for 7 seconds; rest 30 seconds.

4 Repeat 2–3 times as time allows.

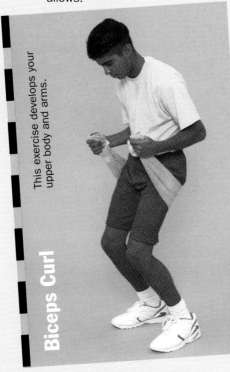

This exercise develops your upper body and arms.

Biceps Curl

Bow Exercise

1 Stand in a position that an archer would take when shooting a bow.

2 Hold a towel with your right arm as if you were holding a bow.

3 Hold the other end of the towel with your left hand near the chin as if holding the string of a bow.

4 Push with your right hand and pull with the left. Hold for 7 seconds; rest 30 seconds.

5 Repeat 2–3 times with each arm forward as time allows.

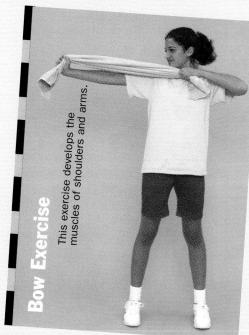

Bow Exercise

This exercise develops the muscles of shoulders and arms.

Leg Curl

1 Stand on your left leg. Hold on to a chair or wall for balance.

2 Loop a towel behind your right ankle and stand on the ends of the towel with your left foot.

3 Keeping your posture erect and your back straight, try to bend your knee against the resistance of the towel. Hold for 7 seconds; rest 30 seconds.

4 Repeat 2–3 times with each leg as time allows.

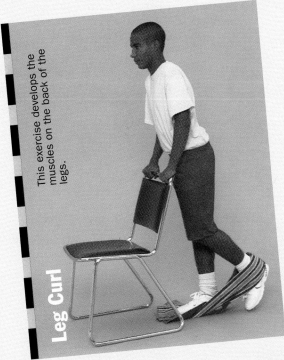

Leg Curl

This exercise develops the muscles on the back of the legs.

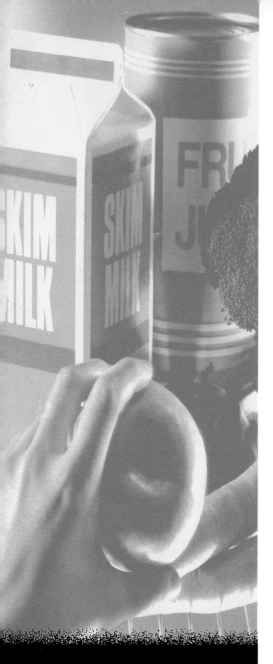

Reviewing Concepts and Vocabulary

Copy the number of each statement on a sheet of paper. Next to each number, write the word or words that correctly completes the sentence.

1. Your body breaks down proteins into simpler substances called _____.

2. Your body can use_____ for energy with little or no change during digestion.

3. You need to limit your intake of _____, a fat-like substance found in animal cells.

4. _____ contain more nutrients than do simple carbohydrates.

5. _____ are food substances required for the growth and maintenance of your cells.

6. A food that is _____ contains a large amount of nutrients for the number of Calories it provides.

Number your paper. Next to each number, choose the letter of the best answer.

Column I	Column II
7. carbohydrate	a. contains some, not all, essential amino acids
8. proteins	b. cannot be digested by the body
9. fiber	c. provides you with energy
10. complete protein	d. contains all eight essential amino acids
11. incomplete protein	e. building blocks of your body

On your paper, write a short answer for each statement or question.

12. Describe and refute a myth some athletes have about eating before physical activity.

13. Explain how complete proteins are important for your health.

14. Explain how calcium is important to your health and tell what you can do to help keep your bones strong.

15. Why is water considered an important nutrient, and why might a person who is exercising need extra amounts of it?

Thinking Critically

Write a paragraph to answer the following question.

Your friend asks your advice about her diet. She wonders if the food choices she makes are important or if she only needs to count Calories. She has started to increase her physical activity and wonders how that will affect her Caloric and nutritional needs. What advice would you give your friend?

Project

Collect labels from six foods that you frequently eat. Compare the nutritional values of the foods represented. Which of the foods are the most nutritious? the least nutritious? Which foods are lowest in sugar, fat, saturated fat, cholesterol, and sodium? Plan one or more healthful meals around some of the foods represented by the labels.

18

Managing Stress

Frisbee® Golf

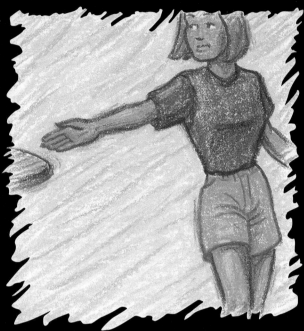

People of all ages can enjoy Frisbee golf. It is an enjoyable activity that can help you relax and reduce stress. To play the game, you try to throw the Frisbee from each "tee" into each goal, or "hole." You can design your own course using rope, baskets, hula hoops, or chalk lines on the ground as holes.

Each hole has a "par" of the recommended number of throws to get the Frisbee in the goal. The object is to achieve par or less for each hole. Your score is the total number of throws for 18 holes of Frisbee golf.

If you are playing for relaxation, it is best not to be too competitive. You might want to compare your score to par and try to improve, rather than comparing your score to someone else's.

Your instruction sheet describes exercises to do at each tee to improve your fitness.

18.1 Lesson · Facts About Stress

Lesson Objectives
After reading this lesson, you should be able to:
1. Define stress and list its causes.
2. Explain how eustress and distress differ.
3. Discuss the effects of stress.
4. Describe competitive stress.

Lesson Vocabulary
stress response, stress, stressor, eustress, distress

How would you feel if a bear were running toward you? Most likely, you would feel frightened. Your heart rate would increase; your muscles would tense. Your body would release a chemical called adrenaline to give you energy to run away. These changes and those shown on the next page are part of the **stress response,** your body's way of preparing you to deal with a demanding situation. If danger presents itself, your stress response prepares your body for bursts of energy you can use to face danger or avoid it.

Encountering a bear is an unusual situation. However, you probably face some stressful situations every day that affect you both physically and emotionally. In fact, two-thirds of Americans report feeling "stressed out" at least once a week.

In this lesson, you will read more about stress. You will learn about its many causes and you will find out how it can affect you.

What Is Stress?
Stress is the body's reaction to a demanding situation. A series of physical changes takes place automatically when you are in a highly stressful situation. Some of these physical changes are shown in the drawing on the next page.

What causes stress? Anything that causes you to worry or get excited or anything that causes other emotional and physical changes can cause stress. Something that causes or contributes to stress is called a **stressor**. For adults, stressors might include bills, vacation plans, work responsibilities, and family conflicts. Stressors for teenagers include grades and schoolwork, family arguments, and peer pressures. Other common stressors for teenagers include moving to a new home, serious illness or death in the family, poor eating habits, lack of physical activity, feelings of loneliness, a change or loss of friends, substance abuse, and trouble with school or legal authorities.

Eustress and Distress

Not all stressful experiences are harmful. Scientists use the term **eustress** to describe positive stress. Situations that might produce eustress include riding a roller coaster, successfully competing in an activity, passing a driving test, playing in the school band, and meeting new people. Eustress helps make your life more enjoyable by helping you meet challenges and do your best.

On the other hand, unpleasant situations also cause stress. Negative stress is sometimes called **distress**. Situations that cause worry, sorrow, anger, or pain produce distress.

A situation that causes eustress for one person can be distressful for another. For example, an outgoing person might look forward to joining extracurricular activities at school or attending social events; a shy person might dread the same situations. A similar experience can be eustressful or distressful for you at different times. For instance, if you are well-prepared for a test, taking that test might cause eustress. On the other hand, taking a test for which you are not prepared might cause distress.

Small amounts of stress may help you prepare for more stressful situations in the future. For example, doing physical activity may be a stressor. Yet regular physical activity can help make you fit, healthy, and better able to handle future stressful situations. Ideally, you need to strive for the right amount of stress — neither too much nor too little.

Causes of Distress

Distress can have a negative effect on your total health and fitness. In order to control stress in your life, you need to understand the cause of the stress you are experiencing.

Physical Stressors Conditions of your body and the environment that affect your physical well-being are physical stressors. Examples include thirst, hunger, overexposure to heat or cold, lack of sleep, illness, pollution, noise, accidents, and catastrophes such as floods or fires. Even excessive exercise can be a stressor. Athletes who "overtrain" experience this kind of negative effect. Healthy people who are fit are better able to adapt to the changes produced by physical stressors.

Emotional Stressors Emotions such as worry, fear, anger, grief, depression, or even "falling in love" are powerful stressors and can strongly affect your physical and emotional well-being.

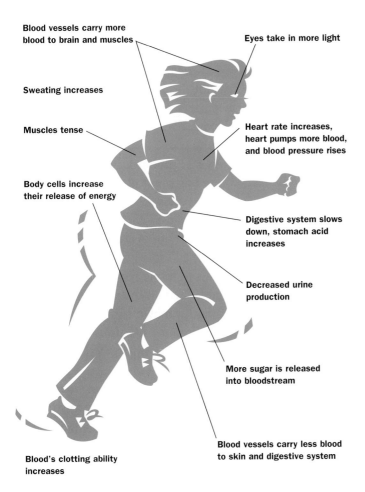

Blood vessels carry more blood to brain and muscles

Eyes take in more light

Sweating increases

Muscles tense

Heart rate increases, heart pumps more blood, and blood pressure rises

Body cells increase their release of energy

Digestive system slows down, stomach acid increases

Decreased urine production

More sugar is released into bloodstream

Blood vessels carry less blood to skin and digestive system

Blood's clotting ability increases

The stress response: your body's way of preparing

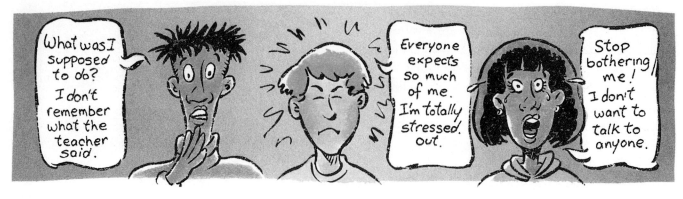

Emotional signs of stress

Social Stressors Social stressors arise from your relationships with other people. Each day, you have experiences that involve your family members, friends, teachers, employers, and others. As a teenager, you probably are exposed to many social stressors. Think about stressors in social situations in your life. Much of the stress you experience may be caused by social stressors.

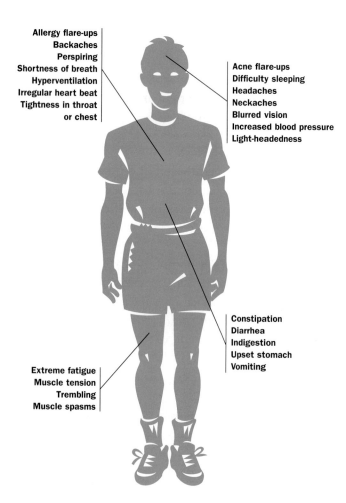

Allergy flare-ups
Backaches
Perspiring
Shortness of breath
Hyperventilation
Irregular heart beat
Tightness in throat
or chest

Acne flare-ups
Difficulty sleeping
Headaches
Neckaches
Blurred vision
Increased blood pressure
Light-headedness

Constipation
Diarrhea
Indigestion
Upset stomach
Vomiting

Extreme fatigue
Muscle tension
Trembling
Muscle spasms

Physical signs of stress

Effects of Stress

Stress can lead to both emotional and physical changes. Emotional effects of stress can include: upset or nervous feelings; anger, anxiety, or fear; frequently criticizing others; frustration; forgetfulness; difficulty paying attention; difficulty making decisions; irritability; lack of motivation; boredom, mild depression, or withdrawal; or change in appetite. Some of these signs are illustrated in the picture above.

Have you ever experienced extreme fatigue, light-headedness, or upset stomach due to stress? These and other reactions shown in the picture at the left are common physical reactions to stressors. These reactions vary from one person to another. They usually last a short period of time, disappearing once the source of the stress is removed.

High levels of stress and prolonged periods of stress can be related to many physical conditions. For example, increased stomach acid resulting from stress can aggravate ulcers. High blood pressure can be related to stress and can lead to serious cardiovascular diseases and disorders. Prolonged stress can lower the effectiveness of the body's immune system, making a person more susceptible to certain diseases. Some doctors think that many health problems in the United States requiring medical attention are stress-related. The motivation to deal effectively with stress, especially distress, is clear.

Use your Self-Assessment record sheet to find out how prone you are to stress. If you are prone to stress, consider using the procedures for managing stress that are described in the next lesson.

Competitive Stress

In the next lesson, you will learn that doing regular noncompetitive physical activity can help you reduce

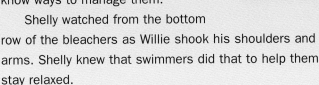

No Excuses

Controlling Competitive Stress

A little stress can give you more energy and help you meet a challenge. However, the effects of too much stress can interfere with your performance, especially during a competition. To do your best, you need to recognize the symptoms of stress and know ways to manage them.

Shelly watched from the bottom row of the bleachers as Willie shook his shoulders and arms. Shelly knew that swimmers did that to help them stay relaxed.

"You're the best, Willie! You're going to win." Shelly had to yell so Willie would hear her. The crowd around them was cheering the swimmers.

Willie thought to himself, "I'm not so sure." He shook his shoulders and legs again.

"You can do it!" Shelly screamed. "You're faster than anyone. We're all behind you." She wasn't sure if Willie heard her.

Willie had heard, and he thought, "That's the problem! The whole school is watching! My parents, too! If I

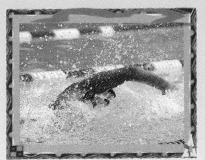

don't get at least second place, our team might not go on to the Regionals. The way my stomach feels, these people are more likely to see me throw up than win the 200."

Willie knew it was just stress. He had felt the same way at the last meet. Shelly had told him she felt the same kind of stress during a debate last week. The debate coach had shown her how to slow down her breathing to help her relax, and she had shown Willie.

Shelly stood up and took a deep breath. Willie saw her and did the same thing, and then grinned to let her know he felt better. Willie was ready.

For Discussion
How were Willie's muscles affected by the stress he felt? What were his other symptoms? How was Willie's stress similar to the stress Shelly felt before her debate? Fill out the questionnaire to find out how competitive stress affects you.

stress levels. However, competitive sports and other competitive activities, such as performing a music solo or giving a speech, can cause stress. Some factors that make these activities stressful are competition, being evaluated by others, performing in front of a crowd, and feeling that the outcome is important.

One way to prevent competitive stress is to avoid competitive situations or situations in which you perform for others. However, as a result, you may miss participating in activities that are fun. You also may fail to accomplish things that you are capable of doing and at which you would be successful.

Another solution is to learn to adapt or cope with competitive stress. The methods of managing stress that are discussed in the next lesson can help you cope with stressful situations. Remember that most people feel stressed the first few times they compete or perform

in public. With experience, competing and performing does become easier. Practice and preparation, as well as good stress management, will help you experience eustress when competing and performing and will help you to achieve your full potential.

Lesson Review
1. **List three common causes of stress.**
2. **How do eustress and distress differ?**
3. **Describe the physical and emotional effects stress can have on the body.**
4. **What are some reasons that competitive activities are stressful?**

Self-Assessment 18
Identifying Signs of Stress

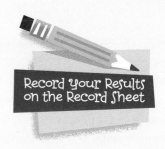

Record Your Results
on the Record Sheet

All people experience some negative stress in their lives. Your body sends off certain signals when you are experiencing such distress. In this Self-Assessment, you will learn to identify some of the body's stress signals.

The chart at the right lists some signs that commonly accompany stress. You may notice some of these signs when you are not under excessive stress. However, in times of great stress, these signs are often especially apparent.

One way to determine if an activity is stressful to you is to self-assess signs and signals of stress before and after the activity. Work with a partner. Help each other look for some of the signs and symptoms of stress indicated in the chart.

• Lie on the floor, close your eyes, and try to relax. Have your partner count your pulse and your breathing rate. Ask your partner to observe for irregular breathing and unusual mannerisms. Then ask your partner to evaluate how tense your muscles seem. Report "butterflies" or other indicators of stress to your partner. Write your results on your record sheet. Have your partner lie down while you record your observations about him or her.

• When directed by your instructor, all members of the class should write their names on a piece of paper and place the papers in a hat or a box. The teacher will draw names until only three remain in the container. The students whose names remain must give one-minute speeches about the effects of stress. Observe your partner before and during the name-drawing. Look for the signs and signals of stress. Record your results on the record sheet. Also, try to remember your feelings during the drawing. Finally, observe the people who were required to make the speech. Record this information on the record sheet.

• Finally, walk or jog for five minutes after your second stress assessment. Once again, work with a partner to assess your signs of stress. Write them in the third column of the record sheet. Notice that the exercise causes heart rate and breathing rate to increase. However, it may help reduce earlier signs of the emotional stress related to performing in front of the class.

Signs of Stress

Heart Rate

Is it higher than normal?

Muscle Tension

Are the muscles tighter than usual?
• arms and shoulders
• legs

Mannerisms

Are unusual mannerisms present?
• frowning/twitching
• hands to face (nail biting)

Nervous feelings

Do you feel differently?
• "butterflies" in stomach
• tense or anxious feelings

Breathing

Have you noticed differences?
• irregular
• rapid/shallow

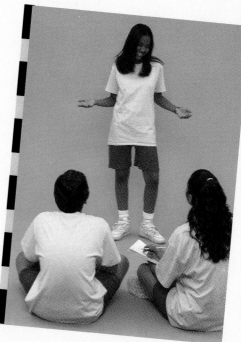

18.2 Lesson Dealing with Stress

Lesson Objectives
After reading this lesson, you should be able to:
1. Discuss how to manage stress in everyday life.
2. Describe health practices that can help a person deal with stress.

Lesson Vocabulary
none

Perhaps you feel overwhelmed by the many causes of distress and its effects. Distress in life is unavoidable. These suggestions can help you deal effectively with it:

Effective Ways to Manage Stress
Fortunately, you can take steps to manage the stress in your life. When a situation seems distressful, try some or all of the following suggestions:

• **Rest in a quiet place.** Relax indoors or outdoors. The teenager in the picture is relaxing by reading a book in a quiet place.

• **Reduce breathing rate.** Sit or lie quietly. Take several long, slow breaths in through your nose and breathe out through your mouth.

• **Reduce mental activity.** Sometimes, it is best to get rid of distressful thoughts until a later time. Try imagining a pleasant outdoor scene or listening to music.

• **Reduce muscle tension.** Relaxing your muscles can effectively help reduce distress. You will learn helpful techniques for this in the Activity on pages 241-243.

• **Use exercise as a diversion.** An excellent way to relieve distress is through physical activity. Try sports or another physical activity you enjoy.

• **Identify the cause of the stress.** Clearly identify the stressor. For example, if anger is causing you stress, try to identify what is making you angry.

• **Tackle one thing at a time.** If several problems pile up, ask yourself, "What can I do now to change things?" "What can wait?" "What cannot be changed?"

• **Take action.** Rather than worrying about a problem, try to solve it. Make decisions and carry them out. When making a decision, look at several choices, consider the results of each, and choose the best.

• **Manage time effectively.** Prioritize your activities so that you have time for the most important things. Learn to say "no" to new responsibilities or activities if you cannot give them the time required.

• **Accept what cannot be changed.** Not all problems can be solved as you would like, but you can still deal with them effectively. For example, suppose you made an error. You cannot change the past, but you can deal with the stress by recognizing that all people make errors and by learning from your mistakes.

• **Think positively.** Positive thoughts can help reduce distress. For example, try thinking that you WILL get a hit in the softball game instead of worrying about striking out. Also, make an effort to perceive a stressor as a challenge rather than as a problem.

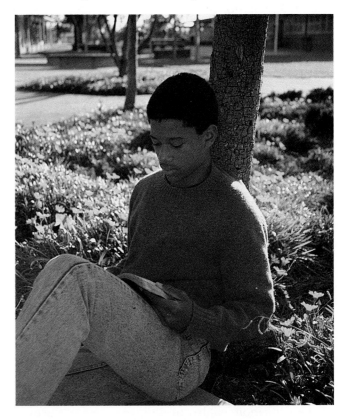

Relaxing in a quiet place can help reduce stress.

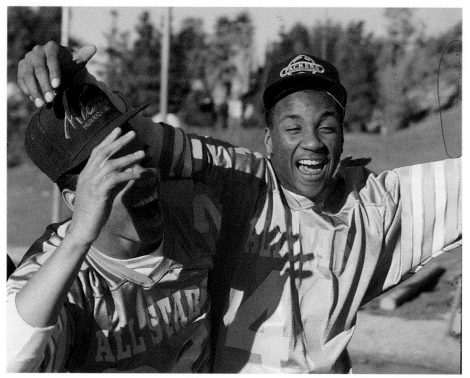

Regular fun physical activity can help reduce distress.

• **Do not mask your problems.** Sometimes people who are experiencing distress try to avoid the problem. Usually, masking the problem leads to more distress.

• **Try not to let little things bother you.** Many events in life are simply not worth stressful feelings. For example, if you are disappointed, remember that a situation might be better the next time.

• **Be willing to make adjustments.** Learning to bend a little, or adjust to changes, can be helpful. You use this ability to help handle distress.

Stress Management, Fitness, and Good Health

Keeping your body in good health and physically fit can help you manage stress. Following these health practices can help you deal with stress in your life:

• **Eat a nutritious, well-balanced diet.** Good nutrition helps lead to good health, which can help you deal better with stress. Chapter 17 discusses the importance of good nutrition.

• **Avoid unnecessary, distressful situations.** If you know a situation will be stressful, you often can avoid it. For example, you can choose to avoid an event at which alcohol might be served.

• **Get enough sleep.** Lack of sleep can contribute to distress. In fact, lack of sleep is itself a stressor. Some problems might be easier to handle when you feel rested. Try to sleep at least eight hours each day.

• **Pay attention to your body.** Pay attention to how your body reacts in different situations. If you experience physical signs of distress, use some of the stress-management techniques described in this lesson.

• **Have fun.** Laughter can help lessen distress. Take time to laugh and have fun. Enjoy life!

• **Do regular physical activity.** Doing some form of regular physical activity can help you reduce your stress. For example, people who jog regularly report a "runners high" that comes from their activity. As you learned in Lesson 1, sometimes competitive activities can cause stress. Taking "time out" in the form of a non-competitive activity can help you get your mind off stressful situations.

Getting Help

Often people need help in managing their stress. Parents, family members, teachers, members of the clergy, and friends can be sources of help and support. School counselors, school nurses, physicians, and other specially trained people can provide advice about stress management. In addition, many communities have health professionals to help people manage stress. A doctor, a school counselor, or a hospital referral service can direct you to sources of help in your community.

Lesson Review

1. List five ways to deal with a stressful situation.
2. What are some health practices that can help you deal with stress in your life?

Activity 18
Relaxation Exercises for Stress-Management

Did your Self-Assessment indicate that you have a high amount of stress? Most people need to deal with stress at one time or another. You might find that doing some of these exercises can help you manage stressful feelings.

Notice that you can do some of these exercises at almost any time and almost any place. You might do them when you sit and study or while you are riding or waiting for a bus. You can do most of them lying down or from a sitting position. You can even adapt some of these exercises so you can do them while you are standing. When you do these exercises, be sure to write your results on your record sheet.

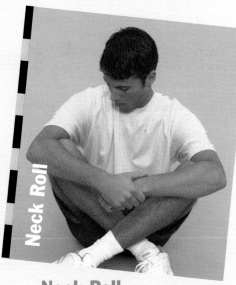
Neck Roll

Rag Doll

1 Sit in a chair (or stand) with your feet apart. Stretch your arms and trunk upward as you inhale.

2 Then exhale and drop your body forward. Let your trunk, head, and arms dangle between your legs. Keep your neck and trunk muscles relaxed. Remain relaxed like a rag doll for 10–15 seconds.

3 Slowly roll up, one vertebra at a time; repeat the stretch and drop.

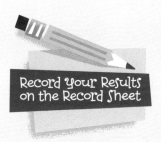
Record your Results on the Record Sheet

Neck Roll

1 Sit in a chair (or on the floor with your legs crossed).

2 Keeping your head and chin tucked, inhale as you slowly rotate your head to the left as far as possible. Exhale and slowly return your head to the center.

3 Repeat to the right.

4 Rotate 3 times in each direction, trying to rotate farther each time, so you feel a stretch in the neck.

5 Now, drop your chin to your chest and inhale as you slowly roll your head in a half circle to the left shoulder and then exhale as you roll it back to the center. Repeat to the right shoulder.
Caution: Do not roll your head backward or in a full circle.

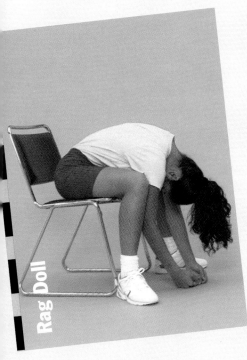
Rag Doll

Body Board

1 Lie on your right side. Hold your arms over your head.

2 Inhale and stiffen your body as if you were a wooden board. Then exhale as you relax your muscles and collapse completely.

3 Let your body fall without trying to control whether it tips forward or backward.

4 Lie still as you continue letting the tension go out of your muscles for 10 seconds. Then repeat the exercise starting on your left side.

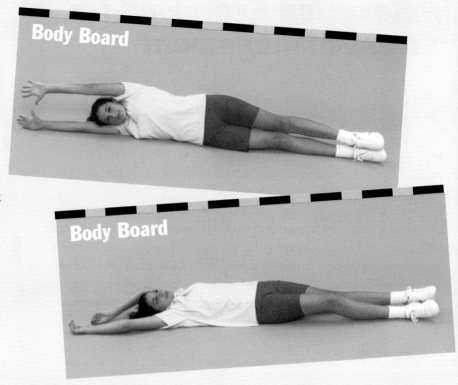

Body Board

Body Board

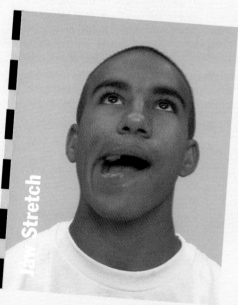

Jaw Stretch

Jaw Stretch

1 Sit in a chair (or on the floor), head erect, arms and shoulders relaxed.

2 Open your mouth as wide as possible and inhale. (This may make you yawn!). Relax and exhale slowly.

3 Open your mouth and shift your jaw to the right as far as possible; hold 3 counts.

4 Repeat to the left. Repeat on both sides 10 times.

...ress   Managing Stress

Contract-Relax Relaxation Exercise Routine

Lie on your back with a rolled-up towel placed under your knees. Contract your muscles in the order that they are named below. Hold each contraction for 3 counts. Then relax the muscles and keep relaxing for 10 counts. Each time you contract, inhale. Each time you relax, exhale.

Do each exercise twice. Try this routine at home for a few weeks. With practice, you should eventually progress to a combination of muscle groups and gradually eliminate the "contract" phase of the program.

1 Hand and forearm—Contract your right hand, making a fist; Relax and continue relaxing. Repeat with your left hand. Repeat with both hands.

2 Biceps—Bend both elbows and contract the muscles on the front of your upper arm. Relax and continue relaxing. Repeat.

3 Triceps—Bend both elbows, keeping palms up; straighten both elbows and contract the muscles on the back of the arm by pushing the back of your hand into the floor. Relax.

4 Hands, forearms, and upper arms—Concentrate on relaxing these body parts altogether.

5 Forehead—Make a frown and wrinkle your forehead. Relax and continue relaxing. Repeat.

6 Jaws—Clench your teeth. Relax. Repeat.

7 Lips and tongue—With teeth apart, press your lips together and press your tongue to the roof of your mouth. Relax. Repeat.

8 Neck and throat—Push your head backward while tucking chin. Relax. Repeat.

9 Relax your forehead, jaws, lips, tongue, neck, and throat. Relax hands, forearms, and upper arms. Keep relaxing all of these muscles.

10 Shoulder and upper back— Hunch your shoulders to your ears. Relax. Repeat.

11 Relax lips, tongue, neck, throat, shoulders, and upper back. Keep relaxing these muscles altogether.

12 Abdomen—Suck in your abdomen, flattening your lower back to the floor. Relax. Repeat.

13 Lower back—Contract and arch your lower back. Relax. Repeat.

14 Thighs and buttocks—Squeeze your buttocks together and push your heels into the floor. Relax. Repeat.

15 Relax shoulders and upper back, abdomen, lower back, thighs, and buttocks. Keep relaxing these muscles altogether.

16 Shin—Pull your toes toward your shins. Relax. Repeat.

17 Toes—Curl your toes. Relax. Repeat.

18 Relax every muscle in your body altogether and keep relaxing.

* Adapted from *Concepts of Fitness and Wellness* (1994) by Charles Corbin and Ruth Lindsey. Brown and Benchmark Publishers.

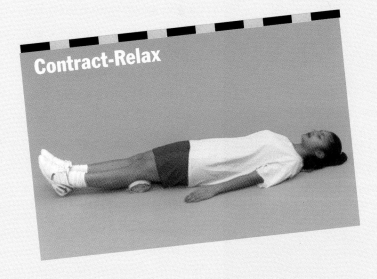

Contract-Relax

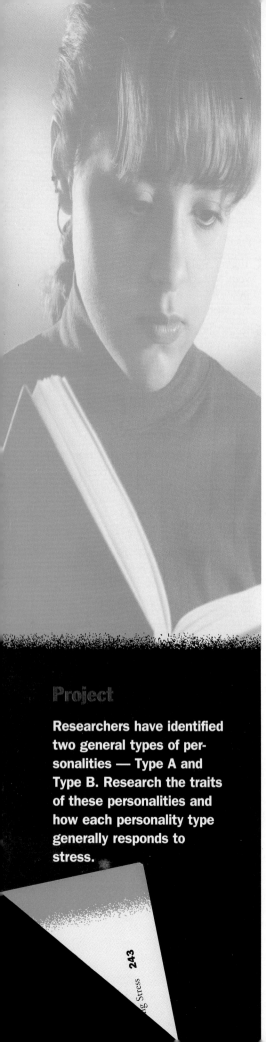

g Stress

18 Chapter Review

Reviewing Concepts and Vocabulary

Copy the number of each statement on a sheet of paper. Next to each number, write the word or words that correctly completes the sentence.

1. To help reduce stress, contract and then _____ your muscles.

2. Excessive exercise, such as that done by athletes who "overtrain," is a _____ stressor.

3. The _____ is your body's way of preparing you to deal with a demanding situation.

4. Worry and fear are examples of _____ stressors.

5. Stress can affect the immune system, making a person more susceptible to certain _____.

6. Getting enough _____ every night can help prevent fatigue and help you deal effectively with stress.

Number your paper. Next to each number, choose the letter of the best answer.

Column I	Column II
7. stress	a. positive stress
8. eustress	b. negative stress
9. stressor	c. the body's reaction to a stressful situation
10. distress	d. causes or contributes to stress

On your paper, write a short answer for each statement or question.

11. Describe some negative effects of competitive stress and explain how to deal with such stress in a positive manner.

12. Describe some ways of thinking that can help you deal with stress.

13. How can physical activity help you deal effectively with stress?

14. How can an activity cause both eustress and distress?

15. Name five sources of guidance and support for those who need help dealing with a stressful situation.

Thinking Critically

You have been invited to give a speech in front of your class. You are concerned that if you refuse the opportunity, you may feel disappointed in yourself. However, you are afraid that you will be too nervous to give a speech in front of a large group. What are the positive and negative consequences of each choice? What decisions would you make? How can you manage stress associated with whichever decision you make?

Project

Researchers have identified two general types of personalities — Type A and Type B. Research the traits of these personalities and how each personality type generally responds to stress.

Glossary

A

abdominal muscles, the muscles on the front of the body between the chest and the pelvic area

Achilles tendon, tendon on the back of the leg that connects the muscles in the calf to the bone of the heel

activity neurosis, a condition that occurs when a person is overly concerned about getting enough exercise

aerobic activity, steady activity in which the heart can supply all the oxygen the muscles need

aerobic dance, a combination of dance steps and calisthenics done to music

agility, the ability to quickly change the position of the body and to control the body's movements

amino acids, substances that make up proteins

anabolic steroid, strong drug similar to the male hormone testosterone that can make muscles bulky but that can be extremely dangerous to health

anaerobic activity, physical activity done in short, fast bursts in which the heart cannot supply blood and oxygen as fast as muscles use it

anorexia athletica, an eating disorder that has symptoms similar to those of anorexia nervosa in which a person severely restricts food intake in order to maintain a very low body weight

anorexia nervosa, an eating disorder in which a person severely restricts food intake in an attempt to be exceptionally underfat

artery, a blood vessel that carries blood from the heart to other parts of the body

arthritis, a disease in which the joints become inflamed

atherosclerosis, a disease in which certain substances, including fats, build up on the inside walls of the arteries

attitude, a person's feelings about something

B

balance, the ability to keep an upright posture while standing still or moving

ballistic stretching, a series of quick but gentle bouncing or bobbing-type motions

basal metabolism, the amount of energy the body uses just to keep living

biceps, the large muscle in the front part of the upper arm

biomechanical principle, a rule related to the study of forces that can help a person move the body efficiently and avoid injury

blood pressure, the force of blood against the artery walls

body composition, all of the tissues that together make up the body

body fatness, the percentage of body weight that is made up of fat

body mass index, a method of assessing body composition

bulimia, an eating disorder in which a person does binge eating, followed by purging

C

caliper, an instrument that is used to measure skinfold thickness

calisthenics, exercises done using all or part of the body weight as resistance

Calorie, a heat unit that refers to the energy available in food and the energy used by body activities

cancer, a disease characterized by uncontrollable growth of abnormal cells

carbohydrate, a nutrient contained in starches and sugars that provides energy

cardiac muscle, heart muscle

cardiovascular fitness, ability of the heart, lungs, and blood vessels to function efficiently when a person exercises the body

cardiovascular system, body system that includes the heart, blood vessels, and blood, and functions by moving oxygen and nutrients to body cells and removing cell wastes

cholesterol, a fat-like substance found in animal cells and some foods such as meats, dairy products, and egg yolks

committed time, time spent on necessary activities or pledged to specific activities

complete protein, a protein that contains all eight essential amino acids

complex carbohydrate, a nutrient found in starches such as breads, vegetables, and grains that provides the body with energy; made of long chains of simple sugars

controllable risk factor, a risk factor a person can act upon to change

cool-down, a series of activities to help the body recover after a workout; usually consists of a heart cool-down and a muscle cool-down and stretch

coordination, the ability to use the senses together with the body parts or to use two or more body parts together

D

dehydrated, lacking the necessary amount of body fluid

deltoid muscle, muscle of the shoulder by which the arm is raised

diabetes, a disease in which a person's body cannot regulate the level of sugar

Dietary Guidelines, suggestions developed by the U.S. Department of Agriculture for following healthful eating practices

distress, negative or unpleasant stress

E

eating disorder, a health problem that manifests itself through starvation, eating binges followed by purging, or overeating

essential amino acid, one of the eight amino acids that the body needs to take in from food

essential body fat, the minimum amount of body fat a person needs

eustress, positive stress

exercise, physical activity done especially for the purpose of becoming physically fit

F

fad diet, a nutritionally unbalanced diet that falsely promises quick weight loss

fast-twitch muscle fibers, muscle fibers that contract at a fast rate and have great strength but very little endurance

fats, nutrients that provide energy, help growth and repair of cells, and dissolve and carry certain vitamins to cells

fiber, a type of indigestible carbohydrate

fitness profile, a brief summary of fitness

FITT formula, formula in which each letter represents a factor important for determining the correct amount of physical activity: F, frequency; I, intensity; T, time; T, type

flexibility, the ability to move the joints through a full range of motion; part of the FITT formula

flexor, a muscle that when contracted bends a joint in the body

food supplement, a product intended to add to a person's nutrient consumption

form, placement of body parts during an exercise

free time, time left over when time for work, school, and other commitments has been accounted for

frequency, how often physical activity is done

frostbite, a condition that results when body tissues become frozen

G

goal setting, a plan to determine ahead of time what is expected to be accomplished and how it can be accomplished

gluteal muscle, one of the muscles of the buttocks

H

hamstring muscle, muscle located on the back of the thigh

health, the state of optimal physical, mental, and social well-being

health-related fitness, parts of physical fitness that help a person stay healthy; includes cardiovascular fitness, flexibility, muscular endurance, strength, and body fatness

heart attack, sudden failure of the heart to function properly that occurs when the blood supply into or within the heart is cut off

heart rate, the number of times the heart beats per minute

heat exhaustion, a condition caused by excessive exposure to heat and characterized by cold, clammy skin and symptoms of shock

heat stroke, a condition caused by excessive exposure to heat and resulting in a high body temperature and dry skin

heredity, characteristics that are passed from parents to their offspring

high-density lipoprotein (HDL), substance often referred to as "good cholesterol" because it carries excess cholesterol out of the bloodstream and into the liver for elimination from the body

hyperkinetic condition, a health problem caused by doing too much physical activity

hypermobility, the ability to extend the knee, elbow, thumb, or wrist joint past a straight line

hypertension, a disorder in which the blood pressure is consistently higher than normal

hypertrophy, increase in muscle size

hyperventilate, breathe too quickly

hypokinetic condition, a health problem caused partly by lack of exercise

hypothermia, a condition often related to cold weather in which the body temperature becomes abnormally low

I

incomplete protein, a protein that contains some, but not all, of the essential amino acids

intensity, how hard a person performs physical activity; part of the FITT formula

intermediate muscle fibers, muscle fibers that have characteristics of both slow- and fast-twitch fibers

interval training, physical activity in which short bursts of high intensity exercise are alternated with rest periods

involuntary muscle, muscle that a person cannot consciously control

isometric contraction, muscle contraction in which no movement occurs because of an equal force in the opposite direction

isometric exercise, exercise that involves isometric contractions in which body parts do not move

isotonic contraction, muscle contraction that pulls on the bones and produces movement of body parts

isotonic exercise, exercise that involves isotonic contractions and in which body parts move

J

joint, a place in the body where bones come together

L

latissimus muscle, large muscle attached to the back and arm

laxity, looseness of the joints that allows the bones to move in ways other than intended

ligament, a band of strong tissue that connects bones

lipoprotein, substance that carries cholesterol through the bloodstream

lordosis, a back condition characterized by too much arch in the lower back; sometimes called swayback

low-density lipoprotein (LDL), substance often referred to as "bad cholesterol" because it carries cholesterol that is most likely to stay in the body

low-impact aerobic exercise, exercise in which one foot contacts the floor at all times

M

maturation, the process of becoming fully grown and developed physically

microtrauma, an injury so small that it is often difficult to see or recognize, especially when it first occurs

mineral, a nutrient that performs many functions in regulating the activities of cells

muscle fibers, muscle cells, which are long, thin, and cylinder-shaped

muscle cramp, a spasm or sudden tightening of a muscle

muscle-bound, having tight, bulky muscles that prevent a person from moving freely

muscular endurance, ability to contract the muscles many times without tiring or to hold one contraction for a long time

N

noncontrollable risk factor, a risk factor a person cannot change or control

nutrient, a food substance required for the growth and maintenance of body cells

nutrition, the study of foods and how they nourish the body

nutritionally dense, containing large amounts of nutrients for the number of Calories provided

O

obesity, the condition of being very overfat or having a very high percentage of body fat

orienteering, a combination of walking, jogging, and map-reading

osteoporosis, a disease in which the bones deteriorate and become weak

overfat, having too much body fat

overload, see: principle of overload

overuse injury, a body injury that occurs when a repeated movement causes wear and tear on the body

P

parcourse, an outdoor course containing exercise stations with signs suggesting the number of repetitions for each exercise

peak bone mass, a person's greatest bone mass, usually present when a person is young

pectoral muscle, muscle of the chest

physical activity, movement using the larger muscles of the body; includes sports, dance, and activities of daily life; may be done to accomplish a task, for enjoyment, or to improve physical fitness

physical fitness, the ability of the body systems to work together efficiently

physical skill, specific physical task that a person performs

PNF stretching, a variation of static stretching that is more effective for improving flexibility

power, the ability to use strength quickly

primary risk factor, a risk factor that is considered a major contributor to a disease

principle of overload, rule that states that in order to improve fitness one needs to do more physical activity than he or she normally does

principle of progression, rule that states that the amount and intensity of physical activity needs to be increased gradually

principle of specificity, rule that states that specific types of exercise improve specific parts of fitness or muscles

progressive resistance exercise, the gradual increase of resistance used in strength training exercises

protein, a nutrient that builds and repairs body cells

pulse, the regular beating felt in the arteries caused by contractions of the heart muscle

Q

quackery, method of advertising or selling that uses false claims to lure people into buying products that are worthless or even harmful

quadriceps muscle, muscle on the front of the thigh

R

range of motion, the amount of movement one can make in a joint

range of motion (ROM) exercise, flexibility exercises that are used to maintain the range of motion already present in the joints

reaction time, the amount of time it takes a person to move once he or she realizes the need to act

registered dietitian, expert in nutrition who is qualified to give advice about food and diet

rehydrate, to drink liquids to replace those lost during physical activity

repetitions, the number of consecutive times one does an exercise; usually referred to as "reps"

resistance training, exercises using resistance, in the form of free weights or machines, to develop muscular endurance or strength; also called weight training

resistance, a force that acts against the muscles

respiratory system, body system that includes the lungs and air passages and that functions by bringing oxygen into the bloodstream and eliminating carbon dioxide from the blood

resting heart rate, the number of heartbeats during a period of inactivity

RICE formula, formula in which each letter represents a step in the treatment of a minor injury: R, rest; I, ice; C, compression; E, elevation

risk factor, anything that increases a person's chances of a health problem occurring

RM, repetition maximum; 1RM refers to the maximum amount of weight a group of muscles can lift at one time

S

saturated fat, a nutrient that is found mostly in animal products

self-management skill, skill by which a person can take control of his or her lifestyle or behavior in order to stay physically active

set, one group of repetitions

shin splint, a pain in the front of the shins caused by overuse

side stitch, a pain in the side of the lower abdomen that occurs as a result of vigorous activity

simple carbohydrate, a nutrient found in sugars that can be used by the body for energy with little or no change during digestion

skeletal muscle, muscle attached to bones that makes movement possible

skill-related fitness, parts of fitness that help a person perform well in sports and activities that require certain skills; includes agility, balance, coordination, power, reaction time, and speed

skinfold, the fat under the skin

slow-twitch muscle fibers, muscle fibers that contract at a slow rate and have great endurance

smooth muscles, muscles that make up the walls of hollow internal organs such as the stomach and blood vessels

speed, the ability to perform a movement or cover a distance in a short period of time

sports, activities that generally are done competitively and have well-established rules

sports supplement, a product sold to enhance athletic performance

sprain, an injury to ligaments and muscles

static stretching, stretching slowly as far as possible without pain, and then holding the stretch for several seconds

strain, an injury to a tendon or muscle

strength, the amount of force a muscle can produce

stress, the body's reaction to a demanding situation

stress response, the body's way of preparing a person to deal with a demanding situation

stressor, something that causes or contributes to stress

stretching exercise, flexibility exercise that works to increase the range of motion by stretching farther than the current range of motion

stroke, injury to the brain that occurs when the blood supply to the brain is severely reduced or shut off, often as a result of a blood clot or other obstruction

T

target ceiling, a person's upper limit of physical activity

target fitness zone, the correct range of physical activity to build fitness

target weight, the weight at which a person has the proper amount of body fat

tendon, a band of strong tissue that connects a muscle to a bone

threshold of training, the minimum amount of overload one needs to build physical fitness

time, how long a person does physical activity; part of the FITT formula

triceps muscle, muscle located on the back of the upper arm

U

underfat, having too little body fat

underwater weighing, a technique used to assess body fat levels in which a person is immersed in water and then weighed

unsaturated fat, a nutrient found in plant products such as vegetable oils

V

vein, blood vessel that carries blood filled with waste products from the body cells back to the heart

vitamin, a nutrient needed for growth and repair of body cells

voluntary muscle, muscle over which a person has conscious control

W

warm-up, a series of activities, usually consisting of a heart warm-up and a muscle warm-up and stretch, that prepares the body for more vigorous exercise and helps prevent injury

weight training, the lifting of weights to build strength; also called resistance training

wellness, a state of being that enables a person to reach his or her highest potential; includes intellectual, social, emotional, physical, and spiritual health

workout, the part of the physical activity program during which a person does activities to improve fitness

Index

Acknowledgments

Photographs

Unless otherwise acknowledged, all photographs are the property of ScottForesman. The abbreviations indicate position of pictures: (t)top, (b)bottom, (l)left, (r)right, (c)center.

Page 3(l): © David Young-Wolff/PhotoEdit. **3(c):** © David Young-Wolff/PhotoEdit. **3(r):** © Michael Newman/PhotoEdit. **5(r)** © Michael Newman/PhotoEdit. **10:** © G. Glod/Superstock. **11:** © David Young-Wolff/PhotoEdit. **12:** © Mike Powell/AllSport USA. **21:** © David Young-Wolff/Tony Stone Images. **24:** © T. Rosenthal/Superstock. **39:** © Brian Bailey/Tony Stone Images. **49:** © David Young-Wolff/PhotoEdit. **52(l):** © Tony Freeman/PhotoEdit. **52(r):** © R. Heinzen/SuperStock. **63(l):** © 1994 CMSP All Rights Reserved. **63(r):** © 1994 CMSP All Rights Reserved. **65:** SuperStock. **74:** © Tony Freeman/PhotoEdit. **78(l):** © David Young-Wolff/PhotoEdit. **78(r):** © David Young-Wolff/PhotoEdit. **83:** © Tony Freeman/PhotoEdit. **89:** SuperStock. **90:** © G. Glod/Superstock. **92:** © David Young-Wolff/PhotoEdit. **105(l):** © David Young-Wolff/PhotoEdit. **105(c):** © Dennis Hallinan/FPG. **105(r):** © T. Rosenthal/SuperStock. **107:** © Tony Freeman/Photo Edit. **113:** © David Young-Wolff/Photo Edit. **135:** © Robert Brenner/PhotoEdit. **137:** © Tony Freeman/PhotoEdit. **142:** © Richard Hutchings/PhotoEdit. **149:** © Simon Bruty/AllSport USA. **150(l):** © Mary Kate Denny/PhotoEdit. **150(r):** © Tony Freeman/PhotoEdit. **154:** © T. Rosenthal/SuperStock. **155:** © David Young-Wolff/PhotoEdit. **161:** © David Young-Wolff/Photo Edit. **163:** © Michelle Bridewell/PhotoEdit. **165(l):** © David Young-Wolff/PhotoEdit. **165(r):** © T. Rosenthal/SuperStock. **168:** © David Young-Wolff/PhotoEdit. **170:** © B. Howe/Photri. **177(l):** © Myrleen Ferguson/PhotoEdit. **177(r):** © Tony Freeman/Photo Edit. **180:** © David Young-Wolff/PhotoEdit. **189:** © Tony Freeman/PhotoEdit. **197:** © Alan Oddie/PhotoEdit. **198:** © David Young-Wolff/PhotoEdit. **200:** © Marshall Prescott/Unicorn Stock Photos. **210:** © Jeff Greenberg/Unicorn Stock Photos. **213:** © Brian Bailey/Tony Stone Images. **214:** © David Young-Wolff/PhotoEdit. **222:** © 1994 Dallon Design ALL RIGHTS RESERVED/Custom Stock Medical. **228:** © G. Fritz/SuperStock. **237:** © Daniel J. Olson/Unicorn Stock Photos. **239:** © Myrleen Ferguson/PhotoEdit. **240:** © Myrleen Ferguson/PhotoEdit.

Text

Pages 25-26, 40-41, 53-54: from *The Prudential FITNESS-GRAM®*. Printed with permission of the Cooper Institute for Aerobics Research, Dallas Texas.
Page 53: "Body Mass Index Chart" from FITNESS & YOUR HEALTH by David C. Nieman, Dr. P.H., FACSM. Copyright © 1993 Bull Publishing Co. Reprinted by permission of the publisher.
Page 94: "Triceps Plus Calf Skinfolds: Males" and "Triceps Plus Calf Skinfolds: Females" reprinted by permission of Dr. Tim G. Lohman, Department of Exercise and Sport Sciences, University of Arizona.
Page 126: "Predicted 1RM Based on Reps to Fatigue" This chart is used as modified from the JOURNAL OF PHYSICAL EDUCATION, RECREATION, AND DANCE, January 1993, page 89. JOPERD is a publication of the American Alliance for Health, Physical Education, Recreation and Dance, 1900 Association Drive, Reston, VA 22091
Page 174: Credit is extended to Michelle Stewart for developing the basics of these step aerobics routines.
Page 211: Adapted from the *One Mile Walk Test* with permission of the author, James M. Rippe, M.D.